Pharmacodynamic Models of Selected Toxic Chemicals in Man

Volume 2: Routes of Intake and Implementation of Pharmacodynamic Models

Pharmacodynamic Models of Selected Toxic Chemicals in Man

Volume 2: Routes of Intake and Implementation of Pharmacodynamic Models

Prepared for the
Directorate-General of Employment,
Social Affairs and Education
of the Commission of the European Communities

by

A. D. Smith and M. C. Thorne

Associated Nuclear Services
60 East Street, Epsom, Surrey, England

 MTP PRESS LIMITED
a member of the KLUWER ACADEMIC PUBLISHERS GROUP
LANCASTER / BOSTON / THE HAGUE / DORDRECHT

for the Commission of the European Communities

Published in the UK and Europe by
MTP Press Limited
Falcon House
Lancaster, England

British Library Cataloguing in Publication Data
Smith, A. D.
  Pharmacodynamic models of selected toxic
  chemicals in man.
  1. Toxicology—Methodology
  2. Chemicals—Physiological effect
  3. Pharmacokinetics
  I. Title   II. Thorne, M. C.
  615.9'07   RA1199

ISBN 0-85200-953-4 v. 2

Published in the USA by
MTP Press
A division of Kluwer Boston Inc.
101 Philip Drive
Norwell, MA 02061, USA

Library of Congress Cataloging-in-Publication Data
Thorne, M. C.
  Pharmacodynamic models of selected toxic
  chemicals in man.

  (ANS report; no. 512-2)
  Includes bibliographies and index.
  Contents: v. 1. Review of metabolic data—
  v. 2. Routes of intake and implementation of
  pharmacodynamic models/A. D. Smith and M. C. Thorne.
  1. Carcinogens—Metabolism.   2. Pharmacokinetics.
  3. Carcinogens—Metabolism—Mathematical models.
  I. Jackson, D.   II. Smith, A. D. (Anthony David)
  III. Title.   IV. Series. [DNLM: 1. Models, Chemical.
  2. Poisons—pharmacodynamics.   QV 600 T511p]
  RC268.6.S65   1986   616.99'4071   86-124

ISBN 0-85200-952-6 (v. 1)
ISBN 0-85200-953-4 (v. 2)

Publication arranged by
Commission of the European Communities
Directorate-General Telecommunications,
Information Industries and Innovation,
Luxembourg

Printed and Bound by Butler & Tanner Limited, Frome and London

Contents

1 FOREWORD   vii

2 SUMMARY   viii

3 INTRODUCTION   ix

4 REVIEW OF RECENT LITERATURE
  4.1 Arsenic   1
  4.2 Beryllium   16
  4.3 Cadmium   26
  4.4 Lead   40
  4.5 Nickel   51
  4.6 Chromium   55
  4.7 Asbestos   61
  4.8 Benzene   63
  4.9 Vinyl chloride   67
  4.10 Benzidine   72
  4.11 Carbon tetrachloride   78
  4.12 Methyl iodide   85
  4.13 References   85

5 MODEL OF GI TRACT
  5.1 Introduction   106
  5.2 Physiology and anatomy of the GI tract   108
  5.3 Gastrointestinal transit   120
  5.4 Absorption and retention of material by the intestinal wall   129
  5.5 Modelling retention in the gastrointestinal tract   131
  5.6 References   132

6 MODELLING THE DEPOSITION AND RETENTION OF PARTICULATE
  MATERIALS IN THE LUNG
  6.1 Introduction   137
  6.2 The anatomy and physiology of the respiratory tract   138
  6.3 Deposition   158

6.4	Clearance	210
6.5	Model structure	242
6.6	References	246

7 METHOD OF CALCULATION

7.1	General description of the model	270
7.2	The computer code MOSAIC	273
7.3	The computer code GRAPH	291
7.4	References	291

8 IMPLICATIONS OF DIFFERENT REGIONS OF EXPOSURE

8.1	Description of the exposure regimes	293
8.2	Discussion of results	295
8.3	References	299

9 CONCLUSIONS AND RECOMMENDATIONS	300

10 ACKNOWLEDGEMENTS	302

APPENDICES

A	Computer programs for evaluating the implications of different exposure regions	303
B	Graphical output of simulations of the model	351

1
Foreword

       This report contains the results of a study undertaken by Associated Nuclear Services (ANS) for the Directorate General of Employment, Social Affairs and Education of the Commission of the European Communities (CEC). This study was entitled "Dynamics of Selected Toxic Materials in Man".

2
Summary

This report presents results from the second phase of a study on the metabolism of selected actual and potential human carcinogens. In the first phase of this work a comprehensive review of literature relating to the metabolism of these materials was undertaken and pharmacokinetic models were proposed to represent that metabolism. It was suggested that these models, and the reviews on which they were based, would provide information relevant to the development of monitoring programmes and in the interpretation of dose-response data.

In the second phase of the study, attention has been concentrated on the implementation of the models proposed for the various substances reviewed, i.e. arsenic, beryllium, cadmium, lead, nickel, chromium, asbestos, benzene, vinyl chloride monomer, benzidine and its congeners, carbon tetrachloride and methyl iodide. However, this programme has been supplemented by an on-going review of the relevant literature on these substances and a detailed analysis of the applicability of the pharmacokinetic models used for the organs of intake, i.e. the lung and gastrointestinal tract.

Reviews of the literature have led to some minor modifications to the models proposed previously and the development of a model for carbon tetrachloride, but not to major conceptual or structural changes in previously proposed models. The review of literature on the gastrointestinal tract has demonstrated that the ICRP model used previously is generally appropriate. The review of literature for the lung has demonstrated the need for a new lung model which incorporates competition between solubilisation and macrophage-mediated transport and which includes recent data on the regional deposition of particulate materials. This new lung model has been incorporated in the pharmacokinetic models as appropriate.

The various pharmacokinetic models have been implemented as a FORTRAN program running on a microcomputer and this program has been used to produce a large number of graphical outputs relating different regimes of exposure to time-dependent organ and excretory concentrations of the materials and their derivatives. A user's guide to this program is included, while an annotated listing and the graphical output produced form appendices to the main report.

3
Introduction

As was noted in the report on phase 1 of this study (Thorne and Jackson, 1983), there are numerous naturally occurring and man-made substances which can be toxic to man, including elements, small organic molecules and fibrous materials such as asbestos. Once a material has been identified as toxic, and, in particular, carcinogenic, to man, there is a requirement to limit exposure to the substance such that the risks attendant upon exposure are eliminated, or reduced to an acceptable level. In circumstances where use of the substance cannot be eliminated, it is necessary to set levels limiting exposure and to monitor that these levels are being achieved. Such levels may be set in terms of limiting air concentrations of the substance; limiting concentrations of the substance or its derivatives in monitorable materials such as urine, faeces, blood, or exhaled air; or limiting physiological effects of the substance, such as changes in serum enzyme levels.

In formulating standards, there is a requirement for pharmacokinetic models to relate exposure to a substance to levels of that substance, its derivatives, or other induced substances, in tissues, tissue components and excreta.

The report on phase 1 of this study presented a review of the metabolism of twelve materials and proposed pharmacokinetic models for eleven of these. Reviews of further literature have permitted refinement of these models and development of a new model for the last material. Thus, models are now available for arsenic, beryllium, cadmium, lead, nickel, chromium, asbestos, benzene, vinyl chloride monomer, benzidine, carbon tetrachloride and methyl iodide. In addition, a review of literature on the transport of materials through, and their uptake from, the gastrointestinal tract has demonstrated that the ICRP model for the tract (Eve, 1966) is still appropriate for use in pharmacokinetic modelling. In contrast, a review of literature on deposition in, and clearance from, the lung has revealed that the ICRP (1966) lung model is susceptible to considerable improvement. For this reason, a new lung model has been developed. However, because of the established place of the ICRP lung model in literature on this subject, results are presented using both it and the new lung model.

The pharmacokinetic models proposed have all been implemented in a FORTRAN program running on a microcomputer system. This program has been used to calculate time-dependent responses to a wide variety of different exposure regimes and results are presented herein. These exposure regimes encompass the range of interest in both occupational and environmental exposure, viz. single acute intake, continuous intake and shift exposure by ingestion, inhalation and transcutaneously.

In the main report, Section 4 includes an update of the reviews on the individual materials, together with a summary of the pharmacokinetic models as finally used. Sections 5 and 6 contain the reviews of literature on the gastrointestinal tract and lung respectively, with that on lung containing specifications for the new pharmacokinetic model. In Section 7, the implementation of the models is described and in Section 8 the main features of the results are discussed. A summary of the overall conclusions from the study is included as Section 9.

The report is supplemented by two appendices. Appendix A includes an annotated listing of the FORTRAN programs used, so that they are readily available to other organisations. Appendix B contains comprehensive graphical output for all twelve materials and for all exposure regimes investigated to date.

3.1   References

Eve, I.S., 1966. A review of the physiology of the gastrointestinal tract in relation to radiation doses from radioactive materials. Health Phys., 12, 131-161.

ICRP Task Group on Lung Dynamics, 1966. Deposition and retention models for internal dosimetry of the human respiratory tract. Health Phys., 12, 173-207.

Thorne, M.C. and Jackson, D., 1983. Models for the metabolism of chemical carcinogens in man. ANS Report No. 347, September 1983.

4
Review of recent literature

Subsequent to the presentation of the previous report, further literature relevant to the development of pharmacokinetic models of the selected carcinogens has been identified. This is reviewed below.

This review is not intended to replace the earlier work (Thorne and Jackson, 1983), and should be read in conjunction with the relevant appendices to that report.

4.1   Arsenic

Anke et al. (1977) studied the essentiality of arsenic to animals. They fed goats and minipigs on an arsenic-depleted diet (< 50 ppb) and found a reduction in birth rate, in body weight of the new-born and an increase in the mortality rate of the young. Reduced arsenic in the diet had no effect on the growth of the first generation, but the second generation had a lower weight gain. The mortality rate of adult arsenic-deficient goats was also significantly higher than controls. These results suggest that arsenic is an essential element for normal bodily function in animals.

4.1.1   Intake rates

A study of the dietary intake of various metals in a population known to be exposed to lead from water was performed by Sherlock et al. (1983). Their results are summarised below:

Arsenic (mg/week)	0.05	0.6-10	1.1-1.5	1.5-2.0	> 2
No. adults	23	3	3	1	1

The highest dietary intake were found in subjects who had eaten the most fish, as expected from earlier studies. The mean intake of

0.49 mg/week corresponds to a daily intake of 70 µg, confirming the trend for reduced dietary intake of arsenic since the reduction in use of arsenic-containing pesticides on food crops.

A survey of community water supply systems in the United States (McCabe et al., 1970) found that only 0.2% of samples from different regions exceeded the mandatory arsenic limit of 0.05 mg/l and that only 0.4% exceeded the recommended limit of 0.01 mg/l.

A summary of the environmental distribution of arsenic was presented by Bennett (1981) which contained a table of global emissions of arsenic (Table 4.1). An extensive review of the environmental chemistry and global cycle of various metals including arsenic was presented by Merian (1984). Hartwell et al. (1983) investigated the levels of arsenic, cadmium and lead around several zinc and copper smelters in the United States. For arsenic, they found that air, dust and soil concentrations of the element increased with proximity to the smelter, whereas water concentrations were unaffected. The air concentrations varied from 0.1 to 83 ng/m^3, but this depended on various factors, such as wind speed and direction.

TABLE 4.1

GLOBAL EMISSIONS OF ARSENIC TO THE ENVIRONMENT

Source	Emission rate (10^6 kg y^{-1})
Natural	
Volcanoes	7
Biological activity	0.26
Weathering	0.24
Forest fires	0.16
Sea spray	0.14
Total	7.8
Anthropogenic	
Copper production	13
Iron and steel production	4.2
Lead and zinc production	2.2
Agricultural chemicals	1.9
Wood fuel	0.60
Agricultural burning	0.56
Coal combustion	0.55
Waste incineration	0.43
Chemicals production	0.20
Cotton ginning	0.023
Mineral ore mining	0.013
Residual fuels	0.004
Total	23.7

From Bennett (1981)

Tissue & organ	Sex	Number	As(III)	As(V)	MAA	%*	DMAA	%*	Total
Aorta	♂	8	117.0±61.1	335.0± 82.3	ND		17.1± 6.5	100	469.0±131
	♀	8	131.0±74.3	486.0±411	ND		15.8± 4.4	100	633.0±480
	Total	16	124.0±66.1	411.0±297	ND		16.4± 5.4	100	551.0±350
Adrenal gland	♂	10	33.5±11.5	134.0±135	ND		26.2±10.0	100	194.0±140
	♀	9	59.9±57.3	390.0±433	ND		25.4±20.1	100	475.0±479
	Total	19	46.0±41.3	255.0±331	ND		25.8±15.2	100	327.0±364
Cerebellum	♂	15	28.7±13.9	99.5± 60.2	ND		ND		128.0± 71.9
	♀	15	31.8± 9.9	107.0± 33.7	ND		ND		138.0± 41.5
	Total	30	30.0±12.2	102.0± 50.0					132.0± 60.2
Cerebrum	♂	15	20.8±10.7	56.1± 38.7	ND		ND		77.3± 49.0
	♀	15	17.0±11.9	59.8± 30.4	ND		ND		75.3± 39.1
	Total	30	19.0±11.3	57.8± 34.5					76.3± 43.9
Kidney	♂	14	31.2±15.5	88.2± 74.8	3.8±2.7	71	27.2±12.3	71	142.0± 89.1
	♀	10	21.9± 7.5	45.6± 11.0	3.4±2.7	80	28.2± 9.2	80	94.8± 21.4
	Total	24	27.3±13.4	70.4± 60.6	3.6±2.6	76	27.6±10.7	76	129.0± 72.3
Liver	♂	12	30.9±18.0	99.5± 38.0	6.8±6.8	75	13.4± 3.8	67	145.0± 45.4
	♀	11	17.9± 5.3	82.3± 24.3	4.6±6.2	55	14.7± 7.6	73	112.0± 24.3
	Total	23	24.7±14.8	91.3± 32.7	5.9±6.5	65	14.0± 5.7	70	129.0± 39.7

Levels of arsenic (ng of As per g wet weight)

Values denote the mean ± SD. As(III) and As(V) was detected in all tissues.
ND: Not detected (the lower detectable limit: 1.0 ng of As per g wet weight).
* Ratio of tissue/organ samples where MAA or DMAA was detected.
From Yamauchi and Yamamura (1983).

TABLE 4.2

LEVELS AND CHEMICAL SPECIES OF ARSENIC IN THE NORMAL TISSUES
AND ORGANS OF THE JAPANESE

Levels of arsenic (ng of As per g wet weight)

Tissue/organ	Sex	Number	As(III)	As(V)	MAA	%*	DMAA	%*	Total
Lung	♂	12	17.1± 7.0	74.2± 20.1	ND		6.7± 3.8	100	98.0± 26.1
	♀	10	17.4± 9.2	87.0± 32.3	ND		8.9± 5.9	100	113.0± 32.9
	Total	22	17.2± 7.8	79.7± 26.1			7.6± 4.8	100	104.0± 29.5
Muscle	♂	12	24.5±11.1	65.5± 34.0	ND		20.2± 8.7	92	109.0± 42.7
	♀	10	24.5± 6.0	61.4± 13.3	ND		17.7± 9.0	100	104.0± 18.2
	Total	22	24.5± 8.8	63.6± 25.7			18.9± 8.7	96	106.0± 32.7
Pancreas	♂	10	35.3±18.0	107.0± 64.0	ND		13.7± 9.4	100	156.0± 82.0
	♀	8	25.0±10.6	111.0± 49.6	ND		16.0± 6.6	100	152.0± 60.4
	Total	18	30.7±15.6	109.0± 56.5			14.7± 8.1	100	154.0± 71.4
Skin	♂	11	19.6± 7.3	111.0± 45.4	ND		4.5± 5.0	91	134.0± 51.9
	♀	11	27.6±17.7	141.0±113.0	ND		2.9± 4.1	91	172.0±129.0
	Total	22	23.6±13.9	126.0± 85.5			3.7± 4.5	91	153.0± 97.7
Spleen	♂	10	24.6±15.8	66.3± 41.5	ND		11.8± 7.8	90	101.0± 58.7
	♀	10	24.5± 9.0	67.4± 34.5	ND		13.7± 3.8	70	101.0± 41.2
	Total	20	24.5±12.5	66.9± 37.2			12.6± 6.2	80	101.0± 49.4

Values denote the mean ± SD. As(III) and As(V) was detected in all tissues.

ND: Not detected (the lower detectable limit: 1.0 ng of As per g wet weight).
 * Ratio of tissue/organ samples where MAA or DMAA was detected.
  From Yamauchi and Yamamura (1983).

TABLE 4.2 (Contd)

4.1.2   Distribution of arsenic in human tissues

Further studies of arsenic concentration in human tissues were identified. The first, by Yamauchi and Yamamura (1983), used autopsy samples from humans who had died of cerebral bleeding, pneumonia or cancer.

The samples were assayed for arsenic species and total arsenic. The subjects had no known exposure to high occupational or environmental levels of arsenic. The results are shown in Table 4.2. In general, the total arsenic concentration for each tissue, is some-what higher than previously reported values (see Thorne and Jackson, 1983). For the four chemical species detected, As (III) and (V) were predominant in all tissues, comprising 20.4% and 72.0% of all tissue arsenic, respectively. Methylarsonic acid (MAA) was only detected in liver and kidney, whereas dimethylarsonic acid (DMA) was found in all tissues, but at much lower concentrations than the inorganic arsenic species.

Dang et al. (1983) obtained tissue samples from subjects who died in accidents in Bombay. These were collected and assayed for arsenic and the results are shown in Table 4.3. They are slightly lower than other reported values (Thorne and Jackson, 1983) except for hair concentrations. Unfortunately, the method of preparation of the hair samples was not stated. This is critical since the arsenic measured in hair may be due to external contamination of the hair by contact, and not due to an excretion process from the body arsenic pool. In an investigation by Pirl et al. (1983), of tissue concentra-tions in two subjects who died from excess arsenic ingestion, it was found that arsenic deposited on hair or nails after contact with an arsenate or arsenite solution (e.g. one case was discovered lying in a pool of vomitus) could not be removed by washing in water or hydro-chloric acid.

In a community where the drinking water was contaminated by arsenic (0.4 mg l^{-1}), arsenic concentrations in blood, urine, hair and nails were significantly higher than in a control population. (Olguin et al., 1983).

In a review of literature values for trace elements in serum or plasma, Versieck and Cornelis (1980) concluded that typical concen-tration in these tissues were in the range 1-5 µg l^{-1}.

Further studies on arsenic concentrations in potential monitoring substances such as blood and urine are included in the discussion of metabolism.

4.1.3   Metabolism

Due to the atypical accumulation of arsenic by rat erythro-cytes, studies of arsenic metabolism in rats are not considered in this review.

4.1.3.1   Retention in the respiratory system

Pershagen et al. (1982) gave hamsters weekly intratracheal instillations of arsenic trioxide, arsenic trisulphide or calcium

Tissue/ Organ	No. of samples	As concentration (ng/g fresh weight)				Geometric mean	Geometric standard deviation
		Range	Median	Arithmetic mean	Standard deviation		
Liver	19	4.5-27.7	12.4	14.5	6.9	13.2	1.2
Kidney	13	1.6-62.8	4.7	12.4	20.7	5.8	2.7
Brain	12	2.5-6.0	4.0	3.9	1.0	3.8	1.0
Lungs	13	2.5-81.8	9.8	19.9	22.7	12.7	1.8
Spleen	18	3.6-46.2	5.8	15.2	16.6	9.5	1.7
Hair	17	63.8-2140	228.0	474.9	596.3	355.2	2.3
Blood	8	3.1-13.8	4.1	5.9	3.9	4.6	1.3
Human milk	25	0.2-1.1	0.8	0.7	0.2	0.6	1.3

TABLE 4.3

ARSENIC LEVELS IN DIFFERENT HUMAN TISSUES

From Dang et al. (1983)

arsenate dust suspensions. Animals were killed at weekly intervals, and arsenic concentrations in lung, liver and hair were determined by atomic absorption spectrophotometry. Animals receiving calcium arsenate exhibited arsenic levels 100 times greater than those recorded in animals receiving arsenic trisulphide and 1000 times those recorded in animals receiving arsenic trioxide. The in vitro solubility of the three compounds corresponded to this trend i.e. arsenic trioxide was most soluble followed by arsenic trisulphide then sodium arsenate. This apparent dependence of lung clearance upon solubility of the inhaled compound could have significance in human exposure situations (see Section 6.4).

4.1.3.2   In vivo studies

Retention, excretion and metabolism of an oral or intravenous (I.V) dose of arsenic, in hamsters, was studied by Charbonneau et al. (1980). They found a biphasic clearance pattern in both instances. With I.V. administration, 65% of the dose was eliminated with a half-time of 0.4 days and 35% with a half-time of 4.5 days. For oral administration, the corresponding values were 98% and 0.3 days for the first phase and 2% and 3.8 days for the second. The main difference in excretion pattern appeared to be due to the increased faecal excretion in orally dosed hamsters, with 70% being excreted in the faeces compared to 6% in I.V. dosed animals. Analysis of the urinary metabolites showed DMA and inorganic arsenic to be present. Inamasu (1983) investigated the excretion of arsenic metabolites following an oral dose of arsenite. Approximately 20% of the dose was excreted in the urine and 50% in the faeces during the 5 days after the administration. Both DMA and MMA were found in the urine, but only MMA was excreted in the faeces.

Renal handling of sodium arsenate in dogs was studied by Tsukamato et al. (1983). When sodium arsenate was infused intravenously, variable arsenite concentrations were found in the plasma and urine. The renal tubule cell was determined to be the probable site of arsenite reabsorption, reduction of arsenate to arsenite and secretion or diffusion of the latter into urine. With high doses of arsenate (15 mg/kg) reabsorption of arsenite to plasma took place. During the experiment, which lasted 100 minutes, only 40% of the arsenate infused was excreted in the urine, with a minimal amount of DMA being detected. In contrast, during the next day, DMA was the major metabolite excreted in urine.

Tsukamato et al. (1983) also observed that low doses of arsenate caused mild pathological changes in the renal tubular epithelium, and that these histological changes were seen before the onset of clinical symptons such as changes in creatinine clearance and potassium reabsorption.

Recent studies in man have been concerned with the excretion of arsenic ingested in seafood. This arsenic is thought to be in the form of arsenobetaine and is not metabolised in the same way as inorganic arsenic (see below). Luten et al. (1983) investigated the excretion of a single oral dose of fish-arsenic in human volunteers. The majority of the arsenic was excreted in urine within the first day after ingestion. Tam et al. (1982) performed a similar experiment and obtained a triphasic excretion pattern with components exhibiting half-times of 0.16 days, 0.75 days and 3.3 days. They also reported that 50% of the administered arsenic was excreted in the first day.

Tissue distribution and retention have been studied using autoradiographic techniques. In studies on mice and hamsters, (Lindgren et al., 1982) tissue retentions were followed after I.V. injection of arsenate and arsenite. The results are shown in Table 4.4. In general, higher organ concentrations were seen for As(III) than As(V) with the only exception being in bone. Initially, highest tissue concentrations are seen in bile, kidney and liver, but clearance from these is fairly rapid.

Tissue distribution and subcellular binding in marmoset monkeys after I.V. injection of arsenite was investigated by Vahter et al. (1982). They found that no methylation of the arsenate occurred, in contrast to all other species studied previously. The elimination of arsenite was much slower than in other studies, lending weight to the suggestion, from similar experiments in other species, that the methylated forms of inorganic arsenic are more mobile than the inorganic forms and are cleared more rapidly from the body.

Transfer of arsenic to the developing organism was studied in mice by Gerber et al. (1982). Three methods were used.

- Arsenic-containing diet was given to the mother after formation of the vaginal plug and tissue distributions were determined in the foetus at various times during the pregnancy, and in the offspring after birth.

- The isotope was injected intraperitoneally during organogenesis (at day 12) and maternal organ concentrations, together with transfer to the foetus, were followed for 7 days.

- The isotope-containing diet was applied throughout the entire pregnancy and for 15 days after. Radioactivity in the mothers was followed for 150 days and in the litter for 15 days. Excretion components with half-lives of less than a day, less than a week and several months could be discerned in the adults. Transfer to the foetus occurred during organogenesis and, after birth, arsenic was taken up by the new born via the mother's milk.

As already noted, the inability of the marmoset monkey to methylate inorganic arsenic lead to a much slower excretion of the substance. The marmoset monkey is the only species so far investigated that does not have this capacity for methylation.

Vahter and Envall (1983) investigated the in vivo reduction of arsenate in mice and rabbits. They followed urinary excretion after I.V. dosing. During the first four hours after administration, approximately 10% of the administered arsenate was excreted in the trivalent form. Arsenic excreted in the first hour was mainly in the unmetabolized pentavalent form, with some trivalent arsenite present. Thereafter, the excretion of the trivalent form and DMA increased. These results indicate that arsenate has to be reduced to arsenite before methylation can occur.

Tissue/fluid	Concentration of ^{74}As-arsenic, ng/g			
	0.5 hr	6 hrs	24 hrs	72 hrs
Blood	164±9.5	16±1.8	1.2±0.1	0.7±0.1
Blood red cells	99±10	14±1.6	1.7±0.2	1.1±0.1
Blood plasma	218±18	16±2.0	0.6±0.1	0.3±0.1
Brain	20±3.6	26±2.5	1.8±0.1	0.6±0.1
Duodenum	553±91	77±14	5.6±0.6	2.0±0.5
Epididymis	127±10	66±11	16±2.3	9.7±1.6
Eyes	74±7.2	22±4.8	6.1±1.2	5.7±0.5
Gallbladder*	1255±298	200±98	<10	<10
Hair*	17±6	1.2±0.5	2.3±0.5	5.0±0.4
Kidney	2355±185	209±33	20±1.5	7.7±0.7
Liver	571±68	77±12	8.1±0.4	3.3±0.2
Lung	291±26	131±19	8.0±0.7	2.3±0.1
Skeleton	388±52	98±24	41±3.8	17±1.5
Skin	184±18	46±3.9	16±1.3	9.1±0.9
Small intestine	214±12	53±8.4	3.9±0.9	1.6±0.3
Spleen	187±19	56±5.4	6.0±0.5	2.6±0.4
Stomach	165±15	81±10	24±1.6	11±0.7
Testis	48±4.8	34±4.0	5.7±0.4	0.9±0.3

Concentration of ^{74}As-arsenic in tissues of mice 0.5-72 hours after single
intravenous injection of ^{74}As-arsenate (0.4 mg As/kg b.wt.). Mean of 5 animals±S.E.

* n = 3
** n = 4

TABLE 4.4
ARSENIC IN MICE

Tissue/fluid	Concentration of ^{74}As-arsenic, ng/g			
	0.5 hr	6 hrs	24 hrs	72 hrs
Blood	106±13	30±1.9	3.8±0.3	2.3±0.1
Blood red cells	121±10	32±1.3	6.3±0.5	4.0±0.2
Blood plasma	85±24	27±2.8	1.1±0.2	0.5±0.1
Brain	21±1.5	41±3.6	3.3±0.3	0.9±0.1
Duodenum	1016±96	150±12	14.±1.9	4.6±0.6
Epididymis	187±15	151±5.6	61±8.1	36.±4.5
Eyes	86±10	41±3.2	14.±1.6	6.9±0.8
Gallbladder*	5172±3022	422±224	<10	<10
Hair*	48±19	11±9.0	4.4±0.9	19.0±4.4
Kidney	1603±211	200±15	20±0.9	7.6±0.5
Liver	1589±222	188±11	29±1.4	12.1±1.0
Lung	540±59	243±37	23±2.9	5.6±0.4
Skeleton	247±34	82±4.5	8.8±1.3	3.6±0.9
Skin	205±22	125±5.5	66±7.8	42±4.3
Small intestine	582±87	124±6.4	9.0±1.1	3.6±0.3
Spleen	412±58	110±6.7	16±1.1	2.8±0.9
Stomach	418±58	118±13	79±5.2	27±3.6
Testis	47±1.7	60±5.0	11±1.0	1.2±0.4

Concentration of ^{74}As-arsenic in tissues of mice 0.5-72 hours after single intravenous injection of ^{74}As-arsenite (0.4 mg As/kg b.wt.). Mean of 5 animals±S.E.

* n = 3
** n = 4

From Lindgren et al. (1982)

TABLE 4.4 (Contd)

In vitro incubation of arsenite, arsenate or DMA with liver, lung and kidney tissue homogenate from rabbits showed that arsenite is the main form of arsenic bound to tissues (Vahter and Marafante, 1983).

In animals injected with arsenate or arsenite, higher tissue concentrations were found as a result of arsenite administration at first, but after four hours, no difference could be detected in concentrations resulting from the two administered forms. This is probably due to in vivo reduction of arsenate to arsenite. Following injection of DMA, excretion is complete within 24 hours, suggesting a low tissue affinity for this compound.

Metabolism and retention studies of the forms of arsenic found in sea-food were performed by Marafante and co-workers (Marafante et al., 1984; Vahter et al., 1983). They found that the compounds arsenobetaine and arsenocholine were almost completely absorbed from the gastrointestinal tract of mice and rabbits. The retention and tissue distribution of these compounds were different from those observed using inorganic arsenic compounds, although the gross excretion patterns were quantitatively similar (70 - 80% of the dose being excreted in urine in 3 days). No degradation of these organic arsenic compounds to inorganic arsenic compounds or to MAA or DMA was observed.

4.1.4   Carcinogenicity of arsenic

The major criticism of epidemiological studies linking occupational exposure to arsenic with induction of cancer is that it is impossible to evaluate the effects of other factors in the occupational environment. To start to answer this criticism, several groups have tried to assess the interrelationships between smoking, arsenic exposure and lung cancer. Pershagen et al. (1981) investigated the above interactions using data on deceased Swedish copper smelter workers. The age standardized mortality ratio for lung cancer was 3.0 for arsenic-exposed non-smokers and 4.9 for smokers with no occupational exposure to arsenic, compared with non-exposed non-smokers. For arsenic exposed smokers the ratio was 14.6, indicating a multiplicative effect of the two agents, (suggesting that a strong preventative effect on lung cancer incidence could be obtained by decreasing either one of the exposures or by disaggregating them). Welch et al. (1982) obtained a clear dose-response relationship for arsenic exposure and respiratory cancer incidence in smokers at a copper smelter. Men in the highest exposure category ($\geq$ 5 mg/m^3) had a sevenfold excess of cancer, those in the low and medium classes (< 500 µg/m^3) had a risk close to that expected. Maximum levels of arsenic exposure appeared to be more important that did time-weighted average exposure. Smoking did not appear to be as important as arsenic exposure in inducing respiratory cancer in this particular population. These findings suggest that if exposure is kept below 500 µg/m^3 little or no excess lung cancer should be seen. However, the estimates of arsenic exposure were based on department averages, rather than concentrations for individual jobs. Also, in a preliminary report on this work (Higgins et al., 1981) it was found that among the heavily exposed workers, there was a lower proportion of non-smokers (suggesting some interaction between smoking habits and arsenic exposure). Furthermore, comparison of smoking habits reported by smelter workers suggested that, as a group they smoked more heavily than average for the population from which they were drawn.

It seems likely that smoking and arsenic exposure interact in the causation of lung cancer. However, there is sufficient evidence to suggest that occupational exposure, with arsenic present in the environment, can lead to respiratory cancer in non-smokers. There is still no evidence that arsenic alone is responsible, since other carcinogenic substances, such as sulphur dioxide, are usually found in the same environments.

Wicks et al. (1981) observed that 38% of lung cancers from patients who worked at a copper smelter were found to be adenomas, compared with 12% among controls. This statistically significant enhancement of adenocarcinomas relative to all lung cancers, was associated with arsenic exposure. However, once again, it was impossible to ascertain whether arsenic was the only potential carcinogen in the environment. Many of the studies undertaken to elucidate the mechanisms of toxicity of arsenic have used in vitro methods. McCabe et al. (1983) investigated the action of arsenic on human and bovine lymphocyte mitogenesis. At low arsenate concentrations, they found a potentiation of the effect of phytohaemaglutinin (a mitogenic agent in its own right) on mitogenesis. At higher concentrations, a more generalised toxic effect was seen, and mitogenesis was completely inhibited. It was suggested that, by potentiating mitogenesis, arsenic compounds could increase the possibility of errors in DNA replication, some of which could be potentially carcinogenic. In addition, interference with the immune system could enable potentially cancerous cells to escape immune surveillance.

Jung et al. (1970) observed that arsenic could inhibit DNA repair enzymes which adds weight to the hypothesis of excess errors in DNA replication being produced by arsenic-induced mitogenesis.

A review of arsenic mutagenesis and carcinogenesis was presented by Leonard (1984). He concluded that the negative findings on experimental animals suggest that observations of occupational exposure-related cancers may be due to arsenic acting as a co-carcinogen with other agents present in the work environment, i.e. the primary carcinogenic agent causing the abnormality in DNA, with arsenic inhibiting DNA repair mechanisms. However, DNA abnormalities must occur during normal replication. These are usually dealt with by the repair mechanisms. If this is inhibited by arsenic, then it is reasonable to expect arsenic to be carcinogenic in its own right.

Finally, it is noted that in an in vivo experiment, Ishinishi et al. (1983) instilled arsenic trioxide intratracheally into Syrian golden hamsters once a week. The control animals were treated with the vehicle, phosphate buffer solution. During the total life span, 3 lung adenomas were manifested in 10 hamsters and, in another study, 2 lung adenomas were manifested in another 20 hamsters after 15 instillations of arsenic. In contrast, no lung tumours were detected in 35 hamsters in 2 control groups. These results show that arsenic trioxide induces lung tumours in Syrian golden hamsters.

Exposure ($\mu g/m^3$)		Blood Arsenic ($\mu g/l$)	Urine Arsenic ($\mu g/l$)σ						
			InAs	MMAA	DMAA	MethAs	InAsMet	OF[a]	Total-As[b]
4.5-619	x̄	30.7	17.5	13.7	50.0	63.7	81.2	7.5	88.7
	SD	(16.8)	(10.5)	(8.9)	(34.2)			(13.9)	(34.0)
	range	8-48	7-31	5-26	23-100			0-29	60-138
0.6-2.9	x̄	12.5	6.3	4.1	15.9	20.0	26.3	7.6	33.9
	SD	(10.5)	(4.3)	(3.0)	(13.4)			(13.1)	(23.4)
	range	0.5-38	0.5-15	0.5-12	0.5-61			0-59	1-103
<0.5	x̄	13.4	4.9	2.2	13.4	15.6	20.5	5.2	25.7
	SD	(15.0)	(5.1)	(1.1)	(7.9)			(7.7)	(19.8)
	range	0.5-37	1-16	0.5-4	7-31			0-18	8-67
Total	x̄	15.7	7.1	4.7	18.9	23.6	30.7	7.0	37.7
	SD	(13.2)	(6.5)	(8.4)	(19.2)			(10.9)	(29.9)
	range	0.5-48	0.5-31	0.5-26	0.5-100			0-59	1-138

[a] OF = other forms of As, calculated as the difference between total-As and InAsMet.

[b] Determined by ashing of the urine samples in toto.

From Foa et al. (1984)

TABLE 4.5

BLOOD AND URINE As CONCENTRATION IN GLASS WORKERS OCCUPATIONALLY EXPOSED TO As_2O_3

4.1.5   Occupational exposure

Urinary excretion of arsenic is the most convenient method of monitoring exposure to the element. However, there is disagreement in the literature as to whether urinary arsenic levels reflect levels of occupational exposure. Schrenk and Schreibis (1958) reviewed the early literature and concluded that urinary arsenic levels were not a reliable index of industrial exposure.

In workers exposed to arsenic-based wood preservatives, Takahashi et al. (1983) found a significantly higher urinary arsenic concentration than in a non-exposed group. Also, Cant and Legendre (1982) found a progressive reduction in urinary arsenic levels subsequent to improvement in industrial hygiene standards.

The main problem in monitoring urinary arsenic is in the chemical speciation of the arsenic compounds in urine. It has already been noted that inorganic arsenic and the organic forms of arsenic present in foods are metabolised independently by the body. The purpose of monitoring is to assess occupational exposure to the substance. In the past, workers have tried to correlate total urinary arsenic with exposure. However, total urinary arsenic will also contain the contribution due to arsenobetaine from dietary intake. As there is no possibility of occupational exposure to this chemical form of arsenic, a better correlation would probably be obtained if the urinary excretion of inorganic arsenic and its metabolites MMA and DMA was measured and related to occupational exposure, which will almost invariably be to inorganic arsenic.

The organic arsenic compounds in sea-food are not biotransformed in the body and are excreted in the form in which they were ingested. Unlike the organic metabolites of inorganic arsenic, MMA and DMA, they do not produce arsine gas (AsH_3) when treated with reducing agents. Norin and Vahter (1981) utilised this property to develop an assay for inorganic arsenic and its derivatives in urine, with no contribution from sea-food derived arsenic compounds.

A similar method was used by Foa et al. (1984) to investigate the chemical speciation of the chemical form of arsenic in urine. They found in a normal population, average total urinary arsenic levels of 17.2 $\mu g \ l^{-1}$ comprising of 10% each of inorganic arsenic, MMA and DMA, and 70% of other organic forms of arsenic. Average blood arsenic levels were 5.1 $\mu g \ l^{-1}$ and correlations with the urinary concentration of inorganic arsenic and with the total arsenic (inorganic arsenic plus DMA plus MMA) were found. Data were also reported on blood and urinary levels of arsenic in a subject after an attempted suicidal ingestion of sodium arsenite. Unfortunately, these data could not be used to derive kinetic parameters for the retention of arsenic in normal subjects, since 45% of the subject's blood was replaced in an exchange transfusion and peritoneal dialysis was used in treatment.

Data were presented by Foa et al. (1984) for urinary concentrations of the various forms of arsenic in glass workers exposed to arsenic trioxide. These are shown in Table 4.5. The total arsenic concentration in blood is proportional to exposure and correlates only with DMA excretion. DMA in urine seems to be the most appropriate single indicator of exposure. At high exposure levels (total arsenic excretion > 200 $\mu g \ l^{-1}$), arsenic accumulates in the organism, and DMA excretion reflects this accumulation. At low exposure levels (total arsenic excretion < 50 μg l^{-1}) short term accumulation does not occur, and the best biological indicator is inorganic arsenic excretion.

A confirmation of the finding that sea-food ingestion causes a marked increase in total urinary excretion of arsenic, unaccompanied by a rise in inorganic arsenic-related excretion was presented in the above study.

Arsenic concentration in hair has also been reported to reflect total arsenic exposure. However, as already mentioned, hair is very susceptible to external contamination, which is difficult to remove. Until an accepted washing and sample preparation procedure is developed, results from studies in which exposure is monitored by assays of hair concentration should be treated cautiously.

However, Hartwell et al. (1983) (see Section 4.1.2) used a very thorough washing procedure, and found that the most useful indication of environmental metal levels, at various distances from zinc and copper smelters, was hair, rather than urine or blood.

4.1.6   Development of a metabolic model

A review of the most recent literature on the subject of arsenic metabolism revealed no information sufficient to justify

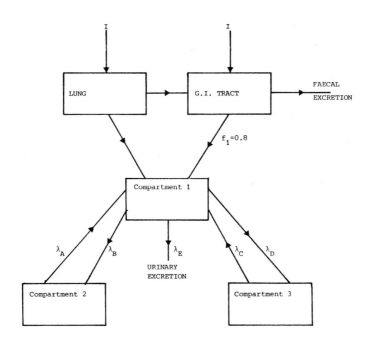

Note: for parameter values see text.

FIGURE 4.1 SYSTEMIC MODEL OF ARSENIC METABOLISM

altering the model developed by Thorne and Jackson (1983), and this model has been implemented. The model is based primarily on a study by Mealey et al. (1959), who interpreted their results in terms of three compartments.

This model structure is shown in Fig. 4.1 and is used in conjunction with following parameters.

Parameter	value (d^{-1})
λ_A	0.336
λ_B	18.48
λ_C	0.012
λ_D	9.24
λ_E	9.24

Individual tissue concentrations are computed as follows:

Liver = 0.64 (COMPARTMENT 1) + 0.05 (COMPARTMENT 2) + 0.052 (COMPARTMENT 3)

Kidney = 0.12 (COMPARTMENT 1) + 0.01 (COMPARTMENT 2) + 0.008 (COMPARTMENT 3)

Blood = 0.24 (COMPARTMENT 1) * 1.6

Other tissue = 0.94 (COMPARTMENT 2) + 0.94 (COMPARTMENT 3)

Arsenic is absorbed readily from the GI tract, and an f_1 value of 0.8 is assumed. With a typical dietary intake of 150 µg day^{-1} and no occupational exposure, the following values are calculated as the equilibrium contents of the compartments of the model.

compartment (1) = 0.013 mg
compartment (2) = 0.714 mg
compartment (3) = 9.987 mg

4.2   Beryllium

No further data on rates of intake or human tissue concentrations of beryllium (Be) were identified.

4.2.1   Metabolism

Vacher and Stoner (1968a) studied the transport of beryllium sulphate administered intravenously. They concluded that when beryllium sulphate enters the blood, beryllium phosphate is produced, and that most of the aggregates are probably bound to plasma α-globulin. In a further paper, Vacher and Stoner (1968b) investigated the removal from the body of beryllium administered intravenously in different

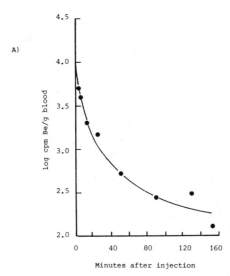

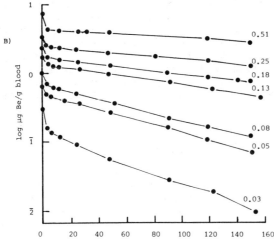

Note:
Redrawn from Vacher and Stoner (1968a)

FIGURE 4.2.   CLEARANCE OF BERYLLIUM FROM THE BLOOD OF RATS
A) AFTER INJECTION OF CARRIER FREE ^{7}Be Cl$_2$
B) AFTER INTRAVENOUS INJECTION OF DIFFERENT DOSES OF Be SO$_4$
THE DOSES (mg. Be per kg. body wt.) ARE INDICATED BY THE
FIGURES ABOVE EACH CURVE

chemical forms. Different kinetics were observed when [7]Be was administered as carrier-free Be or as [7]BeSO$_4$. As can be seen from
Fig. 4.2, disappearance of [7]Be from blood is much more rapid when
carrier-free [7]Be is administered. When [7]Be SO$_4$ is administered the
clearance curve is biphasic. The difference between the two curves
was tentatively explained as follows. The clearance of carrier-free
[7]Be was mainly governed by the disappearance of diffusable beryllium.
However, with the addition of a carrier, this component is much
reduced, and clearance of the resulting beryllium phosphate aggregates
by the reticuloendothelial system becomes more important. For the
second phase of the clearance of [7]BeSO$_4$, an inverse, non-saturable
relationship between dose and rate of removal was observed. This has
been observed for clearance of other commonly used particles such as
carbon. However, these agents are administered with suspending
materials such as gelatin, which are not neutral in the reactions
concerned with the clearance of the particles. The beryllium phosphate particles are formed in situ in the plasma, with no suspending
agents, suggesting that the biphasic clearance of particles by the
reticulendothelial system is not dependent on the presence of a suspending agent.

Vacher and Stoner (1968b) also presented data on tissue
concentrations of [7]Be, 2.5 hours after I.V. injection (Table 4.6).

These data show an inverse relationship between dose and
fractional uptake by skeleton and kidney (implying that this transfer
involves the freely diffusable beryllium component) whereas there is a
direct relationship between dose and fractional uptake of liver,
spleen (reticuloendothelial system) and muscle (suggesting clearance
of particulate beryllium phosphate).

Clary et al. (1975) investigated the effect of reproduction
and lactation on the onset of latent chronic beryllium disease. They
administered radio-labelled beryllium intratracheally to female rats
which were then separated into two groups. One group was bred continuously, whereas the second group were not bred. This was done to
study the effects of adrenal stimulation (resulting from repeated
pregnancy and lactation) on the onset of beryllium disease. No
difference in the time of onset, as indicated by lung granuloma, was
noticed between the bred and un-bred rats, suggesting that adrenal
stress is not an inducer of latent chronic beryllium disease. The
distribution of beryllium in tissues was similar in the two groups.
Beryllium appeared to have no detrimental effect on reproduction, but
radioactivity was detected in some of the foetuses, suggesting that
trans-placental movement of beryllium does occur.

4.2.2   Cellular actions of beryllium

Vacher et al. (1975) studied the hepatoxicity of beryllium.
Plasma β-glucuronidase and transaminase were used as indices of cell
damage. The intravenous injection of sub-lethal doses of beryllium
phosphate produced a biphasic variation in plasma levels of the
β-glucuronidase with two peaks 7 h and 96 h after administration. The
96 h peak was accompanied by a large rise in plasma transaminase
(implying cell lysis). Doses below 100 μg kg^{-1} produced the first
phase only, with no observable change in levels of transaminase after

Dose mg. Be per kg. body weight	Liver	Spleen	Lungs	Kidneys	Musculature	Skeleton
			Percentage of dose (Mean ± S.E.)			
0.51 (17)	18.1±1.2	2.0±0.1	3.5±0.4	1.1±0.1	8.8±0.7	9.6±0.8
0.25 (6)	19.8±3.4	2.1±0.2	5.0±2.1	0.9±0.1	5.6±1.4	7.3±0.7
0.18 (3)	14.8±0.5	1.6±0.1	13.0±3.4	1.1±0.1	5.8±0.9	11.7±2.0
0.13 (5)	19.9±2.8	2.2±0.4	7.7±3.2	1.4±0.1	5.4±0.7	11.0±1.3
0.08 (7)	22.8±3.8	1.9±0.5	3.6±1.0	1.9±0.2	3.8±0.4	14.8±2.2
0.05 (4)	13.4±1.7	1.1±0.2	2.1±0.7	2.4±0.3	4.0±0.9	24.0±2.5
0.03 (4)	6.5±1.2	0.3±0.1	0.6±0.3	4.6±1.1	3.0±1.1	29.7 (24.7, 34.6)
^{7}Be (3)	5.7±1.3	0.1±0.03	0.2±0.03	2.6±0.19	1.1±0.2	30.2 (31.3, 29.0)

No. of rats shown in parentheses. Where there were only 2 samples available the individual values are given in parentheses after the mean. From Vacher and Stoner (1968b).

TABLE 4.6

THE DISTRIBUTION OF BERYLLIUM 2.5 hr. AFTER ITS I.V. INJECTION
AS $BeSO_4$ OR AS CARRIER-FREE ^{7}BE

Author	Year	Species	Compound	Mode of Administration	Total dose (mg Be)	Incidence of Osteosarcoma
Gardner	1946	rabbits	Zn-Be-silicate		60	7 in 7
			BeO		360	1 in 7
		guinea pigs	Zn-Be-silicate	i.v. in 20 doses	60	0
			BeO		360	0
		rats	Zn-Be-silicate		60	0
			BeO		360	0
		rabbits	Zn-Be-silicate		17	4 in 5
			BeO		140	0
Cloudman	1949	mice	Zn-Be-silicate	i.v. in 20-22 doses	0.26	"some"
			BeO		0.55	0
Barnes	1950	rabbits	Zn-Be-silicate	i.v. in 6-10 doses	7.2	4 in 14
			BeO		15	2 in 3
			BeO		180	1 in 11
			Zn-Be-silicate (BeO - 2.3%)		3-7	3 in 6
			Zn-Be-silicate (BeO - 14%)			
Hoagland	1950	rabbits	Be phosphate	i.v. in 1-30 doses	10-12	3 in 4
			BeO		1307	0 in 5
					350	1 in 8
Nash	1950	rabbits	Zn-Be-silicate	i.v. "repeated"	12+	5 in 28
				i.v. in 17-25 doses	54-90	2 in 3
				i.v. in 20-26 doses	360-700	6 in 6
Dutra	1951	rabbits	BeO	inhalation	1*	0 in 5
				25 hrs/wk	6*	1 in 6
				9-13 months	30*	0 in 8
Janes	1954	rabbits				
	1956	splenectomized rabbits				5 in 10
Kelly	1961	rabbits	Zn-Be-silicate	i.v. in 20 doses	12	7 in 7
Higgins	1964	rabbits			12	10 in 14
					3300	"many"

* atmospheric concentration in mg Be/m^3

From Reeves (1979)

TABLE 4.7

OSTEOSARCOMA FROM BERYLLIUM

96 h.   This dissociation was not seen with carbon tetrachloride, another hepatotoxic agent, and was thought to illustrate a specific lysosomal effect of beryllium.   The changes in β-glucuronidase activity were thought to be related to the postphagocytic intralysa-somal storage of beryllium phosphate.   The first phase was attributed to selective exocytosis of lysosomal enzyme while the second was attributed to toxic cell damage.

Recent research on the biochemical basis of beryllium carci-nogenity has been directed toward interactions with the components of the cell nucleus.   Perry et al. (1982) studied the effects of bery-llium on hormonal regulation of gene expression in vitro.   They found that exposure to 1 μM $BeSO_4$ had no effect on cell growth, but the induction of tyrosine aminotransferase (TA) synthesis, by glucoc-corticoids was specifically impaired.   Glucocorticoids are steroid hormones produced by the adrenal cortex, and these compounds pass through the cell membrane to exert their effect directly upon DNA. Induction of TA synthesis by insulin (a peptide hormone which binds to the cell surface and mediates its effects via a second messenger),or by cyclic adenosine 3'-5' monophosphate (the second messenger) was not affected.   This implies that low concentrations of beryllium select-ively interfere with regulatory mechanisms controlling transcriptional events in gene expression.

A similar study was performed by Ord and Stocker (1981) who administered an LD_{50} dose of beryllium to rats.   They also found a decrease in glucocorticoid induction, but in addition observed "super-induction".   It has been suggested that after an enzyme is induced, a corresponding regulatory or degrading enzyme for the first enzyme is also induced.   Assuming that both induction processes are inhibited by beryllium, if the administration of beryllium gave rise preferren-tially to the induction of the inhibitory enzyme, an enhanced or "super" induction would be observed.   This again points to the specific action of beryllium at a site regulating gene expression, possibly by interaction with the steroid receptor protein, which binds with the hormone in its normal state, with the complex mediating the effects of the hormone.

An extensive review of the biochemical properties of bery-llium potentially relevant to its carcinogenially was presented by Skilleter (1984).

4.2.3   Beryllium carcinogenesis

No further data were found with respect to beryllium car-cinogenesis, but an excellent review of previous animal studies was identified (Reeves, 1979).   Summary tables for osteosarcoma (Table 4.7) and pulmonary carcinoma (Table 4.8) are presented.

With regards to cancer induction in man, Reeves concluded that "the presently available evidence is incomplete, and allows contradictory interpretations regarding the carcinogenicity of bery-llium in man".

Author	Year	Species	Compound	Mode of Administration or Duration of Exposure	Dose or Atm. Concn. (Be)	Incidence of Pulmonary Carcinoma
		rabbits rats	Zn-Be-Mn silicate		2.3-6.9 mg	0
					0.46 mg	0
					3.4 mg	0
	1950	guinea pigs	Be stearate Be(OH)2 Be metal	intratracheal injection	5 mg	0
					31 mg	0
					54 mg	0
					75 mg	0
	1953		BeO	intratracheal inj. in 3 doses	338 γ	1 in 4
					33 γ	1 in 5
				12-14 mo.		4 in 8
	1955			13-18 mo.	33-35 γ/m³	17 in 17
				3-18 mo.	55 γ/m³	55 in 74
				12 mo.	180 γ/m³	11 in 27
Vorwald	1962*	rats	BeSO₄	3-22 mo.	18 γ/m³	72 in 103
				8-21 mo.		31 in 63
				9-24 mo.		47 in 90
				11-16 mo.		9 in 21
				8-21 mo.		25 in 50
	1966		BeO	9-24 mo.	1.8-2.0 γ/m³	43 in 95
				13-16 mo.		3 in 15
				3-12 mo.	9 mg/m³	22 in 36
			BeSO4	18 mo.	21-42 γ/m³	"almost all"
				18 mo.	2.8 γ/m³	13 in 21
	1968	monkeys	BeSO4	inhal av.15 3 + yrs. hra/wk	38.8 γ/m³	8 in 11
			BeO	bronchomural implant + intra-bronchial inj.	18-90+ mg	3 in 20

TABLE 4.8

* unpublished

Author	Year	Species	Compound	Mode of Administration or Duration of Exposure	Dose or Atm. Concn. (Be)	Incidence of Pulmonary Carcinoma
	1957		$BeSO_4$	6-9 mo.	32-35 γ/m^3	58? in 136
						ca. 35-60 in 170
		rats	Be phosphate	1-12 mo.	227 γ/m^3	ca. 7 in 40
			BeF_2	6-15 mo.	9 γ/m^3	ca. 10-12 in 200
	1961	rabbits	Zn-Be-Mn silicate	1-9 mo.	0.85-1.25 mg/m^3	ca. 4-20 in 220
				24 mo.	1 mg/m^3	0
Schepers		guinea pigs		22 mo.		0
	1964	monkeys	$BeSO_4$	12 mo.	35 γ/m^3	0 in 4
			BeF_2		35-200 γ/m^3	0 in 4
					180 γ/m^3	0 in 4
			Be phosphate	8 mo.	0.2 mg/m^3	1 in 4
					1.1 mg/m^3	0 in 4
					8.3 mg/m^3	0 in 4
	1967			13 mo.	34.25±23.66 γ/m^3	43 in 43
				3 mo.		19 in 22
				6 mo.		33 in 33
Reeves	1969	rats	$BeSO_4$	9 mo.	35.66±13.77 γ/m^3	15 in 15
				12 mo.		21 in 21
				18 mo.		13 in 15
	1972	guinea pigs		18-24 mo.	3.7-30.4 γ/m^3	0 in 58
	1976*	rats			~ 15 γ/m^3	0 in 110
			beryl		620 γ/m^3	18 in 19
			bertrandite		210 γ/m^3	0 in 30-60
Wagner	1969		beryl	17± mo.	620 γ/m^3	0 in 48
		hamsters	bertrandite		210 γ/m^3	0 in 48
		monkeys	beryl		620 γ/m^3	0 in 12
			bertrandite		210 γ/m^3	0 in 12

TABLE 4.8 (Contd.)

* unpublished
From Reeves (1979)

4.2.4   Occupational studies

In this section, studies dealing with occupational exposure are reviewed, where they may have relevance to monitoring exposure levels, or toxicity of the substance.

Cotes et al. (1983) published the results of an extensive study of workers at a factory manufacturing beryllium products. The exposure data show that overall mean air concentrations of beryllium oxide were reduced from 1 $\mu g\ m^{-3}$ in 1952 to 0.4 $\mu g\ m^{-3}$ in 1960.. On average, 10% of samples taken exceeded the threshold limit value of 2 $\mu g\ m^{-3}$. Even with an improved industrial hygiene record, there were four reported cases of beryllium disease. In subjects with no clinical or radiological evidence of beryllium disease, no convincing evidence was obtained of an association between tests of lung function and the estimated exposure to beryllium, implying that lung function tests cannot be used as a monitoring procedure.

The lymphocyte transformation (LT) test has been used by several groups, to ascertain its potential as a monitoring technique for beryllium exposure. Briefly, this test involves incubating a blood sample from a subject with $BeSO_4$ present in the culture medium, and then pulsing radio-labelled thymidine into the culture after 4 days. An increased uptake of thymidine is observed in the "transformed cells". Rom et al. (1983) investigated the relationship between LT and beryllium exposure over a three year period. There were 16% positive LT tests in 1979 and 8% in 1982. Of eleven positive LT's in 1979, eight were negative in 1982, concomitant with a significant reduction in exposure. A positive LT test was not associated with radiological signs of beryllium disease. A similar type of study was performed by Williams and Williams (1983). Sixteen patients with chronic beryllium disease, 10 subjects with suspected disease and 117 healthy beryllium-exposed workers were LT tested. The tests gave a positive response in all patients with confirmed beryllium disease and a negative response in the suspected group. Two of the healthy workers had a positive response indicating both exposure and sensitization. It is not known whether sensitized workers are more liable to develop the disease (see Hooper, 1981). Both Rom et al. and Williams and Williams considered positive LT tests to be related to beryllium exposure, and advocated its use in monitoring of the health of potentially exposed workers. The work of Rom et al. also suggests that the response to the LT test in beryllium workers is reversible when exposure levels are reduced, implying it could be a good long-term monitor of industrial hygiene standards.

4.2.5   Development of a metabolic model

No further references to the in vivo metabolism of beryllium, relevant to the development of a metabolic model for the metal, were identified. For this reason, the model proposed by Thorne and Jackson (1983) is implemented. This model is represented diagramatically in Fig. 4.3. The following parameters are used in conjunction with the model:

Parameter	Value (d^{-1})
λ_A	0.046
λ_B	0.32
λ_C	0.00046
λ_D	0.88
λ_F	0.22
λ_G	0.66

The compartmental contents are as follows:

compartment (1) = 1.136 x 10^{-4} mg

compartment (2) = 7.905 x 10^{-4} mg

compartment (3) = 0.217 mg

I in Fig. 4.3 refers to intake via the relevant route and λ_L λ_T and λ_s are dependent on the models of lung and GI tract retention used with this model of systemic metabolism. The value of λ_s is partly determined by the fractional uptake f_1 of the substance. An f_1 value of 0.005 is adopted here (ICRP, 1979).

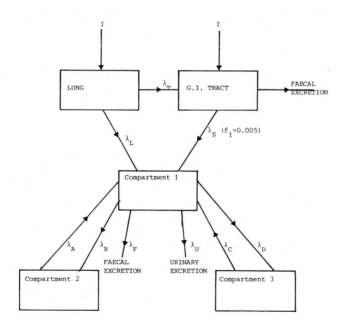

Note: for paramter values see text.

FIGURE 4.3 SYSTEMIC MODEL OF BERYLLIUM METABOLISM

Individual tissue contents are calculated as follows:

Bone = 0.075 (compartment (1)) + 0.795 (compartment (3))

Liver = 0.025 (compartment (1)) + 0.19 (compartment (2))
        + 0.02 (compartment (3))

Kidney = 0.005 (compartment (1)) + 0.19 (compartment (2))
        + 0.02 (compartment (3))

Muscle = 0.4 (compartment (1)) + 0.125 (compartment (2))
        + 0.06 (compartment (3))

Other tissue = 0.495 (compartment (1) + 0.5 (compartment (2))
        + 0.105 (compartment (3))

4.3   Cadmium

4.3.1   Intake as a result of smoking

The trend for local authorities to deal with the problem of municipal waste by using the sludge as fertiliser has caused some concern over the release into the environment of the large amounts of heavy metals, principally cadmium, found in the sludge, and their possible entry into the food chain. Gutenman et al. (1982) compared the concentration of cadmium and nickel in smoke from cigarettes made from tobacco cultivated on sludge-amended soils with that from tobacco cultivated on untreated soil. Tobacco from contaminated soils had a cadmium concentration of 67.4 ppm whereas tobacco from non-contaminated soils had a concentration of 3.2 ppm, the latter value being within the previously reported range for uncontaminated conditions (see Thorne and Jackson, 1983). The quantities of tobacco (μg/cigarette) found in the mainstream particulate fraction of the smoke were 6.7 and 0.2 respectively, confirming that 10% of tobacco-bound cadmium is volatized to an inhalable form. Clearly, smokers of tobaccos grown on sludge-contaminated soils will possibly be inhaling 30 times as much cadmium as smokers of tobacco grown on untreated soils. On this basis, "pack a day" smokers of tobacco grown on contaminated soils have an intake of cadmium comparable with the daily dietary intake and the systemic uptake from smoking would almost certainly dominate over the uptake from the diet. Whether this concentration difference applies to all crops grown on sludge-treated soils is a matter of some debate, since it is known that tobacco produces a cadmium-binding protein which may enhance the retention of cadmium by the crop. However, the possibility of transfer of cadmium from sludge-treated soils to human food chains should be a cause for concern.

The cadmium content of cigarettes purchased in eight different countries was reported by Elinder et al. (1983). The average concentration ranged from 0.19 to 3.0 ppm with a general tendancy toward lower values in cigarettes from developing countries. Once again, 10% of cadmium in a cigarette was found to be present in mainstream smoke.

Sharma et al. (1983) compared the effect of dietary intake and smoking on blood and urine levels of cadmium. They compared dietary intake of a widely consumed oyster-species with a high cadmium content (5 µg/g wet wt) in groups of smokers and non-smokers. It was found that smoking had a much greater effect on blood cadmium concentrations than did dietary intake, presumably because of the low fractional absorption of ingested cadmium (see Section 4.3.3). Dietary cadmium only gave rise to a small elevation in blood and urine cadmium concentration.

This confirms the finding of Moreau et al. (1983), who reported that blood cadmium was strongly elevated in current smokers. They also found that ex-smokers had significantly higher blood cadmium levels than non-smokers, suggesting that blood cadmium levels partly reflect previous or accumulated exposure to cadmium.

Blood levels in non-occupationally exposed Japanese were found to be related to the high cadmium content of rice eaten in the region, but smoking did give rise to a further increase (Watanabe et al. 1983).

4.3.2   Distribution of cadmium in human tissues

Body and individual tissue burdens of cadmium were measured in autopsy samples from Finnish accident victims (Salmela et al., 1983). The results are shown in Table 4.9. Total body burden reached its maximum values in the 30-39 year age group. The highest value (8.3 mg) is less than previously reported values (Thorne and Jackson, 1983), but this could be due to low cadmium exposure of the population. At these exposure levels, kidneys and liver contain 85% of the total body burden of cadmium. This value differs from earlier reported figures of 45-50%. The cadmium contents of cancellous bone were also determined in autopsy samples from Finnish accident victims (Knuutila et al., 1982). The mean cadmium concentration was 0.27 ppm on a wet weight basis, which corresponds to a total tissue burden of 2.7 µg. This is again lower than previous values, but the same comments apply as to the study of Salmela et al. (1983). The age dependence of cadmium concentrations in liver, kidney and brain were ascertained by Gross et al. (1976). They used autopsy samples from people who lived in the Cincinatti area. Several foetal samples were also examined, and these showed significant amounts of cadmium in the liver and kidney, implying that trans-placental transfers had occurred. Liver concentrations increased until the seventh decade, whereas kidney concentration peaked in the fourth decade, then decreased steadily from the sixth decade. Concentrations in hair showed no age dependence.

Drasch (1983) measured cadmium contents in old pathology and anatomy specimens from 1877-1939 (year of death) and compared the results with modern values (1968 onwards). The concentration of cadmium in liver was not significantly different in the two sets of samples. However, the renal cortex cadmium concentration was a factor of 47 larger in the recent samples, and the estimated total body burden was increased by a factor of 5 in the modern material. This suggests that the increase in cadmium emissions into the environment during this century, has resulted in increased body burdens of cadmium.

Tissue	Age group (years)							
	0-9	10-19	20-29	30-39	40-49	50-59	60-69	>70
Kidneys	0.17 / 0.02-0.58	1.11 / 0.39-2.56	3.29 / 0.21-11.8	5.03 / 1.46-12.1	4.94 / 1.40-11.1	4.75 / 2.56-12.9	3.49 / 1.89-6.59	2.62 / 0.74-9.44
Liver	0.01 / <0.01-0.48	0.81 / 0.36-2.38	1.44 / 0.15-3.91	1.43 / 0.13-2.89	1.80 / 0.40-4.54	1.38 / 0.16-6.67	1.95 / 1.60-2.26	1.47 / 0.35-4.27
Muscle	<0.01 / <0.01-0.08	0.02 / <0.01-0.77	0.06 / <0.01-2.67	0.04 / <0.01-1.24	0.15 / <0.01-1.85	0.14 / <0.01-3.33	1.89 / 1.65-2.27	0.03 / <0.01-1.61
Lungs	<0.01 / <0.01-0.01	0.02 / <0.01-0.55	0.10 / <0.01-1.75	0.35 / 0.01-1.32	0.09 / <0.01-1.16	0.16 / 0.03-0.58	0.19 / 0.15-0.26	<0.01 / <0.01-0.38
Pancreas	<0.01 / <0.01-0.01	<0.01 / <0.01-0.03	0.05 / 0.01-0.97	0.05 / 0.01-0.16	0.06 / 0.01-0.21	0.03 / 0.01-0.18	0.06 / 0.03-0.08	0.03 / <0.01-0.09
Heart	<0.01 / <0.01	<0.01 / <0.01-0.02	<0.01 / <0.01-0.06	<0.01 / <0.01-0.05	<0.01 / <0.01-0.05	<0.01 / <0.01-0.03	0.02 / 0.01-0.03	<0.01 / <0.01-0.07
Body burden	0.27	2.27	6.17	7.80	9.32	7.86	7.92	4.74
Males/females	3/0	12/4	19/5	11/1	9/5	5/2	3/1	2/4

Note: Smokers and non-smokers mixed. Both sexes are included. Values in mg.

From Salmela et al, (1983).

TABLE 4.9

TISSUE BURDENS, RANGES AND BODY BURDEN OF CADMIUM EXPRESSED AS GEOMETRIC MEANS IN EACH AGE GROUP

The effect of smoking on tissue cadmium concentrations was investigated by Post et al. (1984). Male heavy smokers were autopsied within 3 days of death. Cadmium concentrations in lung, liver and kidney were 0.5, 2.21 and 17.4 ppm, very similar to values reported elsewhere (see Thorne and Jackson, 1983). In liver and kidney, approximately 75% was bound to a low-molecular weight protein. Also, 56% of cadmium in lung was bound to a similar protein, but whether production of this protein is induced by exposure of the lung to cadmium could not be ascertained.

However, Post et al. (1982) found that in the lungs of rabbits exposed to cadmium aerosols, three low molecular weight cadmium binding proteins were present, two of which were electrophoretically similar to liver metallathionein (MT), but the third, which accounted for the majority of cadmium in the soluble fraction of the tissue, did not bind to anionic exchange gels, as does liver MT. This suggests specific cadmium binding proteins are synthesized by the lung.

4.3.3   Metabolism

4.3.3.1   Gastrointestinal absorption

Neonates may be at a higher risk than adults when exposed to the same environmental level of toxic metals. This is at least partly because most toxic metals are poorly absorbed from the gastrointestinal tract in adults, but are more readily absorbed in the new born. Kostial et al. (1983) studied the age dependence of intestinal retention of cadmium in rats. The ileum was found to be the main site of absorption in sucklings, whereas the duodenum and jejunum absorbed more in weaned rats. The percentage retention of the ingested dose in the gut and whole body in the two groups are shown below.

	Age	
	6 days	6 weeks
whole body	29.6	1.51
carcass	9.3	1.29
gut	20.4	0.22
gut, % of whole body	62.1	14.57

Clearly the absorption of cadmium is very much enhanced in the younger rats.

Gruden (1982) used a standard in vitro preparation, the everted gut sac, to study retention and absorption by various segments of the gut. As was found by Kostial et al. (1983), the duodenum and jejunum transported significantly more cadmium than did the ileum. Retention within the gut wall was similar in all three sections (approximately 20%). No active absorption of cadmium was observed.

Coughtrey and Thorne (1983) concluded that cadmium absorption is not under homeostatic control. However, in pregnant and lactating mice, two to three times more cadmium was retained than in control rats exposed to cadmium in drinking water. (Bhattacharyya et al., 1982). The cadmium content of kidney and liver was also markedly increased during pregnancy and lactation and, during lactation, cadmium content of mammary tissue increased nine-fold. It is not clear whether these results were due to homeostatic control of cadmium metabolism, or whether the absorption of cadmium paralleled changes in the absorption of a physiologically important substance (e.g. calcium) which is homeostatically increased by the additional demands of pregnancy and lactation on the body.

Dietary cadmium absorption in man has been measured using a dual isotope method. Cadmium, labelled with Cd-115m, was administered orally with Cr-51 labelled material. The latter radionuclide is very poorly absorbed by the body and is used to mark the passage of the gut contents through the body, into the faeces (McClellan et al., 1978). The total body retention of cadmium, after passage of the faecal marker averaged 4.6% with a range of 0.7 - 15.6%.

Ingested cadmium binds to intestinal cells when it is absorbed. Holt and Webb (1983) found that at low doses (0.1 mg Cd kg^{-1}) administered to 8-day old rats, 70% of the dose is found in the intestine. Most of this is bound to an endogenous copper complex, which normally regulates copper absorption. With larger doses (1 µg kg^{-1}), only 50% of the dose was found in the intestine and 40% was present in the carcass, suggesting that saturation of the binding sites for cadmium had occurred. Most hepatic cadmium was bound to metallothionein. Cadmium injected intraperitonealy (I.P.) was also rapidly bound by the intestinal cells, demonstrating that the transfer between intestinal cells and blood is bidirectional.

4.3.3.2   Systemic metabolism

In rats given daily sub-cutaneous (S.C.) injection of cadmium (0.5 µg kg^{-1}), blood cadmium levels increased continuously. Plasma cadmium was 2% of total blood cadmium initially, rising to 8% after 15 weeks exposure. A significant proportion of plasma cadmium was found in the metallothionein (M.T.) fraction initially, and this fraction increased to 50% of plasma cadmium after 15 weeks exposure. The rest of the plasma cadmium was distributed in the high-molecular-weight protein fraction (Suzuki, 1981).

Garty et al. (1981) studied the redistribution of cadmium in blood after I.V. injection (1 mg kg^{-1}). By 3 hours after injection, blood cadmium concentrations had decreased by two orders of magnitude to 46 µg l^{-1}, then remained constant for 12 h before rising to 75 µg l^{-1} by 60 hours. Between 3 h and 6 h, plasma cadmium fell to 5% of its initial value, cadmium contents of white blood cells did not change and the cadmium contents of red blood cells increased two-fold. In erythrocytes the cadmium was bound to high-molecular-weight proteins initially, but after 60 hours a second cadmium-binding protein, with a molecular weight similar to that of metallothionein, was found to be present. Chowdury et al. (1983a) have reported on the tissue distribution of cadmium in rats after I.V. administration of

Cd-109. During the first two hours, blood cadmium levels declined rapidly with a half-life of approximately 100 minutes. Liver accumulated 5% of the dose in 2 hours, as did the G.I. tract, with the kidneys accumulating 2%.

Hepatic metabolism of cadmium was studied by Frazer and Kingsley (1976), using an isolated perfused rat liver preparation. Their results suggest that cadmium-zinc exchange may be one mechanism for mediating cadmium transport in the liver. When cadmium was added to the perfusate, the metal appeared rapidly, and in a dose-dependent pattern, in bile.

Stowe (1976) found that in anaesthetized, bile ductcannulated, rats, bile flow rates and cadmium concentration in bile were increased after oral administration of 100 ppm cadmium. Administration of zinc caused a reduction in the kidney excretion of cadmium, as would be expected if an exchange mechanism exists.

Elinder et al. (1978) measured cadmium concentrations in liver biopsy, blood and bile samples from gall stone patients. Blood cadmium was found to be a good indicator of cadmium in liver. In bile, an average in cadmium concentration of 2.5 ppb was observed.

Cadmium bound to MT in liver can be released and transferred to other tissues. Tanaka et al. (1981) used carbon tetrachloride to induce liver damage. They found that liver cadmium content decreased and that this decrease was mirrored by an increase in plasma, kidney and urine cadmium concentrations. Cadmium in the hepatic supernatant of carbon tetrachloride-treated rats was mainly bound to MT. This suggests that in some liver disorders, cadmium may be released from the liver and transported to other sites.

The production of M.T. by the liver in response to a cadmium challenge was investigated by Cahill et al. (1983). They found that MT production follows a diurnal rhythm, with MT levels being significantly higher when cadmium was administered during the dark phase. If MT has a protecting influence, this finding may be of relevance in the case of shift workers. In the same study, it was observed that the testes contained six times more cadmium when the cadmium was administered during the dark phase. Kundomal et al. (1983) observed that an elevation of cadmium concentration in the testes leads to testicular atrophy, suggesting that further studies on the testicular uptake, retention and effects of cadmium are necessary.

With the increase in research into trace and essential metal metabolism has grown the realisation that there are extensive interrelationships between the metabolism of these metals. One of these interrelationships, between zinc and cadmium metabolism, has already been mentioned. It is also known that metallothionein binds various metals, such as mercury, copper, zinc and selenium, as well as calcium. However a review of these interrelationships, is beyond the scope of the current work.

The potential of hair samples as a possible monitoring substance for assessing exposure to heavy metals is problematical because of the contrary findings of different studies. External contamination of the hair is a major factor in the observed metal content of a sample. Nordberg and Nishiyama (1972) administered Cd-109 intravenously to mice and tried to correlate whole body retention and hair content. The correlation between the two was very good (correlation coefficient = 0.99). Kollmer (1982) concluded that the internal deposition of cadmium in hair is proportional to the amount absorbed, but is largely masked by external contamination.

4.3.3.3   Transfer to milk

Lynch et al. (1974) measured secretion of cadmium in the milk of cows receiving $CdCl_2$ (9.0 mg/kg) daily, administered orally in gelatin capsules. They found a six-fold increase in cadmium content of milk solids compared with control animals. After cadmium administration ceased, cadmium levels in milk declined to control levels within 54 days. This decrease followed a single exponential, with a half-life of 14 days.

4.3.4   Occupational exposure and potential monitoring substances

In this section, reported levels of various potential monitoring substances are reviewed with concomitant exposure levels, if given. Urine, blood and in vivo tissue monitoring are discussed. Hair is briefly mentioned in section 4.3.3 and very few other data exist.

Cadmium levels in blood

Lilis et al. (1984) measured urinary and blood cadmium levels in employees at a copper smelter (Table 4.10). Smoking habits were also assessed. A significant effect of smoking on blood cadmium levels was observed. However, for all smoking subjects, blood cadmium levels were higher in employees than in ex-employees indicating a contribution of the work environment. Urinary cadmium levels did not exceed 10 µg/g creatinine, the generally accepted "critical" level for chronic renal damage, but values were higher than 2 µg/g creatinine, a level rarely exceeded in the general population. In a study on retired cadmium-exposed workers, Jarup et al. (1983) found that the post-retirement decline in blood concentration of cadmium was best fitted by a two compartment model, the half-times of the two compartments being 75 to 128 days for the shorter-lived compartment and 7.4 to 16.0 years for the longer-lived compartment. These results are similar to those obtained by other workers (see Thorne and Jackson, 1983).

Potential monitoring substances in urine

Normal urinary cadmium levels are below 1 ppm (Thorne and Jackson, 1983). Further studies confirm this value. Thus, Panholzer-et al. (1982) gave a mean value of 0.78 ppm, with a range of 0.22 to 1.7 ppm and Shimizu et al. (1981) gave a mean value of 0.83 ppm with a range of 0.36 to 1.22 ppm.

Other substances found in urine have also been suggested as being potentially useful for monitoring purposes. These are β-microglubulin and metallothionein.

With respect to monitoring of occupationally exposed individuals, it is noted that the kidney is particularly susceptible to

TABLE 4.10

BLOOD AND URINARY CADMIUM LEVELS, INTENSITY OF EXPOSURE,
AND SMOKING HABITS IN ACTIVE COPPER SMELTER EMPLOYEES

		Exposure category			
		Very low	Low	Medium	High
Cd-B (μg/litre)					
Smokers	N	48	102	103	128
	Median	5.03	6.75	7.10	6.90
	Mean ± SD	5.50±4.07	6.79±4.19	7.05±3.66	7.48±4.28
Ex-smokers	N	21	55	52	47
	Median	0.70	0.90	1.00	1.40
	Mean ± SD	0.76±0.34	1.03±0.62	1.53±1.80	1.02±1.61
Non-smokers	N	11	35	33	42
	Median	0.50	0.60	0.80	1.00
	Mean ± SD	0.56±0.27	0.65±0.80	0.99±0.80	1.53±1.28
CD-U (μg/g creatinine)					
Smokers	N	45	86	87	120
	Median	1.00	1.10	1.20	1.40
	Mean ± SD	1.23±0.89	1.21±0.89	1.45±1.26	1.65±1.33
Ex-smokers	N	19	45	48	45
	Median	0.50	0.70	0.70	1.10
	Mean ± SD	0.69±0.55	0.98±0.81	0.88±0.65	1.20±0.81
Non-smokers	N	10	33	29	41
	Median	0.45	0.30	0.40	0.60
	Mean ± SD	0.50±0.28	0.41±0.27	0.62±0.66	0.72±0.47

Note: from Lilis et al. (1984)

chronic cadmium exposure. It is generally accepted that when kidney cadmium concentrations exceed approximately 200 ppm, proximal tubular damage is noticeable. This damage interferes with the ability of the region to reabsorb filtered protein, and, in consequence, a high urinary level of these proteins is observed. Also, cadmium is released from damaged kidneys and a high urinary cadmium level may be indicative of high exposure and/or renal damage.

Normal values of urinary β-microglobulin concentrations are 40-80 μg/l with a mean value of 65 μg/l (Kowal and Zirces, 1983).

Much of the work on chronic cadmium exposure, and urinary monitoring thereof, has been performed in Japan. This is because, as well as having a problem due to occupational exposure, certain regions have exceptionally high environmental levels of cadmium. This leads to a high dietary intake (mainly in rice) and chronic cadmium accumulation, with possible nephrotoxic effects. The prevalence of "itai-itai" disease, (a disease symptomatically identical to osteomalacia) is due to cadmium-induced renal damage and reduced phosphorus reabsorption.

Urinary β-microglobulin (MG) levels were measured in aged Japanese individuals with no known exposure to high dietary or occupational cadmium. Analysis of the relationship between MG and other tests of renal function suggested two distinct phases of renal damage. These were reflected by changes in indices of renal damage which occur at different MG levels (Nomiyama et al., 1983a). These were a slight continuous increase at MG levels of between 160 and 1600 μg l^{-1} and a remarkable increase at MG levels of more than 1600 μg l^{-1}. The latter increase was closely related to depressed tubular reabsorption of MG, but was independent of tubular reabsorption of phosphorus. This suggests that the screening level for renal tubular dysfunction should be a MG level of 160 to 1600 μg l^{-1}. In a second study, Nomiyama et al. (1983b) related urinary MG levels in people from three cadmium polluted areas to urinary cadmium concentrations. Multiple regression analysis showed that the district factor had the highest correlation with urinary MG, age was the second most significant factor, with urinary cadmium being only a relatively small factor for elevating MG.

Since the development of a radio-immuno assay for metallothionein, interest in the potential of this substance as a monitor of exposure has grown. Urinary MT was measured in cadmium-exposed workers by Falck et al. (1983). They found that MT excretion was linearly related, on an individual basis, to protein excretion, urinary MG and cumulative time-weighted exposure (dose), suggesting urinary MT is a useful predictor of cadmium exposure, since it is disputed whether the same can be said of cadmium excretion in urine. Tohyama et al. (1981) measured MT concentration in the urine of women sufferers from "itai-itai" disease, from suspected cases, from an environmentally-exposed population and from a control population (Table 4.11). As can be seen, urinary cadmium levels in "itai-itai" patients were similar to those in a cadmium-exposed population, but urinary metallothionein levels were significantly lower in the cadmium-exposed population, as were urinary MG levels, which can be thought of as a non-specific index of renal proximal tubular damage. It is suggested that a combination of measurements of urinary MT, urinary MG and cadmium may be the most appropriate for monitoring of cadmium-related renal dysfunction.

Group	No. of subjects	Age (years)	Cadmium [2] (μg/g Creatinine)	Metallothionein [2] (μg/g Creatinine)	β_2-Microglobulin [2] (μg/g Creatinine)
i. "Itai-itai" disease patients.	18	75.3 [3] (60–84)	13.5 [3] (9.7–18.8)	1880 [3,4] (1580–2230)	91,200 [3,4] (75,400–110,000)
ii. Suspected patients.	21	72.1 (61–84)	16.4 [3] (13.4–19.9)	2000 [3,4] (1630–2450)	102,000 [3,4] (86,200–112,000)
iii. Inhabitants of Cd-polluted area.	15	74.5 (66–90)	13.8 [3] (10.1–18.7)	880 [3] (588–1320)	5150 [3] (1590–16,700)
iv. Inhabitants of non-polluted area.	13	68.7 (60–83)	5.7 (4.3–7.5)	394 [5] (292–533)	294 (84–1030)

Notes: 1. Statistical expressions used are: age – arithmetic mean and range; cadmium, metallothionein and β_2-microglobulin – geometric mean and 95% confidence intervals.

2. Because of the use of spot urine samples, urinary levels of cadmium, metallothionein, and β_2-microglobulin were corrected by specific gravity (not shown here) and by creatinine. Statistical treatment of the data corrected by specific gravity gave results similar to those obtained after correction by creatinine excretion.

3. Significantly different from Group iv (P < 0.05).

4. Significantly different from Group iii (P < 0.05).

5. The metallothionein level of one sample was below the detection limit (1.46 μg/l); for conservative statistical comparison, the MT level in this sample was assumed to be equivalent to the detection limit.

From Tohyama et al.(1981).

TABLE 4.11

URINANALYSIS OF CADMIUM-EXPOSED FEMALE SUBJECTS [1]

In vivo analysis of tissue cadmium content

Irradiation of a body with fast neutrons leads to various interactions with the elements comprising the body tissues. In particular a neutron may be captured by a nucleus (mass A) to form an isotope of the same element but of higher mass number (mass A + 1). The intermediate is in an excited state and may decay promptly ($\sim 10^{-16}$ s) to its ground state with the omission of γ rays which are characteristic of the isotope involved. The daughter isotope formed in this manner may or may not be radioactive. If it is, it can often be detected, particularly if it emits characteristic photons of energies sufficient to penetrate body tissues without gross absorption ($\geq$ 100 keV).

Cadmium is particularly amenable to detection by the prompt γ-ray method. One of its isotopes, Cd-113 has a 20000 barn absorption cross-section for thermal neutron capture, and exhibits an isotopic abundance of 12.3%. On neutron capture by Cd-113, prompt γ-rays of various energies are emitted, the most prominent peak being at an energy of 0.559 MeV with a yield of 0.7991 gammas per neutron capture. The resultant daughter isotope, Cd-114, is stable and, therefore, cannot be detected by delayed counting techniques. Techniques have now been developed to measure physiological concentrations of cadmium in vivo. An early study by McLellan et al. (1976) developed a method which had a detection limit of 0.5 ppm. In a patient with known chronic cadmium poisoning, a liver concentration in the range 65-110 ppm was obtained using the technique. A liver radiation dose of 5 x 10^{-4} Gy was delivered in achieving the result.

The relationship between liver and kidney cadmium contents was ascertained by Ellis et al. (1980). Liver results were expressed as concentrations because the area of the neutron beam was less than the cross-sectional area of the liver, whereas all the kidney was exposed to the beam, enabling total tissue contents to be measured. Up to a liver concentration of 40 ppm, kidney contents were directly proportional to liver concentration, reaching 31 mg for a liver concentration of 40 ppm. Beyond this point, liver cadmium concentrations continued to rise, whereas kidney cadmium contents fell. It is known that renal damage causes loss of renal cadmium, so a reasonable hypothesis is that renal damage occurred when kidney cadmium reached a threshold content of $\sim$ 30 mg, allowing the release of stored cadmium. Further indices of renal dysfunction such as urinary β-microglobulin levels gave estimates of 31-42 mg for the critical cadmium content of the kidney. Since only one kidney was irradiated, this critical content of 30 mg corresponds to a concentration of 200 ppm, very similar to the critical kidney concentration for renal damage, estimated on the basis of β-microglobulin levels (Roels et al., 1979).

A similar study by Fletcher et al. (1982) obtained a critical liver concentration of 40-50 ppm for renal damage to be observed. This is in close agreement with the above study. The critical kidney concentration was between 160 and 190 ppm. An estimate of tissue half-life was also obtained by comparing repeat measurements separated by 3-4 years, during which the individual concerned was not occupationally exposed to cadmium. A value of 13.5 years for the biological half-life in liver was obtained.

Webb et al. (1982) found that liver and kidney cadmium measurements provided a better guide to cumulative exposure than did β_2-microglobulin, especially at low levels of exposure. However, blood cadmium acted as a more sensitive indicator of current exposure than did other measurements.

A significant difference was found between liver cadmium content of a control population and that of a population occupationally exposed to cadmium (McNeill et al., 1982). A relation was also found between liver cadmium burden and duration of exposure such that

$$Cd_{(liver)} \text{ (ng)} = 6 + 2.6 \text{ t}$$

where t is the duration of exposure in years.

Miscellaneous environmental studies

Ellis et al. (1983) measured cadmium concentrations in monitoring substances (blood, hair and urine) and tried to correlate the values found with liver and kidney contents as measured in vivo. Concentrations in hair were unrelated to body burden. In contrast, blood cadmium seemed to be well correlated with liver cadmium, throughout the whole range of exposure. Ellis et al. (1983) concluded that the relationships between monitoring substances and body burden were not sufficiently quantitative for estimating the body burden of an individual worker.

In a study evaluating the effect of oral intake on the overall uptake of cadmium in exposed workers Roels et al. (1982) found that, compared with office workers, significant contamination of hands by cadmium dust occurred during the working day. Cadmium-exposed workers accumulated amounts as high as 1.2 µg per hand per day in some cases. Faecal cadmium was higher on Friday than on Sunday in these workers, and no such change was observed in office workers not exposed to cadmium. This suggests hand-to-mouth transfer can be an important factor in overall cadmium exposure. Supportive evidence was found in a study of two smelter workers, one of whom wore gloves and had a lower change in faecal cadmium during the working week.

Falck et al. (1983) studied renal dysfunction in workers exposed to cadmium for at least 21 years, but below the permissible exposure limit of 100 µg Cd m^{-3}. Renal dysfunction occurred in 30% of the workers, suggesting that the above statutory limit does not protect against the risk of renal dysfunction after a lifetime's exposure to cadmium fumes.

Smith et al. (1980) found significant renal effects with estimated average inhalation exposures at 63 µg m^{-3} over a 25 year period.

An extensive survey of body burden and monitoring substances was performed by Roels et al. (1981). Their main conclusions were that:

- urinary cadmium levels are related to exposure, but such levels are greatly enhanced when renal dysfunction occurs;

- blood cadmium levels reflect recent cadmium exposure;

- liver cadmium levels are proportional to the product of duration and intensity of cadmium exposure;

- renal cadmium contents are proportional to exposure until renal damage occurs. Subsequent to the induction of renal dysfunction, levels of renal cadmium fall.

The data presented by Roels et al. (1981) indicate that the range of critical kidney concentrations is between 160-285 ppm and that above the top of this range it is highly probable that all persons will show signs of cadmium-induced kidney damage. The corresponding liver concentration is 50-60 ppm. A similar comparison was undertaken by Ellis et al. (1984), who devised a dose-response model for the effects of cadmium. The model predicts a 50% probability of renal dysfunction occurring with kidney and liver cadmium concentrations of 200 ppm and 42.3 ppm respectively.

4.3.5   Metabolic modelling

Whole-body metabolism of cadmium has been modelled by several authors, notably Nordberg and Kjellstrom (1979) and Shank et al. (1977). These latter constructed a multi-compartment model with parameters derived from experiments in mice. This model was adapted by Marcus (1982) to include fast and slow terms for liver and kidney release, but there is no experimental evidence for such a system in man. The model proposed by Nordberg and Kjellstrom (1979) purports to represent cadmium metabolism in man. However, most of the model parameters are either based on data from animal experiments, or are chosen to give the best fit to human tissue concentration studies. This is not an ideal method, since so many inter-related parameters are involved in the model.

The model representing cadmium metabolism in this study is loosely based on the model of Nordberg and Kjellstrom (1979), with respect to the organisation of the compartments. It is shown in Figure 4.4. Inhaled and ingested cadmium passes into the compartment representing "free" cadmium in blood. This actually represents cadmium loosely bound to various blood components such as -SH groups on albumin. This compartment exchanges with a second blood compartment representing metallothionein-bound cadmium.

There are also reversible exchanges with "other tissues" and liver compartments. In vivo, some cadmium in liver binds to metallothionein, and there is also synthesis of this protein in response to a large cadmium influx into the liver. In the model, there is no distinction between MT-bound cadmium and cadmium bound to other molecules in the liver, i.e. there is only one liver compartment, not two. The liver compartment loses cadmium to both blood compartments and also, via biliary excretion, to the faeces. The kidney compartment derives its cadmium entirely from the blood MT-bound compartment. This last assumption is based on data from an animal experiment undertaken by Nordberg and Nordberg (1975), which demonstrated a selective uptake of MT-bound cadmium in kidneys. In vivo, it is likely that, some of the kidney cadmium will initially be obtained directly from the blood "free" cadmium compartment, but this will be a small fraction of the amount transferred in the MT-bound form.

Excretion in urine is solely from the MT-bound fraction in blood, but transfer from blood "free" cadmium to faeces does occur, via the intestinal mucosa.

The transfer between the two blood compartments is assumed to be fairly rapid, but Nordberg and Kjellstrom (1979) suggested that there is a maximum rate for this transfer, since there is normally only a small amount of circulating MT. However, the liver synthesizes more MT when exposed to cadmium, and although this effect may be delayed by a few hours from the start of the exposure, for the purposes of the model it is assumed that sufficient MT is always available to accomodate the transfer to the MT-bound blood compartment.

The assumption of simple exchange between "free" cadmium in blood and the "other tissues" compartments may be open to question, since Post et al. (1982) found that rabbit lung could produce a MT-like cadmium-binding protein. However, in terms of the amount of cadmium in this compartment, on the evidence available, only a small fraction of it will be MT-bound.

The following parameters are used with the model (see Figure 4.4)

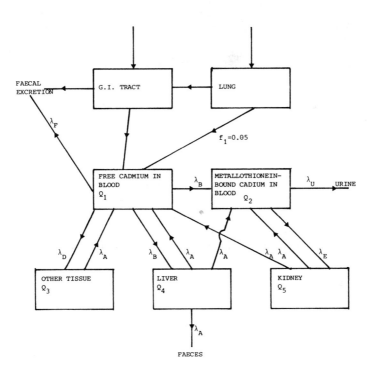

Note: for parameter values see text.

FIGURE 4.4 SYSTEMIC MODEL OF CADMIUM METABOLISM

Parameter	Value (d^{-1})
λ_A	7.6×10^{-5}
λ_B	2.0
λ_D	3.2
λ_E	0.8
λ_F	0.2
λ_U	0.2

"Free" cadmium and MT-bound cadmium are assumed to be bound to the same extent in tissues and are only released very slowly. Biological half-lives of from 10 to 30 years have been quoted in the literature, and in this study a value of 25 years has been used (ICRP, 1980; Underwood, 1977). In the absence of specific data, this value is assumed to apply to all tissues.

A small fraction of body cadmium is available for early excretion. The urinary excretion of cadmium was measured in man by Suzuki and Taguchi (1980). They found a 3-component exponential curve, but it is difficult to distinguish between the first two components. Shaikh and Smith (1980) found a fast excretion component with a half-life of 1.5 days. In the model, this component is represented by the excretion from the relevant blood compartment to faeces and urine. Since faecal excretion from the "free" blood compartment is assumed to be via the cells of the intestinal mucosa, an estimate of this parameter can be derived from the rate of turnover of these cells, which is 5 days (ICRP,1975). Early urinary excretion is assumed to exhibit a half-time of 2 days (Suzuki and Taguchi, 1980).

The value of compartmental contents used with the model are as follows:

Compartment	Content (mg)
liver	4.14
kidney	7.13
other tissue	26.1
blood-"free"	1.1×10^{-3}
blood-MT bound	1.5×10^{-3}

These values are used as the initial conditions of the model. For gastrointestinal absorption, an f_1 value of 0.05 is used.

4.4   Lead

4.4.1   Intake rates

Chamberlain (1983b) estimated the contribution of fallout of lead from vehicles to topsoil lead concentrations, and concluded that an additional 3 ppm in country districts and 10 ppm in town topsoils can be attributed to this source. This is only a fraction of the naturally occurring lead concentration, which has a mean value of 42 ppm for a typical British topsoil (Archer, 1980). From measurements of the naturally-occurring radioisotope Pb-210, Chamberlain estimated that the contribution of lead in fresh vegetables to the dietary intake is of the order of 13 μg day^{-1}. This value is less than a tenth of the typical daily lead intake of 200 to 400 μg (Thorne and Jackson, 1983).

Analysis of the distribution with depth of lead in peat cores (Livett et al., 1979) showed that the annual fallout in the United Kingdom has not changed greatly since the middle of the last century.

This suggests that the increase in fallout due to the use of lead in petrol has been offset by either a decrease in lead smelting, or a more efficient smelting process.

In a study of the relative contribution of various routes of intake of lead to blood lead concentrations, Elwood et al. (1984) concluded that lead in water contributed more to blood lead than did lead in air (Table 4.12). Unfortunately, Elwood et al. did not analyse the dietary lead content, and since the diet is usually the major route of intake of lead, their conclusion may be of limited relevance.

Snee (1982) compared the published models for predicting the effect of concentrations of lead in air on blood lead concentration and concluded that the mathematical models used tended to overestimate the effect of air lead levels for air concentrations of less than 2 μg m^{-3}.

The data from epidemiological studies used to relate blood to air lead concentrations have been described by the following equations (Azar et al., 1975; Williams et al., 1976):

$$\text{Log } C_{BLOOD} = \alpha\text{Log } C_{AIR}$$

or

$$\text{Log } C_{BLOOD} = K + \alpha\text{Log } C_{AIR}$$

where C_{BLOOD} and C_{AIR} are the lead concentrations in blood and air respectively.

Snee (1982) proposed that all possible sources of lead exposures should be taken into account, such that:

$$\text{Log } C_{BLOOD} = K + \alpha\text{Log } I$$

where I is the total rate of intake of lead.

This type of model was found to give a good description of the data of Williams et al. (1975).

Chamberlain (1983a) reviewed published values for ratios of blood lead concentration to air lead concentration, and also reanalysed the data, where he thought appropriate. A range of values of from 0.5 to 3.0 μg/dl per μg/m^3 was found. The range of values was discussed and possible factors giving rise to this range were identified as:

-        non-linearity of the exposure-response relationship;

	Indoor air lead ($\mu g\ m^{-3}$)	Pavement dust lead ($\mu g\ g^{-1}$)	Household dust lead ($\mu g\ g^{-1}$)	Water lead ($mg\ l^{-1}$)	Blood lead ($\mu g\ dl^{-1}$)
Urban area	0.27 0.06–1.15 (34)*	173 22–1341 (29)*	209 44–998 (51)	0.014 0–0.088 (54)	13.2±4.76 (56)
Motorway area	0.17 0.04–0.52 (16)*	185 39–879 (18)*	259 62–1075 (29)	0.004 0–0.029 (17)	9.7±2.69 (31)
Roadside dwelling	0.18 0.05–0.61 (14)*	355 172–731 (42)	200 49–808 (41)	0.007 0–0.041 (39)	8.9±2.48 (42)
Culs de sac dwellings	0.12 0.03–0.37 (14)*	269 83–870 (28)	177 40–788 (27)	0.004 0–0.056 (25)	8.9±2.90 (30)
Village	0.04 0.01–0.13 (9)*	–	177 36–851 (31)	0.003 0–0.021 (28)	7.9±1.86 (33)

Note: Values are geometric mean and total ranges for air lead; means and 95% ranges after log transformation of dust levels, and after cube root transformation of water levels; and mean + s.d. for venous blood lead. Number of samples in parentheses.
* Random sub-samples of dwellings.
From Elwood et al., (1984).

TABLE 4.12

ENVIRONMENTAL AND VENOUS BLOOD LEAD LEVELS OF REPRESENTATIVE POPULATION SAMPLES

- effects of particle size;
- variability in breathing patterns and ventilation rates;
- discrepancies between measured air lead concentration and a subject's actual exposure.

4.4.2   Lead concentrations in human tissues

A comparison of lead contents of bone and soft tissue was undertaken by Barry (1972). Bone samples from women had a 35-40% lower lead content than those from men. Occupational exposure to lead resulted in a three-fold increase in bone lead concentrations, with no comparable increase in soft tissue concentrations.

In a study of the lead content of enamel and dentine in deciduous teeth from Finnish children (Haavikko et al., 1984) a two -fold, and significant, increase was found in the lead concentration of tooth enamel from children born in 1974 compared with corresponding material from children born in 1971. This was interpreted as an increased environmental exposure to lead derived from motor vehicle exhausts.

Brain, liver and muscle autopsy samples from multiple sclerosis and normal subjects were analysed for lead. No significant differences were found between tissue lead concentrations in samples from the two groups. Lead concentrations were typically 0.5 ppm, but, interestingly, cerebellar lead concentrations were four times higher, at 2 ppm. Since one of the symptoms of acute lead poisoning is impairment of motor function which is controlled by the cerebellum, this finding may merit further investigation.

Blood lead concentrations

Ghafourian et al. (1983) collected blood samples from Tehran citizens throughout the year and measured the lead concentration in each. The mean lead concentration throughout the year was 220 ± 100 µg l^{-1}. Higher values were found in autumn than in spring and lead levels in blood from men were 10% higher than those in blood from women. Blood lead concentrations in smokers were also 10% higher than those in non-smokers.

In a study of non-occupationally exposed subjects from Rome, Pallotti et al. (1983) found correlations between blood lead concen- trations and age, sex and smoking habits. A mean value of 173 µg l^{-1} was obtained (198 µg l^{-1} for men and 150 µg l^{-1} for women).

Several groups have published data on lead concentrations in the blood of children (Rehnlund et al., 1979: Ryu et al., 1983; Kaul et al., 1983; Subramanrian and Meranger, 1983; Rabinowitz et al., 1984). All five groups reported very similar values of between 50 and 70 µg/l. Of particular interest is the study by Ryu et al. (1983) who monitored blood lead concentrations in infants who were formula-fed up to 112 days old. At 112 days the mean blood lead concentration was 61 µg l^{-1}. From 112 through 195 days, 10 children received a mean dietary intake of lead of 16 µg d^{-1} and seven received a mean intake of 61 µg d^{-1}. At 196 days of age, mean blood lead concentrations were significantly different (72 and 144 µg l^{-1} respectively).

4.4.3   Gastrointestinal absorption

Heard et al. (1983) measured the absorption of Pb-203 administered in different dietary forms. Fasting subjects absorbed 40 to
50% of Pb-203 taken in distilled water, even with 100 μg of lead
"carrier". When taken with tea or coffee, uptake averaged 14%.
Uptakes of 3 to 7% were found when Pb-203 was taken with a meal, or
incorporated into offal or vegetables eaten as part of the meal, or
when taken with large amounts of calcium or phosphate.

Flanagan et al. (1982) found that 60% of an oral dose of
100 μg of Pb-203 labelled lead was retained. Retention was proportional to dose up to 400 μg of lead. Lead retention was not related
to the capacity to absorb iron, or to the size of the body iron store.
Once again, retention was reduced when lead was taken with a meal.
The absorption of lead in a liquid meal was studied by Blake (1976).
The dose was ingested two hours after breakfast, and values of absorption of from 10 to 70% were obtained. This probably reflects the
amount of food still present in the stomach at the time of ingestion
of the dose. The highest values for absorption may have been associated with the subjects with the fastest rate of gastric emptying, but
data are not available on this point.

In a balance study performed upon young children,
Alexander et al. (1972) found that the children (aged between 3 months
and 8 years) absorbed 50% of the ingested dietary lead. In a similar
type of study, Ziegler et al. (1978) obtained of value of 42% for
absorption of dietary lead. Absorption of lead was inversely correlated with the calcium content of the diet.

The gastrointestinal absorption of lead in man is strongly
dependent upon the form of ingested lead. For dietary lead a value of
between 5 and 15% seems appropriate. However, if children are considered, a value of 50% should be used for modelling purposes.

The inverse relationship between lead absorption and calcium
absorption has been investigated by in vitro techniques, mainly using
the everted gut sac method. Gruden (1975) showed that the active
transport of calcium across the intestinal wall was not inhibited by
lead. Calcium is also transported by a passive process and
Gruden et al. (1974) showed that lead inhibits the transport of
calcium by this route. Experiments using chicks (Mykkanen and
Wasserman, 1982) showed that Vitamin D enhanced lead absorption.
Vitamin D is known to increase the active transport of calcium, and
so, if more calcium is absorbed by this route, less calcium will be
available to compete with lead for the paracellular route.

4.4.4   Metabolism

In a study by Mukai (1981) involving intravenous, intratracheal or oral administration of Pb-210 to guinea pigs, the following observations were made:

-     Concentrations of lead in blood reached their maximum one
      day after intratracheal or intravenous administration where-
      as, with oral administration, blood concentrations after one

day were low, but rose gradually until day 15 when they
began to decrease;

- bone concentrations were high throughout the experiment,
whereas liver showed a high initial uptake followed by a
rapid decrease in content.

The time-dependent distribution of Pb-210 in rats was investigated by Engziek (1981). Bone accumulated most lead, whereas soft
tissues accumulated least. A biological half-life of 60 ± 6 days was
obtained for the whole-body retention of the element.

An extensive study of the uptake of inhaled lead, and its
subsequent elimination was reported by Chamberlain et al. (1979). The
main results from this study were as listed below.

- With a respiratory rate of 15 breaths per minute and a lead
aerosol concentration of 40 μg m^{-3}, there was 40% deposition
in the lung at a mean particle size of 0.04 μm and 70%
deposition with 0.02 μm particles.

- 80% of deposited lead was cleared from the lung within
24 hours.

- The half-time of disappearance of lead from blood was
18.3 ± 1.1 days.

- The ratio of endogenous faecal excretion to urinary excretion was found to be 0.5 (0.4% dose/day in faeces, 0.81%
dose/day in urine).

Endogenous faecal excretion is thought to arise from biliary
and intestinal secretions and from lead bound to sloughed-off intestinal cells. Its existence complicates metabolic balance studies,
since total faecal excretion is the sum of unabsorbed lead and endogenous excretion, making an estimate of the fractional absorption in
man rather difficult.

Biliary excretion of lead by the rat was studied by Cirkt
(1972). After intravenous injection of Pb-210, 6.7% of the administered dose was secreted in bile in 24 h. Excretion via the intestinal
cells was studied after cannulating the bile duct. These experiments
demonstrated that biliary excretion was the major contributer to
endogenous faecal excretion.

A kinetic analysis of lead metabolism in man was undertaken
by Rabinowitz et al. (1976). They supplemented the intake of the
subjects with Pb-204 enriched lead which was ingested with meals for 1
to 124 days. Blood, urine and faecal excretion was continuously
monitored, with hair, nails and intestinal excretions being monitored
at intervals. The data were analysed in terms of a three-compartment
model (Fig. 4.5). This model which was used by Marcus (1979) in
deriving a composite model of lead metabolism, is discussed in
section 4.4.7.

4.4.5   Toxicity studies

Bingham (1969) showed that inhalation of lead oxide by rats, at concentrations of from 10 to 150 $\mu g \, m^{-3}$ for periods of 3 to 12 months resulted in a decrease in the number of alveolar macrophages isolated from the excised lungs. Exposure to 150 $\mu g \, m^{-3}$ for various times from 1 to 20 days revealed that the number of alveolar macrophages that may be washed from the lungs is significantly decreased after 24 h exposure. Upon removal of the animals from exposure, the number of macrophages returned to normal within 3 days.

Two studies were identified which investigated the intracellular compartmentation of lead in two in vitro systems. Rosen (1983) investigated the metabolism of lead in bone cell cultures. Pb-210 was rapidly taken up by osteoclasts whereas osteoblasts showed very little accumulation in comparison. Mediated uptake of lead into osteoclasts also occurred, and this was modified by hormonal agents, such as parathyroid hormone. Parathyroid hormone also caused increased calcium uptake by osteoclasts, but the increased uptake of lead continued after calcium uptake had saturated. It was suggested that modulations in cellular calcium metabolism induced by lead at low concentrations may have the potential for disturbing a variety of cell functions that depend upon calcium as a second messenger.

Isolated hepatocytes were studied by Pounds et al. (1982). Intracellular lead metabolism was interpreted in terms of two compartments, with the majority of the lead being associated with a "deep" compartment, consisting mainly of mitochondria.

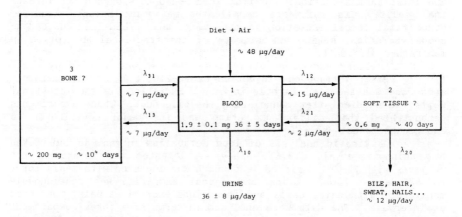

Note:
    From Rabinowitz et al. (1976)

FIGURE 4.5   A three-compartmental model of human lead metabolism derived from tracer and balance data from five healthy men. The lead content and mean life of each pool and the rates of lead movement between the pools (λ) are shown. Numerical values represent the mean values ($\pm$SD) for all subjects for whom data were available. Loss of lead from the body via pool two (λ_{20}) is from integumentary structures (hair, nails, sweat) and alimentary tract losses, such as salivary, biliary, gastric, and pancreatic secretions.

4.4.6   Occupational exposure

Monitoring of lead exposure has been predominantly performed by measuring the lead concentration in blood samples. Dossing and Paulev (1983) observed the change in blood concentration in two groups of smelter workers employed before and after the implementation of an industrial hygiene programme. After three months employment, workers taken on after the start of the programme had blood lead concentrations equal to those found in workers employed before the programme was initiated. The hygiene program was further developed and blood lead levels measured during the ensuing 5 years. Mean blood lead concentrations fell from 450 µg l^{-1} at the beginning of the study to 300 µg l^{-1} in the last year of observation. In this study, it was also found that individual blood lead concentrations had no relationship to air lead concentrations measured with a personal sampler.

In a study of blood lead concentrations in shipyard workers, Grandjean and Kon (1981) found three distinct groups.

- burners and welders (median blood lead concentrations of 390 µg l^{-1});

- other ship repair workers (median blood lead concentration of 260 µg l^{-1});

- retired shipyard workers (median blood lead concentrations of 230 µg l^{-1}).

Labreche and P'an (1981) demonstrated correlation between blood lead levels and the logarithm of urinary δ-aminolaevulinic acid (ALA-U) concentrations and between blood lead levels and the logarithm of free erythrocyte protoporphyrin (FEP) concentrations. Both ALA-U and FEP concentrations rose shortly after blood lead levels reached 450-500 µg l^{-1}.

The dependence of the half-life for reduction of blood lead concentrations on the period of previous lead exposure was investigated by O'Flaherty et al. (1982) who observed the fall in blood lead concentrations in a group of workers on strike. The range of apparent half-lives was from 20 to 130 days and values were correlated with period of exposure to lead (Fig. 4.6).

Brodeur et al. (1983) observed the fall in lead concentrations in saliva and blood after removal from occupational exposure. Blood lead levels fell slowly, whereas salivary lead concentrations fell more rapidly, with a half-life of 5 to 7 days. Temporary return to work by two of the subjects resulted in relatively marked increase of salivary lead concentrations, implying that salivary lead levels are closely related to recent lead exposure.

The pattern of blood lead elimination was studied in workers who had been removed from their jobs as a result of lead in blood concentrations exceeding the legal levels enforced in the USA. For workers removed under a 60/40 trigger i.e. whose blood lead exceeded 60 µg/100 ml and who could not work again until this parameter had fallen to 40 µg/100 ml, 80% had returned to work within 6 months. However, no relationship was found between the rate of decrease in blood lead concentrations and the period of occupational exposure (see also O'Flaherty et al., 1982).

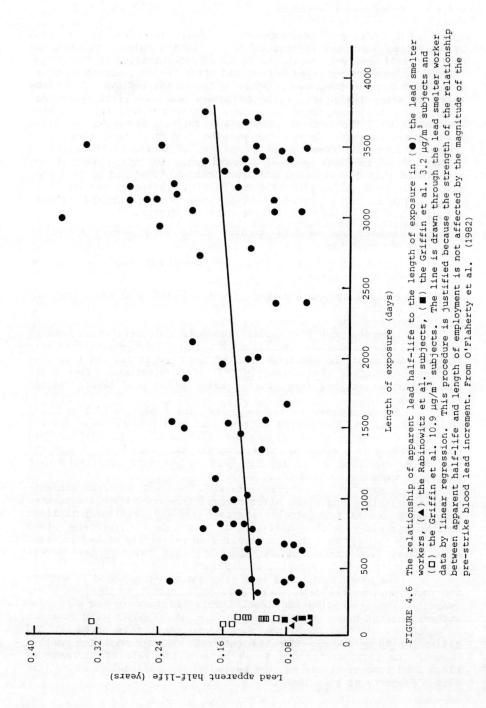

FIGURE 4.6 The relationship of apparent lead half-life to the length of exposure in (●) the lead smelter workers, (▲) the Rabinowitz et al. subjects, (■) the Griffin et al. 3.2 μg/m³ subjects and (□) the Griffin et al. 10.9 μg/m³ subjects. The line is drawn through the lead smelter worker data by linear regression. This procedure is justified because the strength of the relationship between apparent half-life and length of employment is not affected by the magnitude of the pre-strike blood lead increment. From O'Flaherty et al. (1982)

The effect of lead exposure on kidney function was investigated by Lilis et al. (1980). They concluded, that for long-term exposure, occupational groups with a high prevalence of blood lead concentrations in excess of 600 µg l^{-1} and zinc protoporphyrin levels in excess of 1000 µg l^{-1} are at definite risk of impaired renal function.

Sister chromatid exchange (SCE) rates were measured in long-term lead-exposed workers (Grandjean et al., 1983). These rates were significantly correlated with zinc protoporphyrin concentrations in blood. The subjects were examined after a vacation, and it was found that zinc protoporphyrin levels in blood had decreased significantly as had SCE rates. Newly employed workers, with no previous occupational lead exposure, showed an increase in blood zinc protoporphyrin levels but no increase in SCE rates. This implies that a genotoxic effect due to inorganic lead may occur in long-term lead-exposed workers.

4.4.7 Development of a pharmacokinetic model

Several multicompartment models have been proposed to simulate the metabolism of lead by the body (Thorne and Jackson, 1983). The type of model varies from a single compartment model, used to correlate the effect of concentrations of lead in air upon concentrations of lead in blood (Goldsmith and Hexton, 1967), to five compartment models which predict whole-body and individual tissue retention of lead (Bernard, 1977; Marcus, 1979).

Marcus (1979) reviewed several mathematical models of lead accumulation, and proposed a composite five compartment model. This included a central blood compartment, which exchanged lead with four other tissue compartments. These were thought to represent bone, liver, kidney and "other tissue", and had elimination half-times of 1820, 45, 5 and 182 days respectively. The accumulation half-time was assumed to be 35 days.

A similar model is utilised in this study, but different numerical values are used in the calculations, based on the observed tissue concentrations of lead reported by Iyengar et al. (1978). It is assumed that these values are typical for a non-exposed population, and that they represent a steady-state between accumulation and excretion of normal daily lead intake. For a dietary intake of 300 µg and $f_1 = 0.1$, dietary uptake is estimated to be 30 µg d^{-1}. In addition, an intake from air of 1-100 µg d^{-1} (Thorne and Jackson, 1983) in a non-smoking individual, implies an additional uptake ~ 0.5 to 50 µg d^{-1}. Overall, it seems appropriate to assume a typical daily intake of 45 µg. A mean value for urinary lead excretion has been given as 35 µg d^{-1} and a mean value for excretion in bile, sweat and hair has been given as 10 µg d^{-1} (Rabinowitz et al., 1976). This is consistent with the mean estimates of intake given above.

If this is the case, then the ratio of the total amounts of lead in the blood compartment to the total amount in the relevant tissue compartment should be equal to the ratio of the transfer coefficients between the two compartments. This may not be a valid assumption for the bone compartment, which, because of its long half-life of retention, may never reach equilibrium during a person's lifetime.

The model used in this report is represented in Fig. 4.7 and is used in conjunction with the following parameter values (d^{-1}):

$$\lambda_1 = 0.008$$
$$\lambda_2 = 0.693$$
$$\lambda_3 = 0.004$$
$$\lambda_4 = 0.0000866$$
$$\lambda_A = 0.04$$
$$\lambda_B = 0.18$$
$$\lambda_C = 0.05$$
$$\lambda_D = 0.01$$
$$\lambda_E = 0.0027$$
$$\lambda_U = 0.03$$

The parameter values are derived as follows.

The amounts of lead in the various compartments are found by multiplying the relevant tissue or organ lead concentration from Iyengar et al. (1978) by the total organ weight given in "Reference Man" (ICRP, 1975).

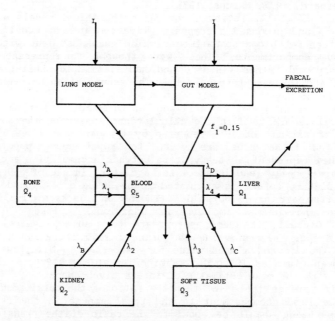

Note: for parameter values see text.

FIGURE 4.7. SYSTEMIC MODEL OF LEAD METABOLISM

Endogenous faecal lead excretion was measured by Chamberlain et al. (1978) and the mean endogenous faecal clearance of this pathway of elimination was found to be 1.8% d^{-1}. This is similar to the value of 2.5% d^{-1} derived from data presented by Rabinowitz et al. (1976). The flux is represented by a transfer from the liver compartment to the faecal compartment. Rabinowitz et al. (1976) and Batschelet et al. (1979) presented data for urinary lead excretion, from which an elimination half-time of 35 days could be derived. Urinary lead excretion was also monitored by Chamberlain et al. (1978) who calculated an elimination half-time of 19 days.

For the compartmental elimination half-times, Bernard (1977) assumed a half-life of 8000 days for bone. Marcus (1979) derived a value of 2640 days but in his conclusions stated that a longer half-life would be appropriate. Rabinowitz et al. (1976) estimated the half-life of their longest-lived compartment to be 10,000 days. For kidney, the half-life value of one day derived by Bernard (1977) seems appropriate. For liver the half-time is assumed to be similar to that for biliary excretion. This gives an elimination half-life from the liver of 43 days (see Marcus, 1979).

The compartment with the second-longest retention half-time has been assumed to represent an "all other tissues" retention compartment. Different values of half-live have been ascribed to this compartment, but the value derived by Marcus (1979) of 183 days is used. This is very similar to the half-life of the second component of the ICRP lead model (ICRP, 1980).

The fractional absorption of lead from the gastrointestinal tract is subject to wide variation, dependent upon the dietary status of the individual. In the fasting state, 60% absorption of ingested lead was observed by Flanagan et al. (1982), whereas when lead is administered with the diet, an absorption of 5 to 10% is observed (Blake, 1976). In calculations presented herein, a value of 15% is assumed.

4.5   Nickel

4.5.1   Intake rates

Studies by Sherlock et al. (1983), Kirkpatrick and Coffin (1974) and Tipton and Stewart (1969) gave values of dietary intake of nickel of 250, 350 and 420 $\mu g \ d^{-1}$ respectively. This tends to confirm the values reported in Thorne and Jackson (1983) (normal value = 400 $\mu g \ d^{-1}$; range = 100 - 800 $\mu g \ d^{-1}$).

4.5.2   Blood and urine levels

Zachariasen et al. (1975) developed a flameless atomic absorption spectrophotometry based technique for measuring nickel concentrations in blood and urine samples. The mean value from 8 subjects were as follows:

plasma nickel $= 4.7 \pm 1.0$ µg l^{-1}

urinary nickel $= 24 \pm 4$ µg l^{-1}

4.5.3   Metabolism

The retention of Ni-63, intratracheally administered to rats as the chloride, was studied by Carvalho and Ziemer (1982). Only 1.3 µg of nickel was administered to each animal. The lungs and kidney exhibited the highest concentrations of Ni-63 and, 21 days after administration, they were the only organs where the radionuclide was still detectable. Urinary excretion was the main route of elimination, with 72% of the initial body burden eliminated in the urine during the first day. By day 21, almost all the Ni-63 had been excreted in the urine (97% of the initial body burden). Retention data could be fitted to a sum of three exponentials:

$$\text{Lung retention} = 60.21\ e^{-26.63\ t} + 36.63\ e^{-0.584\ t} + 4.1\ e^{-0.19\ t}$$

$$\text{Whole body retention} = 61.28\ e^{-2.4\ t} + 38.16\ e^{-0.58\ t} + 4.492\ e^{-0.186\ t}$$

where t is in days.

After intraperitoneal injection of 6 mg of Ni-63 as Ni Cl$_2$ to rats, Tandon (1982) observed that kidneys had the highest uptake of nickel, and that most of the Ni-63 was excreted via urine within 24 h. The daily faecal excretion, though low, was approximately constant up to six days at approximately 1% of the dose per day. At times of more than six days, almost no radioactivity could be detected in the animals.

Schroeder and Nason (1974) demonstrated an increase in zinc content of all organs, except liver, when nickel was adminstered to rats. One possible explanation for this is that increased nickel input causes an increase in metallothionein production by the liver, thus affecting the metabolism of other metals which bind to this protein. Chmielnicka et al. (1982) administered nickel subcutaneously to rats once a day for one week. One day after receiving the final dose, the total amount of zinc in the body had increased by 30% compared with control animals. The tissue concentrations of metallothionein were also significantly increased in nickel-exposed animals, and this increase correlated with the zinc plus nickel content of the tissues.

Hair has been considered as a potential monitoring material for exposure to trace metals, but data from a study in which guinea pigs were exposed to 2.5 ppm nickel in drinking water (Scheiner et al. 1976) suggest that this may not be the case for nickel, since no difference in hair concentrations was found between the exposed and unexposed animals.

4.5.4   Placental transfer of nickel

Two further studies of placental transfer of nickel were
identified, both using mice. In the first, Olsen and Jansen, (1979)
studied the process by autoradiography. A marked uptake of nickel was
seen in the 5-day embryo and foetal accumulation took place up to
16 days gestation. In the early embryo, nickel was distributed uni-
formly throughout all tissues, but the distribution became more diff-
erentiated with increasing gestational age, eventually resembling that
in the mother. Lu et al. (1981) obtained data on maternal tissue and
foetal nickel concentrations, after a single intraperitoneal injection
of nickel on day 16 of gestation. Maximum concentrations in foetal
tissues were reached 8 h after injection, and a slight, gradual,
decrease was observed over the period 8 to 24 h. Thereafter, there
was a rapid decrease in tissue contents.

4.5.5   In vitro studies of the effects of nickel

The intracellular binding of nickel was investigated by
Herlant-Peers et al. (1983). Several different nickel-binding proteins were identified, some of which were only induced after repeated
administrations of nickel to the animal. Lung tissue was always more
highly labelled than the liver, especially in the mitochondrial
fraction.
Johansson et al. (1983) reproduced the pathological effects
observed in lung tissue after exposure to metallic nickel, when
rabbits were exposed to soluble nickel chloride. This implies that
all soluble nickel compounds may produce these tissue effects, which
are similar to those seen in the disease pulmonary alveolar protei-
nosis.
The effects of various culture medium components upon phagocytosis of carcinogenic crystalline, and non-carcinogenic amorphous,
nickel sulphide were investigated by Heck and Costa (1982).
Crystalline nickel sulphide was absorbed by cells in a simple salts/
glucose maintenance solution to an extent similar to that observed in
complex culture media, suggesting that the serum proteins (in culture
media) exert little influence upon the uptake of these particles.
Phagocytosis of crystalline nickel sulphide was shown to be highly
dependent upon calcium in the medium. The opposite surface charge of
crystalline as opposed to amorphous nickel sulphide has been suggested
to account for the differences in phagocytosis and carcinogenicity of
the two forms (Abbrachia et al., 1981) and, by this hypothesis, the
above results imply that the components of culture media do not modify
this charge in such a way as to significantly affect their uptake.
Smialowicz et al. (1984) showed that administration of
nickel chloride significantly inhibited the immune system in mice.
This effect was predominantly upon T-cell mediated immune responses.
The in vitro solubilities of various nickel compounds in
water, serum and renal cytosol was determined by Kuehn and Sunderman
(1982). The majority of compounds were more soluble in serum or
cytosol than in water.

4.5.6   Occupational exposure to nickel

In a study of urinary and faecal elimination of nickel by workers exposed to the metal, significant correlations were obtained between both faecal and urinary excretion and the concentration of nickel in air (Hassler et al., 1983).

Grandjean et al. (1980) found that shipyard workers exhibited a significantly higher mean plasma nickel concentration (5.1 µg l^{-1}) than did a non-exposed control group (1.2 µg l^{-1}). The same was true of urine nickel concentration (4.9 µg l^{-1} in shipyard workers, 2.5 µg l^{-1} in controls). In shipyard workers, 12% had plasma nickel concentrations above 10 µg l^{-1}, the level at which Hogetveit et al., (1977) suggested that workers should be supervised and required to wear masks, or suspended from work, until plasma nickel contrations had fallen to lower values.

In a study of welders of stainless steel, Kalliomäki et al, (1981) found a slight, non-significant, rise in urinary nickel concentrations compared with control values.

Boysen et al. (1984) found that nickel concentrations in plasma and urine of retired nickel-exposed workers were significantly higher among roasting/smelter workers than in electrolysis and non-

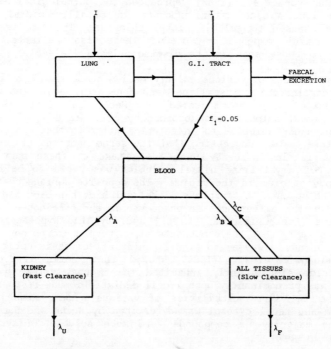

Note: for parameter values see text.

FIGURE 4.8 SYSTEMIC MODEL OF NICKEL METABOLISM

process workers.   The former group have a greater exposure to nickel, and these findings probably reflect the slow release of nickel accumulated during occupational exposure.

4.5.7   Metabolic model of nickel metabolism

No further work on human metabolism of nickel was identified, so the model proposed by Thorne and Jackson, (1983) has been implemented.   This model is shown in Fig. 4.8.   The following parameter values are utilised:

Parameter	Value (d^{-1})
λ_A	1.05
λ_B	0.45
λ_C	5.2×10^{-4}
λ_F	5.8×10^{-5}
λ_U	6.0

An f_1 value of 0.05 is used.   Thus, with a dietary intake of 400 µg day^{-1} the following equilibrium compartmental contents are estimated.   These values are used on the initial condition from the model.

$$\text{blood} = 13.75 \text{ µg}$$

$$\text{kidney (fast clearance)} = 2.41 \text{ µg}$$

$$\text{all tissue (slow clearance)} = 10.71 \text{ mg}$$

Tissue concentrations are calculated as follows:

KIDNEY = [KIDNEY (FAST CLEARANCE)] + 0.005 [ALL TISSUES (SLOW CLEARANCE)]

BLOOD = [BLOOD] + 0.002 [ALL TISSUES (SLOW CLEARANCE)]

OTHER TISSUES = 0.993 [ALL TISSUES (SLOW CLEARANCE)]

4.6   Chromium

There is now sufficient evidence to regard chromium as an essential element in man (Mertz, 1974).   Early studies revealed that chromium deficiency led to impairment of glucose metabolism.   This was linked to deficiency of "Glucose tolerance factor" in the diet. Glucose tolerance factor is a chromium-containing plant protein of molecular weight 2600. The constituent chromium is in the trivalent form (Starich and Blincoe, 1983).   In the gastrointestinal tract of the rat, the compound was found to remain intact through the small intestine, but degradation products were identified in the caecum, possibly as a result of the metabolism by the fauna of the large intestine.   Approximately 30% of the plant material bound chromium was taken up from the gut of the rat (Starich and Blincoe, 1983).

Recent studies have also revealed a link between chromium intake and serum lipid levels. Elwood et al. (1982) studied the effects of dietary supplementation with brewer's yeast (a rich source of glucose tolerance factor) upon the lipid levels in normolipidaemic and hyperlipidaemic subjects. A significant decrease in the total blood cholesterol level was seen in both groups. High density lipo-protein levels were increased in both groups by brewers yeast supp-lementation. Serum triglyceride levels were not affected by supplmen-tation. Anderson et al. (1983) found no effect of dietary chromium supplementation on serum lipid parameters, but the chromium supplement used was chromic chloride which may not affect blood lipids.

4.6.1   Chromium content of body fluids

Versieck and Cornelis (1980) reviewed published data for normal plasma, or serum, chromium concentrations. They concluded that many of the reported values are erroneously high due to inadequate sample preparation or measuring techniques. Typical normal values were reported as 0.1 to 0.5 $\mu g\ l^{-1}$. These values agree with those reported by Kumpulainen et al. (1983) who obtained chromium concen-trations of 0.49, 0.43 and 0.13 $\mu g\ l^{-1}$ in human milk, serum and urine samples.

4.6.2   Biochemical studies of chromium metabolism and effects

After a single intraperitoneal injection of potassium di-chromate to mice, analysis of the soluble fractions of tissue homogen-ates showed that most of the chromium was found in the cytosol (Yama moto et al., 1981). A low-molecular weight chromium-binding compound was identified, using Sephadex gel chromatography. This compound appeared soon after chromium administration and persisted for up to seven days afterwards. Examination of urine and faeces revealed a similar low-molecular weight chromium-binding compound to that found in the eluate from liver homogenates. A significant amount of chrom-ium was found in the same elution fraction of plasma after 2 h although it was not evident 15 minutes after administration of the dose. This suggests that a low-molecular weight chromium-binding substance is formed in liver and that this participates in the reten-tion and excretion of chromium. A similar compound has also been isolated from the liver of rabbits and Wada et al. (1983) also isola-ted similar compounds after dichromate injections in dogs. Two types of compound were identified, which differed in physical and chemical properties. When the compounds were isolated and mice were pretreated with the chromium-free substance there was a marked reduction in mortality rates as a result of subsequent acute poisoning with chromic chloride, reaffirming that this induced compound plays an important role in the detoxification and excretion of chromium in mammals.

Investigation into the cellular events leading to the induc-tion of malignantly transformed cells by chromium have centred on the effects of trivalent and hexavalent chromium on different experimental systems. Hexavalent chromium is a potent inducer of mutations in intact cell assays, whereas trivalent chromium has little or no effect

(Venier et al., 1982). This is thought to be due to to the impermeab-
ility of the cell membrane to trivalent chromium. In tests using
isolated DNA, trivalent chromium is a far more effective inducer of
faults in the DNA replication process than is hexavalent chromium
(Sirover and Loeb, 1976). To explain these findings, it was hypoth-
esized that hexavalent chromium enters the cell and is reduced by the
mixed function oxidase system to trivalent chromium, which can induce
errors in DNA replication leading to a transmissable mutation. In
support of this hypothesis, Gruber and Jennette (1978) demonstrated
the reduction of chromate by rat liver microsomes in the presence of
nicotinamide adenine dinucleotide phosphate (NADPH). The presence of
NADPH alone caused no reduction of chromate.

4.6.3   Metabolism

        The clearance of hexavalent chromium from the lung of the
rat was measured by Weber (1983). At three days after intratracheal
administration, approximately one third of the dose remained in the
lung. In serum, the decline in chromium concentration was monoexpon-
ential, with a half-time of 3 to 4 days.
        A study of the retention of hexavalent chromium in various
organs of the rat was performed by Yamaguchi et al. (1983). After a
subcutaneous administration of chromium, retention in the lung could
be described in terms of two components with half-lives of 60 h and
500 h. Blood levels declined monoexponentially with a half-life of
330 h. A total of 36% of the dose was excreted in faeces over the same
period.
        The renal handling of chromium in rats was concluded to be
flow-independent (Wallach and Verch, 1983), since ADH deficiency had
little effect on Cr-51 retention, despite massive diuresis. This is
probably explained by chromium reabsorption in the proximal tubules,
but incomplete glomerular filtration of chromium due to protein-
binding cannot be ruled out.
        Mice dosed with trivalent chromium retained seven times more
chromium 21 days later than did mice dosed with hexavalent chromium
(Bryson and Goodall, 1983). Analysis of faecal and urinary excretion
confirmed that hexavalent chromium was excreted more rapidly than
trivalent chromium. These differences in retention may partly explain
the observed differences in toxicity between the two forms of the
metal.
        Rats intravenously dosed with Cr-51 labelled hexavalent
chromium excreted more Cr-51 into bile in a 2 h period than did rats
given equal amounts of labelled trivalent chromium. Sephadex gel
chromatography of the bile revealed low-molecular weight chromium
-binding substances (see Section 4.6.2).
        Due to poor absorption of trivalent chromium from the gast-
rointestinal tract (Thorne and Jackson, 1983), radiolabelled chromic
chloride has been used as a marker in studies requiring an indicator
of intestinal transit (Payton et al., 1982; Marx et al., 1980). These
studies are usually dual isotope studies in which the absorption and
excretion of the other nuclide is of primary interest. Faecal
excretion of the element of interest after the excretion of an
empirically-derived fraction of the administered chromium is interpreted as being due to endogenous faecal excretion.

4.6.4   Occupational exposure

Welders, especially of stainless steel, are thought to be at risk of developing lung cancer because of the high levels of chromium in certain welding fumes. A review of 22 epidemiological studies of cancer incidence revealed an overall risk ratio of 1.3 (Stern, 1983).

A linear relationship between chromium concentration in work air and in post-shift urine on the same day was observed by Sjogern et al. (1983) in welders of stainless steel. This suggests that individual measurements can can be used to estimate current exposure. Kalliomaki et al. (1981) measured the amount of lung-retained contaminants in stainless-steel welders by monitoring the residual magnetic field created by ferromagnetic particles in the lung. The magnitude of this field correlated with urinary chromium concentrations.

Tossavainen et al. (1980) proposed a one compartment model to predict the effect of air chromium levels upon urinary chromium concentrations. This model was based on data obtained from welders, and the half-life of chromium in the compartment was calculated as 30 h.

Exceptional pharmacokinetic data were obtained by Kiilunen et al. (1983) from a group of workers exposed to chromium (III) lignosulphate dust. The chromium component of the dust was rapidly absorbed, and a peak of urinary excretion was seen immediately after exposure.

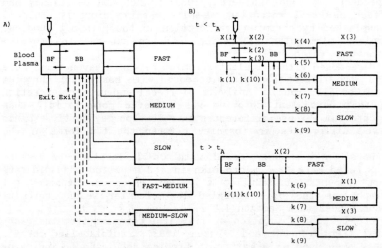

Note:
1. For parameter values see table 4.1
2. Redrawn from Lim et al. (1983)

FIGURE 4.9.   A: FUNCTIONAL COMPARTMENTAL MODEL IN WHICH FAST, MEDIUM AND SLOW COMPARTMENTS ARE TREATED WITHOUT REGARD TO SPECIFIC ORGANS. FAST-MEDIUM AND MEDIUM-SLOW COMPARTMENTS WERE FOUND NOT TO CONTRIBUTE TO THE SOLUTION. ENTRY IS ASSUMED TO BE BY INJECTION OF CR-51 INTO COMPARTMENT BF.
B: FINAL COMPARTMENT MODEL. IN SOLUTION, UPPER MODEL IS CONVERTED TO LOWER ONE BY "COLLAPSING" FAST COMPARTMENT WITH PLASMA-BOUND (BB) COMPARTMENT AT TIME t_A. TIME t_A IS TIME AFTER WHICH EXCHANGE BETWEEN BB AND FAST COMPARTMENT IS SO RAPID COMPARED WITH MEDIUM AND SLOW COMPARTMENTS, THAT THEY CAN BE CONSIDERED AS ONE AND "COLLAPSED" INTO A SINGLE COMPARTMENT

This suggests that chromium taken in this chemical form is behaving metabolically as hexavalent chromium, even though it is trivalent on intake.

Lindberg and Hedenstierna (1983) found that, in chrome-plating workers exposed to an air concentration of 1 µg m^{-3} of chromic acid, complaints of nasal irritation were common. Nasal septum ulceration and perforation were seen in two thirds of workers exposed to peak levels of 20 µg m^{-3} or more. Lung function tests, such as measurements of forced expiratory volume, showed a reduction in lung function between Monday and Thursday in subjects exposed to 2 µg m^{-3}. These results show that, even at the low concentrations of 1 to 20 µg m^{-3} of chromic acid, unpleasant side effects are observed in workers.

4.6.5   Metabolic model

A kinetic model of chromium (Cr) metabolism was developed by Lim et al. (1983). This was based on data obtained by whole body counting, in man, after intravenous administration of Cr-51. Their model is shown in Fig. 4.9.

As this is the only study identified that has modelled chromium metabolism in vivo in normal human subjects, the results are used as the basis of the model developed for this report.

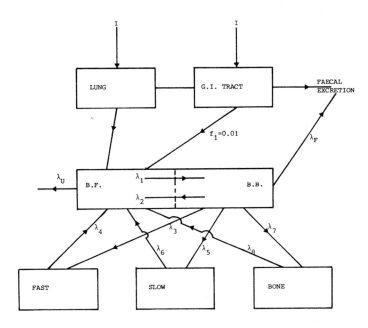

Note: for parameter values see text.

FIGURE 4.10 SYSTEMIC MODEL OF CHROMIUM METABOLISM

In the above study, no long term compartment corresponding to bone was identified. This is probably because the reported half-life of 10,000 d for chromium elimination from the bone compartment (Coughtrey and Thorne, 1983) is much longer than the counting period (84 days). As a large fraction of body chromium is located in bone (ICRP, 1975), a corresponding compartment has to be added to the model. The model adopted in this study is shown in Fig. 4.10.

Absorbed chromium passes into the plasma "free" (BF) compartment, from where it rapidly equilibrates with a plasma "bound" (BB) compartment. In vitro experiments by Lim et al. (1983) suggest that 95% of plasma chromium is in the bound form. Chromium in the BF compartment is filtered through the kidneys and excreted in the urine. From the BB compartment, the chromium equilibrates with the three tissue compartments. The "fast" transfer compartment suggested by Lim et al. (1983) has not been included, since its rate of turnover is very fast compared with the other compartments, and also its contents are less than half those of the plasma compartment.

The "fast" and "slow" compartments are identical to the "medium" and "slow" compartments proposed by Lim et al. (1983). However, an additional compartment, representing metabolism in bone, has been added, for reasons stated above.

Chromium is assumed to be released from the tissue compartments in the unbound form and, therefore, passes into the corresponding plasma compartment. Excretion via routes other than the kidney is represented by a transfer from the BB compartment. This is purely for convenience, since this component of loss is probably dominated by desquamation of intestinal epithetial cells. This is borne out by the observed rate constant, which is of the same order of magnitude as intestinal mucosa cell turnover times (Ganong, 1977).

The rate constants used with the model are given below:

Parameter	Value (d^{-1})
λ_1	219
λ_2	12.1
λ_3	0.34
λ_4	0.053
λ_5	0.5
λ_6	0.0035
λ_6	0.0035
λ_7	0.07
λ_8	6.93×10^{-5}
λ_U	0.36
λ_F	0.1

Consideration of parameters λ_1 and λ_2 leads to the conclusion that equilibration of the two plasma compartments is rapid compared with the times for transfer to the tissue compartments, and so the two plasma compartments can be "collapsed" (Lim et al., 1983) into a single compartment, with appropriate adjustments being made to the excretion rate constants. Thus, the model is very similar to that proposed by Jackson and Thorne (1983), and the remainder of the transfer parameters are derived from that study.

Individual organ concentrations are computed as follows:

$$\text{BONE} = [\text{BONE}]$$

$$\text{LIVER} = 0.02 \, \{[\text{FAST}] + [\text{SLOW}]\}$$

$$\text{SPLEEN} = 0.002 \, \{[\text{FAST}] + [\text{SLOW}]\}$$

$$\text{KIDNEY} = 0.01 \, \{[\text{FAST}] + [\text{SLOW}]\}$$

$$\text{OTHER TISSUE} = 0.968 \, \{[\text{FAST}] + [\text{SLOW}]\}$$

For a typical dietory intake of 75 µg with an f_1 value of 0.01, the following values are calculated for equilibrium compartmental contents and these are used as the initial conditions for the model.

$$\text{BLOOD} = 1.63 \ \mu g$$

$$[\text{SLOW}] = 242 \ \mu g$$

$$[\text{FAST}] = 10.45 \ \mu g$$

$$[\text{BONE}] = 1.65 \ mg$$

4.7   Asbestos

Numerous biochemical studies of the effects of asbestos were identified, but the majority of these were in too specialised a field to be relevant to this review, or repeated work presented in the review by Thorne and Jackson (1983). For this reason, only studies relevant to model development are reviewed in this section.

With respect to the uptake of fibres by the gastrointesinal tract, Meek and Grasso (1983) administered amosite fibres orally to normal rats, and to rats with induced gastrointestinal ulcers. Microscopic examination of the intestinal walls for up to 7 days (long enough for the fibres to have been excreted in faeces) showed no intracellular fibres in intestinal cells from the ulcerated rats, and no pathological lesions in the intestines of normal rats. This evidence supports earlier findings that the gastrointestinal mucosa is an effective barrier to asbestos, but also shows that when this barrier is degenerate, as in the case of ulceration, no cellular uptake is observed.

Samples of hepatic blood from animals ingesting chrysotile fibres were analysed by Weinzweig and Richards (1983) who found that only fibrils (length <1µm) were present. In only 6 out of 15 experiments were the concentrations of fibrils higher in the asbestos exposed rats, once again demonstrating that the fraction of an ingested dose of asbestos that is absorbed is minute. Cunningham et al. (1976) developed an assay for determining the faecal excretion of asbestos. Faecal asbestos was significantly higher in occupationally-exposed subjects than in control subjects, suggesting that monitoring of faecal asbestos excretion may be a useful control technique.

4.7.1   Deposition and clearance from the lung

The effect of static electrification of asbestos upon its deposition in rat lung was investigated by Vincent et al. (1981). An amosite fibre, as dispersed in a typical animal exposure chamber, was found to carry a net charge of magnitude equivalent to approximately 60 electrons. The distribution of charge was bimodal, suggesting that two charging mechanisms were taking place, the main one producing net negative charge and the lesser one producing net positive charge. The presence of this charge enhanced the deposition of asbestos into the deep lung by 40%.

Bolton et al. (1983) measured the clearance of amosite asestos fibres from the lungs of rats, interpreting their results in terms of the model proposed by Morgan et al. (1977). In this model, clearance from the lung is described by the sum of three exponential components with half-lives of 0.6, 11.5 and 170 days respectively. Bolton et al. found that approximately 7% of the inhaled fibres were deposited in each of the medium and slow-clearance compartments, in good agreement with the values of 5% and 8% for the medium and slow compartments respectively proposed by Morgan et al. (1977). In rats exposed to high (>1500µg per rat) doses of amosite, Bolton et al. found that the medium-term clearance compartment became "overloaded". This was interpreted as an overload of the alveolar macrophage clearance mechanism, but as no precise anatomical location and description of the medium and slow clearance compartments exists, this conclusion cannot at present be substantiated.

The translocation of asbestos dust through the bronchiolar wall was investigated by Holt (1982). He observed the location of fibres within the lung, using optical microscopy, at varying times after inhalation of chrysotile fibres by guinea-pigs. Fibres deposited in the larger bronchioles were removed from the lung by the muco-ciliary escalator. Some of the fibres deposited in the pulmonary alveoli were phagocytozed by macrophages which moved towards the periphery of the lung by passing through alveolar walls. Some macrophages aggregated in alveoli near larger bronchioles, penetrated the bronchiolar wall, and were shed into the lumen where they were cleared by the cilia to the trachea. In view of these observations, it is likely that macrophage levels and stimulation of the macrophage response by challenge may modify asbestos clearance (see Section 6).

4.7.2   Development of a metabolic model

In the absence of adequate data on the subjects of gastrointestinal uptake and systemic metabolism of asbestos, these aspects are not included in the model. Though these subjects are obviously of great importance when constructing a model of the toxic actions of asbestos, the number of fibres actually involved in systemic metabolism must be minute when compared with the number of fibres inhaled or ingested.

The proposed model is intended to be used for monitoring purposes. The model of lung retention is that proposed by Thorne and Jackson (1983). This model can be summarised as follows.

- Of inhaled asbestos, 50% can be assumed to be deposited in the lung, including both upper and lower components of the respiratory tract;
- Of inhaled amphibole asbestos, 10% can be assumed to be retained in the lung with a half-life of 200 d and the rest rapidly excreted;
- Of inhaled chrysotile asbestos, 2.5% can be assumed to be retained in the lung with a half-life of 200 d and the rest rapidly excreted;
- For assessment of intakes of asbestos by inhalation the following retention functions are recommended.

Chrysotiles:

$$R(t) = 0.925e^{-0.693t/1} + 0.05e^{-0.693t/10} + 0.025e^{-0.693t/200}$$

Amphiboles:

$$R(t) = 0.85e^{-0.693t/1} + 0.05e^{-0.693t/10} + 0.1e^{-0.693t/200}$$

All three compartments of this lung clearance model are assumed to transfer the asbestos to the gastrointestinal tract, either by direct clearance via the mucociliary escalator or by phagocytosis of the fibres by macrophages, which are then cleared from the lung in the same manner.

Since no uptake or systemic metabolism is considered, the gastrointestinal tract can be represented by a single compartment, the contents of which pass directly to the faeces in a manner governed by the total gastrointestinal transit time. Burkitt et al. (1972) obtained values for this parameter varying from 48 to 96 h depending on the diet of the subject. A value of three days is assumed herein.

A total of 50% of inhaled asbestos is assumed to be deposited in the lung, with a partition between compartments as listed below.

Compartment	Chrysotile	Amphibole
A	0.925	0.85
B	0.05	0.05
C	0.025	0.1

4.8 Benzene

4.8.1 In vitro studies of benzene metabolism

The majority of such studies have been concerned with the elucidation of pathways of benzene metabolism, in particular, the pathways leading to covalent binding to macromolecules. Thus, Tunek and Oesch (1982) ascertained that the metabolic activation of benzene by rat liver microsomes is a multi-stage process involving benzene oxide, phenol and hydroquinone as intermediates and p-benzosemiquinone and/or p-benzoquinone as the major covalently-binding metabolites.

The mixed-function oxidase system is known to be one system in which benzene is metabolized, and several studies have investigated the effects of induction of this system upon the metabolism, and toxicity, of benzene. Post and Snyder (1983a) found that fluoride, but no other halide ions, stimulated the metabolism of benzene by rat liver microsomes. Other mixed-function oxidase reactions were not affected. In a second paper (Post and Snyder, 1983b), they found that two concentration-dependent mixed-function oxidase pathways for benzene metabolism existed. Both pathways were found to be stimulated by pre-treatment with benzene. Saito et al. (1973) found that benzene metabolism of rat liver microsomes was enhanced after pretreatment of the animals with benzene, but not after pretreatment with phenol. Electron microscopic studies of the liver showed proliferation of the smooth endoplasmic reticulum, after 7 and 14 days of benzene treatment.

4.8.2   Carcinogenic action of benzene

The attribution of a carcinogenic action to benzene has been based only on the association between occupational exposure to benzene and the incidence of leukaemia in man. The International Agency for Research on Cancer (1982) concluded that there was only limited evidence that benzene is carcinogenic in experimental animals. However, in a long-term study undertaken at the Institute of Oncology in Bologna, Italy, (Maltoni et al., 1983) it was shown that benzene produced a variety of tumours in rats including Zymbal gland carcinomas, carcinomas of the oral cavity, hepatocarcinomas, lymphoreticular neoplasias and other malignancies. Some of the tumours caused by benzene are uncommon or unusual in the breed of rats used in the study.

Further studies have reaffirmed the link between benzene exposure and leukaemia. Rinsky et al. (1981) conducted a retrospective cohort study of workers who had been exposed to benzene, during the manufacture of rubber. Among 748 workers who had at least one day of exposure to benzene, seven deaths from leukaemia occurred, compared with an expected number of 1.25 (standardized mortality ratio = 560; p < 0.001). Mean exposure to benzene was brief, and 58% of the cohort were exposed for less than one year. Evaluation of leukaemia mortality for those workers exposed to benzene for five or more years showed an SMR of 2100. All leukaemia deaths were myelocytic or monocytic in cell type. Reconstruction of the benzene exposure regimen suggested that in some plants, the air concentration of benzene occasionally rose to several hundred parts per million, but that for the most part, eight-hour time-weighted average exposures fell within the limits considered permissible at the time (25 ppm). The conclusion from this study is that benzene is a human carcinogen at a range of exposures not greatly above the current legal standard of 10 ppm. Arp et al. (1983) and Decouffle et al. (1983) found a standardized mortality ratio of approximately 400 when comparing the incidence of leukaemia in benzene -exposed workers compared with a control group of non-exposed workers.

In a cytogenic evaluation of peripheral lymphocytes from 52 workers exposed to low levels (<10 ppm) of benzene, Picciano (1979) found an increase in aberration rates compared with a non-exposed control group. Statistically significant differences were found in the distribution of specific types of chromosomal aberration, and these induced aberration levels were not related to the age of the workers. This study also suggests that toxic effects of benzene are seen at exposure levels near the present legally permissible limit.

4.8.3   Metabolism

The penetration of benzene through the intact skin of rhesus monkeys was investigated by Maibach and Anjo (1981). Less than 1% of the applied dose was absorbed through the skin, even if the stratum corneum was removed before application of the liquid.

Post-shift urinary phenol concentrations have been used to monitor occupational exposure to benzene (Thorne and Jackson, 1983), but such results should be interpreted with caution. Fishbeck et al. (1975) found that two commonly-used medications could elevate urinary phenol levels above 75 mg l^{-1}. The preparations were found to contain phenyl sulphonate, which is, presumably, metabolized to phenol. In a study of urinary phenol excretion in benzene-exposed workers, Andrzejewski et al. (1981) found that it was advisable to compare urinary phenol concentrations before and after a shift. Braier et al. (1981) suggested that blood benzene concentrations should be determined as well as urinary phenol levels. This was based on measurements of the two parameters in samples from workers exposed to <10 ppm benzene in air. Their results showed that in some samples, urinary phenol levels were not related to blood benzene concentrations.

Two furthur studies on the elimination of benzene in man were identified. Sherwood (1976) studied the elimination of benzene in breath and phenol in urine after the subject was exposed to different concentrations of benzene in inspired air. The elimination of benzene in expired air was interpreted in terms of three compartments with elimination half-lives of 1.3, 4.5 and 27.0 h respectively. The urinary excretion curve exhibited two components, with half-lives of 6.0 and 28.0 h. Sato et al. (1974) resolved the elimination of benzene from blood in a human subject into a sum of three exponentials:

$$Y(t) = 5.93e^{-0.418t} + 8.60e^{-0.0238t} + 2.87e^{-0.00317t}$$

where $Y(t)$ is the concentration in blood ($\mu g \ l^{-1}$) at time t (minutes) after a single brief exposure. The solubility of benzene in various body tissues relative to blood was also investigated. For most tissues, a value of 1 to 3 was found, but in fat, benzene was 30 to 50 times more soluble than in blood. Using mice, Bergman (1979) found a three phase elimination of benzene in breath, with component half-lives of 16.9, 41.1 and 151.6 minutes.

4.8.4   Metabolic model of benzene excretion

        The benzene model used in this study is very similar to that
proposed by Thorne and Jackson (1983), and is shown in Fig. 4.11. The
four main compartments are the same as before , i.e. blood, adipose
tissue, bone marrow and total metabolites, but the interrelationships
between the compartments have been slightly altered. In the original
model, a fraction of the intake of benzene was input to the three
tissue compartments, but in this model, all of the intake of benzene
enters the blood compartment, from where it is redistributed to the
other tissue compartments.
        Reversible exchange via a central blood compartment was
thought necessary, since both Sherwood (1976) and Teisinger et al.
(1958) observed a urinary excretion curve which exhibited two components. The component with the shorter half-life probably represents
clearance of directly produced benzene metabolites by the kidney,
whereas the longer-lived compartment, with a half-life of approximately one day, probably corresponds to the excretion of metabolites
resulting from the metabolism of benzene released from the adipose
tissue compartment.

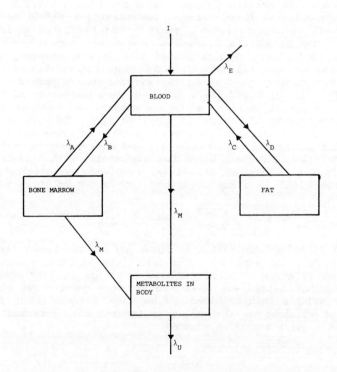

Note: for parameter values see text.

FIGURE 4.11 SYSTEMIC MODEL OF BENZENE METABOLISM

The rate parameters used with the model are as follows.

PARAMETER	VALUE (D^{-1})
λ_a	12.0
λ_b	100.0
λ_c	0.5
λ_d	0.5
λ_e	108.0
λ_m	12.0
λ_u	2.4

Most of the parameters are as in the previous model (Thorne and Jackson, 1983). The parameter values for transfer from blood to bone marrow and to adipose tissue are based on work by Rickert et al. (1979), who found that, for bone marrow, the uptake half-time was "very short", whereas for adipose tissue the value was similar to the elimination half-life for that compartment.

Uptake of benzene is modelled as follows. A fractional absorption of 1.0 from the gastrointestinal tract is assumed, since, as an organic solvent, benzene should cross biological membranes very easily. For intake via the respiratory system, 50% of all inhaled benzene vapour is assumed to be absorbed, with the rest being immediately exhaled (Nomiyama and Nomiyama, 1974). Skin absorption is known to occur and in the absence of relevant kinetic data, benzene absorbed by this route is assumed to pass directly into the blood compartment without delay.

4.9   Vinyl chloride

4.9.1   Toxic actions

With respect to the toxic effects of vinyl chloride, Jaeger et al., (1975) found that, in fasted rats exposed to unsaturated halogenated monomers, the induced liver damage was greater if the glutathione content of the body was pharmocologically depleted. Glutathione levels exhibit a marked diurnal rhythm, and these findings may be important in the case of workers who have just begun night shift work, before these diurnal rhythms have adjusted to the change in habits.

The results of several long-term studies of the carcinogenic properties of vinyl chloride are becoming available. Of particular note are results from a number of long-term experiments conducted on mice, rats and hamsters (Maltoni and Lefemine, 1975). The conclusions drawn from the study were as follows.

- VCM produced tumours in the 3 species studied.
- The range of tumours produced varied from species to species.
- In rats, zymbal gland carcinomas, nephroblastomas, hepatomas, brain neuroblastomas and skin carcinomas were produced. In mice, lung adenomas (frequently undergoing malignant transformation), mammary carcinomas, angiosarcomas and skin

epithelial tumours were observed. In hamster, liver angiosarcomas only were observed, but this species was not studied for as long as were the rats and mice.

- VCM shows a carcinogenic effect in rats at an air concentration of 50 ppm.

- The neoplastic response is affected by the length of exposure to VCM, particularly in the case of angiosarcoma induction.

- Two subcutaneous angiosarcomas were observed in the offspring of rats exposed for 7 days during pregnancy, indicating that transplacental transfer of VCM, or its reactive metabolites, occurred.

- Several ossifying angiosarcomas were observed, which may be of relevance in the interpretation of acro-osteolysis observed in workers exposed to VCM.

In a study of 10,000 workers known to be have been occupationally exposed to vinyl chloride, there appears to be an excess of angiosarcomas and also of brain tumours when compared with an unexposed population (Manufacturing Chemists Association, 1978). However, this study is in its early stages, and the excess of deaths is not statistically significant.

4.9.2   Metabolism

In rats, Watanabe and Gehring (1976) found that there was a correlation between exposures to VCM which induced tumours and those which saturated metabolic, or detoxifying, pathways. They also observed that liver glutathione concentrations fell with increasing dose. The same group had already shown that VCM is excreted at different rates, depending on the exposure (Hefner et al., 1975). At low exposures (< 100 ppm) rats metabolized VCM rapidly, in accordance with first-order kinetics and with a half-time of 86 minutes. At exposures exceeding 220 ppm, a slower metabolic rate was found, with a half-time of 261 minutes.

In rhesus monkeys, Buchter et al. (1980) also observed a saturation of the metabolism of VCM, when the animals inhaled concentrations of the gas in the order of 200 to 300 ppm. Below this concentration, the maximal rate of metabolism was half of that observed in rats, indicating that extrapolation of animal data to man will require careful consideration.

Buchter et al. (1978) presented data on the metabolism of VCM in human subjects. These were interpreted in terms of a one compartment model by Bolt et al. (1981). Two routes of elimination were considered, excretion in expired air and biochemical metabolism in the body. Both routes followed first order kinetics with half-times of 1.4 and 20.5 minutes respectively.

4.9.3   Metabolic model

Various experimental studies, using animals of several species, have demonstrated two phases of vinyl chloride metabolism (Watanabe and Gehring, 1976). Most detailed data are available for the rat and these studies shows first-order pharmacokinetics at atmospheric concentrations up to 250 ppm. This phase is characterized by a low respiratory elimination ($\sim$ 1% of the inhaled dose in 72 hours) and high urinary excretion (70% of inhaled dose in 72 hrs). At high concentrations (5000 ppm), 55% of the dose is eliminated in expired air and 25% is excreted in urine (Watanabe, Zempel and Gehring, 1978). Since Buchter et al. (1980) observed a similar saturation at 250 ppm in rhesus monkeys, it is appropriate to assume that metabolism in man also follows the same pattern. The results indicate that a saturable mechanism is involved in the metabolism of vinyl chloride, and that as this saturates, in the air concentration range 200-300 ppm, unmetabolised VCM accumulates in tissues, and, as a result, a larger fraction is excreted unchanged in expired air. With respect to human exposure, the International Agency for Research on Cancer (IARC) (1979) summarised air concentrations of vinyl chloride monomer (VCM) at various locations in industrial plant as follows:

Location	Air concentration (ppm)
In a polymerization reactor prior to ventilation	3000
In a polymerization reactor during scraping	50-100
Close to the hands during scraping	600-1000
Near polymerization reactors in one factory: 1950-1959	4000
Working places in polyvinyl chloride producing factories	40-312 (peak 33500)
	43-214
	>75
Russian synthetic leather plant	<44
Three UK cable factories	<0.15-0.35

These values should be seen in context of the various limits set on exposure to VCM in various countries and tabulated below:

Country	Concentration (ppm)	Interpretation
USA	1	TWA
	5	Ceiling (15 min.)
Canada	10	TWA
	25	Ceiling (15 min.)
Finland	5	TWA
	10	Ceiling (10 min.)
Italy	50	TWA
	25	TWA (expected)
Japan	10	TWA (expected)
Netherlands	10	TWA
Norway	1	TWA
	5	Ceiling (15 min.)
Sweden	1	TWA
	5	Ceiling (15 min.)
USSR	12	-
France	5	TWA+
	15	Ceiling+
	1	TWA**
	5	Ceiling**
Denmark	1	TWA
Belgium	5	TWA
	15	Ceiling
Federal Republic of Germany	5	TWA
	15	Ceiling+
	2	TWA**
	15	Ceiling**
United Kingdom	10	TWA
	30	Ceiling
Switzerland	10	TWA

Note: * TWA = time-weighted average: + = existing: ** = proposed

From IARC (1979).

In view of these data, although some workers may have been occasionally exposed to concentrations in excess of 100 ppm, current standards should restrict exposure of the most highly exposed personnel to ~ 5 ppm.

Therefore, for the purpose of constructing a pharmacokinetic model, it is assumed that VCM metabolism can be represented by a system which follow first-order kinetics, with the qualification that the model should not be used to simulate exposures where the time-weighted average of air concentration is in excess of 0.5 mg l^{-1} (1200 ppm).

Retention of inhaled vinyl chloride in man was studied by Krajewski et al. (1980). They found that a mean of 42% of inhaled VCM was retained, irrespective of concentration in air up to 60 mg m^{-3} (20 ppm).

If these results are interpreted in terms of the model proposed by Withey (1976), then a model for vinyl chloride metabolism in man can be developed on the basis of the assumption that VCM metabolism in man and in the rat are qualitatively similar. The model is represented diagramatically in Fig. 4.12.

The following parameters are used with the model:

Parameter	Value	Source
A	50%	Krajewski (1980)
λ_A	45.8 d^{-1}	Buchter et al. (1980)
λ_B	91.6 d^{-1}	To maintain 50% retention
λ_C	0.3 d^{-1}	Watanabe et al. (1976)
λ_E	450 d^{-1}	Extrapolated from Withey (1976)
λ_F	0.1 d^{-1}	Watanabe et al. (1976)
λ_M	48.72 d^{-1}	Bolt et al. (1981)
λ_U	1.3 d^{-1}	Watanabe et al. (1976)

The coefficient λ_C represents secondary metabolism of VC metabolites to CO_2. Since excretion of CO_2 via the lung is very rapid ($T_{\frac{1}{2}} \sim 5$ minutes), this transfer is assumed to be directly from the metabolites compartment.

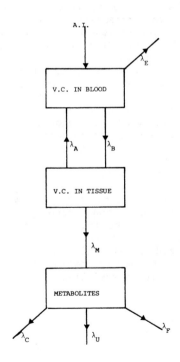

Note: for parameter values see text.

FIGURE 4.12. SYSTEMIC MODEL OF VINYL CHLORIDE METABOLISM

The coefficient λ_U represents urinary excretion of all compounds derived from an intake of VCM and λ_F represents faecal excretion of these metabolites. The value of λ_U is derived from the studies of Watanabe et al. (1976) and the value assumed for λ_F and λ_C are such that 10% and 5% of absorbed VCM are excreted as CO_2 and in faeces respectively (Watanabe et al., 1976).

4.10   Benzidine

Benzidine is potentially a bladder carcinogen in humans. It is an artificial aromatic amine of economic importance for its use in the manufacture of azo dyes. Data on occupational exposure levels are not sufficient for the purposes of estimation of typical levels of benizidine in the workplace air.

4.10.1   Effects

Although benzidine is recognised as a bladder carcinogen in man, and a liver carcinogen in laboratory animals, its toxicological effects seem to include several other endpoints. These were investigated by Littlefield et al. (1983) using mice exposed to benzidine dihydrochloride in their drinking water at concentrations up to 160 ppm. In addition to hepatocellular carcinomas, dose-response trends were noted for pigmentation of the spleen, changes in liver cell structure, hyperplasia of the bile duct, megakaryocytosis of the bone marrow and vacuolization of the brain.

The carcinogenicity of benzidine in man may not be limited to the bladder. Morinaga et al. (1982) investigated the incidence of second primary cancers in 3,322 employees who had worked in the Japanese dyestuffs industry. Among these, there were 244 workers for whom the primary cause of death was recorded as cancer of the genitourinary organs but who also exhibited second primary, histologically confirmed, cancers of the liver and biliary system, the large intestine and the lung. The incidence of the biliary system cancers was significantly greater than expected. These findings appear to confirm previous clinical data (Hueper, 1969) pointing to a pluripotential carcinogenic action of benizidine. One problem is that the workers were exposed to both benzidine and β-naphthylamine, which is also a bladder carcinogen, and thus the observed effects may not have been due to benzidine. Whether the cancer of the large intestine was due to the excretion of benzidine metabolite in bile, or to the metabolism of unabsorbed benzidine by the fauna of the intestine (Cerniglia-et al., 1982) is a matter for speculation.

4.10.2   Metabolic pathways

Zenser and co-workers have presented data related to the potential carcinogenic activation of benzidine by the renal medulla. Prostaglandin endoperoxidase synthetase (PES) is a haemoprotein consisting of two enzymes, fatty acid cycloxygenase and prostaglandin hydroperoxidase. Zenser et al. (1982) showed that aspirin, which inhibits cycloxygenase, had no effect on benzidine metabolism by the peroxidase part of the molecule. This allowed a model of benizidine activation by the enzyme to be formulated. Inspection of the model suggests several stages where application of pharmacologic agents could inhibit activation of benizidine and reduce or even eliminate its carcinogenic effects. The model is shown in Fig. 4.13 and the site of potential pharmacologic intervention are indicated. Zenser et al. (1983) investigated the inhibition of PES-activated binding of benzidine by several agents. The agents they used exerted their effect at different stages of the proposed process (see Fig. 4.13). Thus, vitamin C reduced binding by acting at site 3 (reducing the activated molecule back to the parent molecule). Phenidone was thought to act at site 2, preventing interaction between the enzyme and substrate. Binding by benzidine metabolites was found to be inhabited by Phenidone. Glutathione was found to form a conjugate with benzidine and hence must act at site 4 to reduce binding. The study demonstrated the existence of multiple sites for inhibiting PES activation of benzidine and the possibility of pharma-

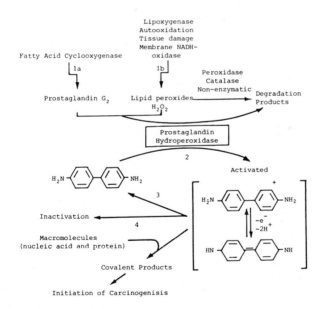

Note:
    From Zenser et al.

FIGURE 4.13.   A WORKING MODEL BASED ON THE HYPOTHESIS THAT PHS IS INVOLVED
                IN THE INITIATION OF CANCER INDUCED BY BENZIDINE AND BENZIDINE
                ANALOGS. THIS MODEL PROPOSES THAT BENZIDINE IS METABOLIZED
                WITHIN THE TARGET TISSUE BY THE PROSTAGLANDIN HYDROPEROXIDASE
                PORTION OF PHS TO A REACTIVE INTERMEDIATE THAT CAN COVALENTLY
                BIND TO PROTEIN AND NUCLEIC ACIDS, INITIATING THE CARCINOGENIC
                PROCESS. THIS MODEL ALLOWS ONE TO PROPOSE SPECIFIC SITES
                (NUMBERED 1,2,3 AND 4) AT WHICH STRATEGIES MAY BE DEVELOPED
                TO PREVENT CARCINOGENESIS: 1) SYNTHESIS OF PEROXIDE COSUB-
                STRATES; 2) ACTIVATION OF CARCINOGEN BY PROSTAGLANDIN HYDRO-
                PEROXIDASE; 3) CONVERSION OF THE ACTIVATED INTERMEDIATE BACK
                TO THE PARENT COMPOUND; AND 4) INACTIVATION OF REACTIVE
                INTERMEDIATE(S) BY FORMING CONJUGATE(S)

cologic prevention of cancer. The activation of benzidine by PES and subsequent excretion of these activation products in the urine has been suggested to be responsible for bladder cancers observed in workers exposed to benzidine. However, if benzidine is a pluripotent carcinogen, as suggested by Morinaga et al. (1982) then this pharm- acologic blocking may still not prevent occupation-induced cancers at other sites due to benzidine exposure.

4.10.3   Metabolism

        Benzidine metabolism in the isolated perfused rat liver was studied by Lynn et al. (1983). They found that ^{14}C-labelled benzidine was rapidly removed from the perfusate, with a half-time of removal of 5 minutes. Acetyl benzidine was produced initially and this was further metabolized to diacetyl benzidine. Biliary excretion was also followed, with 22% of the activity appearing in bile in the first 2 hours. The major biliary metabolites were benzidine glucuronide and acetyl-benzidine glucuronide initially, with diacetyl benzidine glucuronide becoming the major metabolite 1 hour after the labelled benzidine was added to the perfusate.

        Additional data concerning the transcutaneous absorption of benzidine were presented by Shah and Guthrie (1983). They studied the absorption and subsequent elimination of ^{14}C-labelled benzidine, dichlorobenzidine and dimethoxybenzidine applied to the shaved skin of the mid-back region of the rat. Plastic collars were fitted to pre- vent licking, and consequent ingestion of the compound.

        Retention of radioactivity in various organs was obtained at 1, 8 and 24 h after application and amounts in faecal and urinary excretion were also measured at these times.

        Both benzidine and its dichloride analogue were found to be readily absorbed through the skin, with 5% of the applied radioactivity being absorbed in the first hour, and 50% absorbed by 24 hours. Dimethoxybenzidine was less well absorbed, to the extent of 30% in 24 hours. With respect to organ contents, liver and intestine showed the greatest uptake of radioactivity, with blood and lung accumulating slightly less. The data presented are not sufficient to construct a pharmacokinetic model, but do provide a qualitative picture of uptake and retention in various organs.

        The pattern of faecal and urinary excretion seems to vary with the benzidine analogue used. For benzidine and dimethoxybenzi- dine, approximately 50% of excreted material is lost from the body via each pathway, but for the dichloro-derivative, 33% is excreted in urine and 67% in the faeces.

        An extensive study of the metabolism of 3-3' dimethoxyben- zidine in the rat was undertaken by Rodgers et al. (1983). Metabolism was rapid and 30 minutes after I.V. administration, < 2% of the dose could be recovered as the parent compound. Substantial biliary excretion occurred, but resorption must also have taken place, since over the first 3 days, 70% of the dose was excreted in bile, but only 50% was eliminated in the faeces, with a further 35% excreted in the urine. Of the radioactivity remaining in the body, 50% was covalently bound to liver. The retention of radioactivity in each organ could be described by a 3 exponential retention curve, with the longest-lived phase having a half-life of 55 hours.

With respect to human exposure, Lowry et al. (1980) found benzidine and monoacetyl benzidine in the urine of workers exposed to benzidine-based azo dyes, a situation which gave cause for concern. Hatfield et al. (1982) observed no elevation of urinary aromatic amines as a result of occupational exposure. The technique was a non-specific colorimetric method, and "positive" (> 1 ppb) results were only obtained from subjects with high background excretion level, or, in one case, as a result of medication.

4.10.4 Development of a mathematical model

Very little, if any, data exist from which a pharmacokinetic model of benzidine metabolism could be proposed on the basis of experimental findings in human subjects. However, sufficient data were available from experiments using animals to enable a general mammalian model to be devised. Two assumptions were made before the model was prepared.

- All analogues of benzidine are treated identically by the body. There is evidence, from experiments on rats, (Shah et al., 1983) that this is not the case, but in the absence of more detailed experimental data, this assumption must be made.

- Benzidine is metabolized identically in different mammalian species. In this context, it is noted that Kellner et al. (1973) in studies on rats, dogs and monkeys observed inter-species differences in the pattern of excretion, but that difficulties were experienced with collection of faecal samples from monkeys and dogs.

Data from retention studies after administration of benzidine and its analogues by various routes suggest that the compounds accumulate in the following tissues: blood, liver, GI tract and contents (Baker and Deighton, 1953) and lung (Kellner et al., 1973; Hsu and Sikka, 1982). However, all of these studies were concerned with the retention of radioactivity in the tissues and so no distinction between the parent compound and metabolites can be made on the basis of the data presented.

Benzidine is metabolised very rapidly by the isolated liver in vitro (Lynn et al., 1983; Rogers et al., 1983), and so, in the model, benzidine, and its analogues, are assumed to be absorbed into a central distribution compartment representing blood. From this compartment, the majority is transferred to liver where it is metabolised. The metabolites produced by this process are assumed to either be excreted in bile and urine or exchanged with a "covalently bound metabolites" compartment. The proposed model is represented diagrammatically in Fig. 4.14.

Metabolism of benzidine by prostaglandin synthetase in the kidney is represented by a transfer directly from blood to the free metabolites compartment. Rate constants for the model can be derived either from direct experimental measurements (e.g. Kellner et al., 1973; Hsu et al., 1982; Rogers et al. 1983) or from the observed behaviour of benzidine in the body (see below).

Kellner et al. (1973) observed that 5% of intravenously administered benzidine was excreted unchanged in the urine of a monkey within 4 hours of application. The remainder was presumably distributed throughout the body, predominantly to the liver, but some would also have passed to the kidney to be metabolised as already described.

Excretion of metabolites was studied by Rogers et al. (1983). They found that 3 days after an I.V. or an oral dose of ^{14}C-dimethoxybenzidine, 50% of the administered radio-label had been excreted in the faeces and 30-40% excreted in the urine. The radioactivity remaining in the animal was assumed to be covalently bound to tissues. Of this residual radioactivity 45% was found in the liver. Rogers et al. (1983) also noted that recirculation of radioactivity excreted in bile must occur, since in animals with the bile duct cannulated, 70% of the administered radioactivity was excreted in the bile, whereas in the intact animal only 50% was recovered in the faeces. This implies that 29% of the material excreted in bile is reabsorbed.

Metabolism of benzidine in the rat has already been noted as being extremely rapid. Rogers et al. (1983) found that 30 minutes after administration, less than 2% of radioactivity could be recovered in the form of the parent compound. Lynn et al. (1983), using the isolated perfused rat liver preparation, found that benzidine was rem-

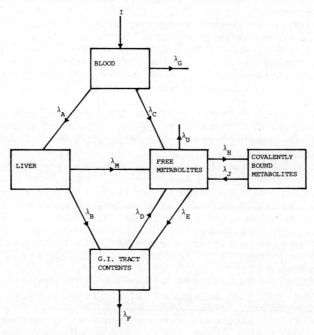

Note: for parameter values see text.

FIGURE 4.14 SYSTEMIC MODEL OF BENZIDINE METABOLISM

oved from the perfusate with a half-life of 10 mins. They also found that biliary excretion of the metabolites exhibited a half-life of 6 hours.

Retention studies of various ^{14}C-labelled benzidine analogues in the rat revealed three- and two-phase exponential retention curves for several organs (Rogers et al., 1983; Kellner et al. 1973; Hsu et al., 1982). The half-life of these curves tend to fall into two groups, one with characteristic half-life of 3-10 hours the other with half-life ranging from 40-100 hours.

This latter group probably represented release of covalently bound metabolites, whereas the former has values of half-life similar to those derived for urinary and faecal excretion of metabolites. For example, Bos et al. (1980) analysed the time course of mutagen production in the urine of rats to which benzidine had been intraperitoneally administered. If it is assumed that this represents the urinary excretion of benzidine metabolites, these data can be used to infer that such metabolites were excreted by a process which followed first-order kinetics, with a half-life of 6 hours. It is of interest to note that if β-glucuronidase was present in the incubation medium for the mutagen test, then a higher level of mutagenesis was detected than in the control sample. This implies that some of the metabolites are bound in the form of glucuronides, and that in this form they are not mutagenically active.

The model shown in Fig. 4.14 is used in conjunction with the following parameters.

Parameter	Value (d^{-1})
λ_A	15.0
λ_B	2.8
λ_C	5.0
λ_D	0.4
λ_E	2.8
λ_F	1.0
λ_G	2.8
λ_H	1.4
λ_J	0.25
λ_M	30.0
λ_U	2.8

Intake of benzidine into the body is assumed to be directly into the blood compartment. Benzidine can enter the body via three routes; inhalation, ingestion or transcutaneous absorption. Unfortunately, there is very little information on the kinetics of these processes. Transcutaneous absorption is thought to pose the greatest potential hazard for occupationally exposed workers. Meigs et al. (1954) found that urinary excretion of benzidine could not be accounted for by inhalation of the substance. They also found that skin absorption tended to be greater on hot, humid days implying that perspiration facilitates absorption in some way. For modelling purposes and in the absence of detailed kinetic data, the quantity entering the body via skin exposure is assumed to pass directly into blood.

Similarly, with respect to respiratory retention, in the absence of data, it is appropriate to make the conservative assumption that all benzidine inhaled is transferred to blood.

An f_1 value of 1.0 is assumed for gastrointestinal absorption. Thus, all ingested material is absorbed directly into the blood. It is not passed into the GI tract contents compartment of the model and then absorbed, since material in this compartment represents that which has already been metabolized, and the metabolized and unmetabolized forms must be kept separate for modelling purposes.

The model does not deal with individual metabolites of benzidine and its analogues, as relevant pharmacokinetic data are not available. Thus, the benzidine analogues in the urine are comprised of both unmetabolized benzidine (from the blood compartment), and metabolites. This is analogous to the "quinonizable" material measured in urine by Meigs et al. (1954).

4.11   Carbon tetrachloride

No further references were found on the subject of background exposure, nor were any further reports of tumour induction, in man or animals, identified.

4.11.1   Metabolism

As previously noted by Thorne and Jackson (1983), very few experiments using carbon tetrachloride (CCl_4) as a toxic agent are relevant to the development of a pharmacokinetic model of CCl_4 metabolism. However, several references have been found which make the construction of such a model possible.

Inhalation

Bergman (1979) performed an extensive study on the distribution and metabolism of several organic solvents in mice, after exposure, by inhalation, to ^{14}C-radiolabelled vapours.

Distribution of each solvent was obtained both by whole body autoradiography and by individual organ analysis. Thirty minutes after cessation of inhalation of $^{14}CCl_4$, radioactivity was mainly concentrated in body fat, the central nervous system (presumably in the insulating sheath which surrounds myelinated nerve fibres) and in the liver.

Elimination of $^{14}CCl_4$ in exhaled breath was also studied. The elimination curve is shown in Fig. 4.15. This curve was fitted by a three-phase exponential, the three terms having half-lives of 7.2 mins, 44.1 mins and 126.4 mins. Total uptake and metabolism of the inhaled $^{14}CCl_4$ is as follows:

inhaled amount (μl)	eliminated in the exhaled air		eliminated in urine (% dose)
	unchanged CCl$_4$ (% dose)	as CO$_2$ (% dose)	
5	70.4 ± 3.3	4.5 ± 0.3	0.48 ± 0.03

Elimination values are totals during eight hours after inhalation. Values represent mean ± s.e. for four mice (from Bergman, 1979).

A technique for measuring changes in blood CCl$_4$ concentration was developed by Stewart et al. (1960). In testing this method, they exposed rabbits 5000 ppm CCl$_4$ by inhalation and followed the changes in blood concentration. Whilst the results could not be used for modelling purposes, the form of the concentration curve was characterised by a rapid fall during the first hour after exposure, followed by a more gradual decline in concentration during the next three hours. It is interesting to note that feeding ethanol, which is

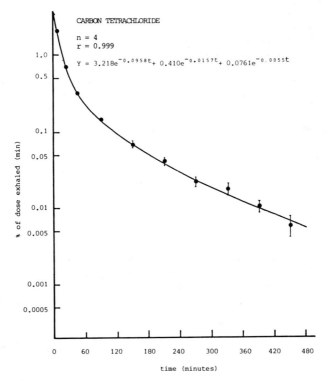

CARBON TETRACHLORIDE

n = 4
r = 0.999

$$Y = 3.218e^{-0.0958t} + 0.410e^{-0.0157t} + 0.0761e^{-0.0055t}$$

% of dose exhaled (min)

time (minutes)

Note:
    Redrawn from Bergman (1979)

FIGURE 4.15. ELIMINATION OF CARBON TETRACHLORIDE IN EXHALED AIR BY MICE
    PREVIOUSLY EXPOSED AT AN AIR CONCENTRATION OF 1 mg/m^3

known to increase the toxicity of CCl_4 when administered simultaneously, caused a higher peak CCl_4 blood concentration in animals exposed to the same vapour concentration.

Most studies on inhalation toxicology are performed on animals exposed to a more or less constant concentrations of the compound of interest. Van Stee et al. (1982), exposed rabbits to different exposure regimes characterised by a constant total product of concentration and time and studied the effect of these different regimens on hepatotoxicity of CCl_4. They found that two equal exposures 60 minutes apart were less hepatotoxic than if they were 180-240 minutes apart. Indices of necrosis (vacuolation) varied in a more complex manner, but the conclusion was that a single time-weighted average concentration may not be the ideal index of the toxicity (and possibly carcinogenicity) of CCl_4, or indeed any other metabolically activated compound.

Ingestion

All data on human ingestion are derived from accidental or deliberate (suicidal) intakes of the solvent. Blood CCl_4 levels were measured by Fischl and Labi (1966) who found that, 1 hour after ingesting approximately 40 g of CCl_4, the blood concentration of the substance was 1000 ppm. In a sample taken 3 days later, no CCl_4 was detectable in blood. However, the minimum detection level of the technique was 500 ppm.

The treatment of CCl_4 ingestion has also been studied. Since the major route of elimination is by exhalation, Gellert et al. (1983) examined, in the rat, the effect of hyperventilation on tissue CCl_4 levels after ingestion. Liver, fat and blood exhibited the highest CCl_4 concentrations, but these levels were reduced when the animal was made to hyperventilate. In a case study of attempted suicide, treatment by CO_2 induced hyperventilation was used (Goldermann 1983). Blood CCl_4-levels fell from 120 ppm to 30 ppm within 6 days. However, two weeks later, the patient developed pneumonia and the resulting decrease in respiratory rate gave rise to an immediate increase in blood CCl_4, suggesting that the hyperventilation had been responsible for the previous lowering of the blood CCl_4 level.

4.11.2   Development of a metabolic model

Sufficient data exists for the tentative proposal of a pharmacokinetic model of CCl_4 metabolism. Several studies of CCl_4 distribution in tissues agree that the substance accumulates most in adipose tissue, followed by liver then blood. Bone marrow also accumulates CCl_4, but this is assumed to be in the fat present in that tissue. Distribution ratios of 8:3:1 (fat:liver:blood) were found in rabbits exposed by ingestion (McCollister, 1951).

If CCl_4 is assumed to be distributed into various body compartments, then, as for any volatile organic solvent, analysis of the respiratory elimination curve should yield information as to the rates of release of the substance from the various compartments into the blood, and from blood into the air.   Bergman (1979) followed the elimination of CCl_4 in expired air and found a tri-phasic curve, with half-times of 7.2, 44.1 and 126.4 minutes.

Using the tissue distribution already reported, this could be conceptualized as corresponding to the release of CCl_4 into the air from blood, from liver to blood and from fat to blood respectively. Fat is assumed to be the largest storage compartment and the slowest releasing, since CCl_4 is very lipid soluble.

In monkeys, McCollister et al. (1951) obtained a biphasic respiratory excretion curve with component half-times of 0.6 days and 12 days.   However, excretion was measured only at two or more days after the exposure, so any short-lived components would not have been identified.

Few experiments have been performed to elucidate the respiratory elimination of CCl_4 in man, due to the understandable reluctance of investigators to administer a known toxic substance to subjects.   Morgan et al. (1970) and Stewart et al. (1961) both interpreted the available respiratory excretion data in terms of the function

$$E = A \, t^{-B}$$

where B = 0.1 (Morgan) and 0.6 - 1.0 (Stewart).

Reanalysis of both sets of data reveals an exponential decay curve with half-lives of 1.2 hours (Morgan) and 1.7 hours (Stewart). Excretion was only followed for 4 hours, so longer-lived components would not have been identified.   In a study of cutaneous absorption of CCl_4, Stewart and Dodd (1964) found, after cessation of exposure, a monophasic decay in breath concentrations, with a half-life of 2 hours.

In a case of attempted suicide by ingestion of a mixture of methanol and CCl_4, (Stewart et al., 1963) measured the change in CCl_4 breath concentration during the patient's recovery.   Discarding results from the first two days, since methanol was still present in the body and has a stimulating action on CCl_4 metabolism, the decay curve from day 2 to day 20 was biphasic with components exhibiting half-life of 1.4 and 4.5 days.

The uptake of CCl_4 by the lungs in monkeys was found to be 30% (McCollister, 1951).   Although Bergman (1979) found an uptake of 80% in mice, this was for a relatively short exposure period.

The preceding data suggest that respiratory uptake and elimination of CCl_4 by man can be simulated by a three compartment model representing blood, liver and adipose tissue.   30% of inhaled CCl_4 is assumed to be absorbed and pass directly into the blood compartment where it is distributed to the other two compartments, to achieve the observed concentration ratios 8 (fat): 3 (liver): 1 (blood).   The remaining 70% of inhaled CCl_4 is assumed to be eliminated in the first few breaths subsequent to inhalation.   Respiratory elimination of CCl_4 is taken to be triphasic, with the three compartments exhibiting half-lives of 0.06, 1.4 and 4.5 days respectively.

There are no data relevant to CCl_4 metabolism within the human body.   For this reason, modelling has to be based on data from animal experiments.   The rate of metabolism of CCl_4 can be assumed to

be similar to that of other organic compounds, since the mixed function oxidase system is involved in the metabolism of most such
materials.

In monkeys, McCollister et al. (1951) found that 5% of the
administered radioactivity was recovered in the expired air as carbon
dioxide (CO_2). This represents complete oxidation of CCl_4, and presumably is a secondary stage of metabolism. The CO_2 concentration in
expired air was found to decrease monotonically with a half-life of
1.75 days. Production of CO_2 from CCl_4 has also been observed in
subsequent studies. Thus, Bergman (1979) found that during the first
8 hours of the post exposure period, 5% of the administered radioactivity was recovered as CO_2 in exhaled air in mice.

As with metabolism, urinary and faecal excretion of CCL_4 and
its metabolites has not been studied in man.

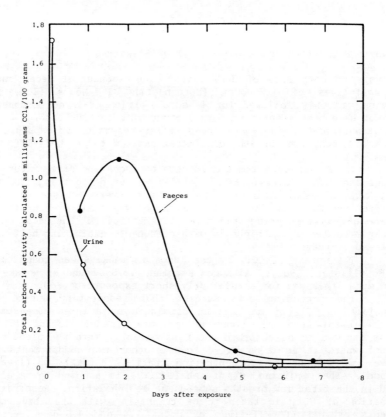

Note:
    Redrawn from Mc Callister (1951)

FIGURE 4.16. EXCRETION OF CARBON TETRACHLORIDE BY MICE
PREVIOUSLY EXPOSED AT AN AIR CONCENTRATION OF 1 mg/m^3

Faecal elimination by monkeys was studied by McCollister (1951) and results are shown in Fig. 4.16. Peak faecal excretion did not occur until 2 days after cessation of exposure. Unfortunately, only spot samples were taken, so the elimination kinetics cannot be analysed in detail. In rats, Reynolds et al. (1982) found that 3% of the administered radioactivity was eliminated in the faeces in 24 hours, and 1% was excreted in urine in the same period. In mice, 0.5% of the administered dose was recovered in urine in 8 hours.

With regards to modelling the internal metabolism of CCl_4, it may be assumed that the liver is the major organ involved, although extrahepatic sites of metabolism, such as renal cortex and upper respiratory and gastrointestinal tract mucosa have been identified by Tjalve and Lofberg (1983). No reference could be found identifying specific metabolites, but it is assumed that there is an initial stage in metabolism, presumably catalysed by the mixed function oxidase system, and that the metabolites thus formed are either excreted in urine or faeces, or undergo further metabolism to CO_2 which is eliminated in expired air.

The complete metabolic model is shown in Figure 4.17. This should be used with the following parameter values:

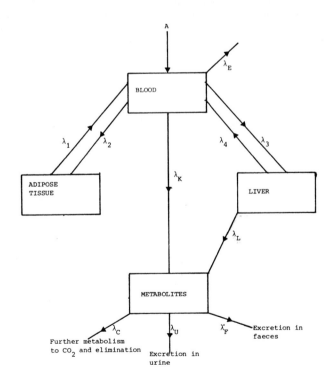

Note: for parameter values see text.

FIGURE 4.17. SYSTEMIC MODEL OF CARBON TETRACHLORIDE METABOLISM

Parameter	Value (d^{-1})	Reference
λ_1	2.4	
λ_2	0.15	Stewart et al (1963)
λ_3	0.5	
λ_4	0.5	Stewart et al (1963)
λ_E	14.2	Morgan et al (1970)
λ_K	1.2	
λ_L	10.0	
λ_C	0.4	McCallister et al (1951)
λ_U	0.1	
λ_F	0.005	
A	30%	McCallister (1951)

For gastrointestinal administration an f_1 value of 1.0 is appropriate, and the substance is assumed to pass straight into the blood compartment. Skin exposure was studied by Stewart and Dodd (1964). Transcutaneous absorption was shown to occur, but detailed kinetics for this absorption were not obtained. For the purpose of the model, CCl_4 entering the body as a result of skin exposure is assumed to pass directly into the blood compartment.

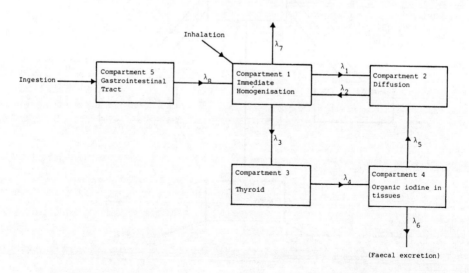

Note: adapted from Coughtrey et al.(1983)

FIGURE 4.18. PROPOSED FIVE COMPARTMENT MODEL FOR THE METABOLISM OF IODINE

4.12   Methyl iodide

No further literature was identified that had reference to the metabolism of methyl iodide. For this reason, the model prepared by Thorne and Jackson (1983) is used here. This is shown diagramatically in Fig. 4.18.

The following parameter values are used with this model:

Parameter	Value (d^{-1})
λ_1	48
λ_2	18.7
λ_4	0.00875
λ_5	0.0525
λ_6	0.00583
λ_7	6.9

The value of λ_3 is calculated such that homeostatic equilibrium is maintained, i.e.

$$\lambda_3 = \lambda_7 \, (\lambda_5 + \lambda_6) \, Q_4/(I-\lambda_6 \, Q_4)$$

where Q_4 is the mass of organic iodide in tissues; and
I is the average daily intake of iodine.

A value of 1.2 mg is taken for Q_4 and I is calculated as a running 6 h average, since 6 h is the biological half-life of iodide in the body (Riggs, 1951).

4.13   References

Alexander, F.W., Delves, H.T. and Clayton, B.E., 1972.   The uptake and excretion by children of lead and other contaminants.   Int. Symp. Env. Health Aspects. Lead. (Amsterdam), 319-331.

Alexeeff, G.V. and Kilgore, W.W., 1983.   Learning impairment in mice following acute exposure to dichloroethane and carbon tetrachloride.   J. Toxicol. Environ. Health, 11, 569-581.

Anderson, R.A.,   Polansky, M.M.,   Bryden, N.A.,   Roginsky, E.E., Mertz, W. and Linsman, W.G., 1983.   Chromium supplementation of human subjects: effects on glucose, insulin and lipid variables. Metabolism, 32, 894-89.

Andrzejewski, S., Paradowski, A., Lis, E. and Rojewska, E., 1981. Analysis of the methods of evaluation of occupational exposure to benzene and phenol of petrochemical industry workers.   Med. Pr., 32, 91-98.

Anehus, S., Enger, T., Engelbrecht, C., Hafstrom, L. and Herty, O., 1983.   Urinary polyamine excretion as related to cell death and cell proliferation induced by carbon tetrachloride intoxication. Exp. Mol. Pathol., 38, 255-263.

Anke, M., Grün, M. and Partschefeld, M., 1977.   The essentiality of arsenic for animals.   Trace substances in Environmental Health, 10, 403-409, University of Missouri, Ed. D.D. Hemphill.

Ansari, G.A., Treinen-Molen, M. and Reynolds, E.S., 1982.   Evidence for in vivo covalent binding of CCl_3 derived from CCl_4 to cholesterol of rat liver.   Biochem. Pharmacol., 31, 3509-3510.

Arp, E.W., Wolf, P.H. and Checkoway, H., 1983.   Lymphocytic leukaemia and exposure to benzene and other solvents in the rubber industry.   J. occup. Med., 25, 598-602.

Baker, R.K. and Deighton, J.G., 1953.   The metabolism of benzidine in the rat.   Cancer Res., 13, 529-531.

Barry, P.S.I., 1972.   A comparison of lead concentrations in human bones and in soft tissue.   Int. Symp. Environ. Health Aspects Lead. (Amsterdam), 415-426.

Batschelet, E., Brand, L. and Steiner, A., 1979.   On the kinetics of lead in the human body.   J. Math. Biol., 8, 15-23.

Bennet, B.G., 1981.   Exposure of man to enviromental arsenic - an exposure commitment assessment.   Sci. Tot. Environ., 20, 99-107.

Bergman, K., 1979.   Whole body autoradiography and allied tracer techniques in distribution and elimination studies of some organic solvents: benzene, toluene, xylene, styrene, methylene chloride, chloroform, carbon tetrachloride and trichlorethylene. Scan. J. Work Environ. Health, 5, (Suppl. 1), 1-263.

Bernard, S.R., 1977.   Dosimetric data and metabolic model for lead. Health Phys., 32, 44-46.

Bhattacharyya, M.H., Whelton, B.D. and Peterson, D.P., 1982.   Gastrointestinal absorption of cadmium in mice during gestation and lactation.   Toxicol. Appl. Pharmacol., 66, 368-375.

Bingham, E., 1969.   Trace amounts of lead in the lungs.   In: Trace substances in environmental health (III), (Ed. E.E. Hemphill), 83-90.

Blake, K.C., 1976.   Absorption of Pb-203 from gastrointestinal tract of man.   Environ. Res., 11, 1-4.

Bolt, H.M., 1981.   Inhalation pharmacokinetics based on gas uptake studies. III.   A pharmacokinetic assessment in man of 'peak concentrations' of vinyl chloride.   Arch. Toxicol., 48, 213-228.

Bolton, R.E., Vincent, J.H., Jones, A.D., Addison, J. and Beckett, S.T., 1983. An overload hypothesis for pulmonary clearance of UICC amosite fibres inhaled by rats. Br. J. Ind. Med., 40, 264-272.

Bos, R.P., Bruons, R.M.E., Van Doorn, R., Theuws, J.L.G. and Henderson, P.Th., 1980. The appearance of mutagens in urine of rats after the administration of benzidine and some other aromatic amines. Toxicol., 16, 113-122.

Boysen, M., Solberg, L.A., Torjussen, W., Poppe, S. and Hogetviet, A.C., 1984. Histological changes, rhinoscopical findings and nickel concentrations in plasma and urine in retired nickel workers. Acta Otolaryngol. 97, 105-115.

Braier, L., Levy, A., Dror, K. and Pardo, A., 1981. Benzene in blood and phenol in urine in monitoring benzene exposure in industry. Am. J. Industr. Med., 2, 119-23.

Brodeur, J., Lacasse, Y. and Talbot, D., 1983. Influence of removal from occupational lead exposure on blood and saliva lead concentrations. Toxicol. Lett., 19, 195-199.

Bryson, W.G. and Goodall, C.M., 1983. Differential toxicity and clearance kinetics of chromium III or VI in mice. Carcinogenesis, 4, 1535-1539.

Buchter, A., Bolt, H.M., Filser, J.G., Goergens, H.W., Laib, R.J. and Bolt. W., 1978. Pharmakokinetik und karzinogense von vinylchlorid arbeitsmedizinische risikoheurteilung. Verh. Dtsch. Ges. Arbeitsmedizin, 18, 111-124.

Buchter, A., Filser, J.G., Peter, H. and Bolt, H.M., 1980. Pharmacokinetics of vinyl chloride in the rhesus monkey. Toxicol. Lett., 6, 33-36.

Cahill, A.L., Nyberg, D. and Ehret, C.F., 1983. Tissue distribution of cadmium and metallothionein as a function of time of day and dosage. Environ. Res., 31, 54-65.

Cant, S.M. and Legendre, L.A., 1982. Assessment of occupational exposure to arsenic, copper and lead in a western copper smelter. Am. Ind. Hyg. Assoc. J., 43, 223-226.

Carvalho, S.M. and Ziemer, P.L., 1982. Distribution and clearance of Ni-63 administered as 63NiCl$_2$ in the rat: intratracheal study. Arch. Environ. Contam. Toxicol., 11, 245-248.

Cerniglia, C.E., 1982. Metabolism of azo dyes derived from benzidine, 3,3'- dimethyl benzidine and 3,3'- dimethoxybenzidine to potentially carcinogenic aromatic amines by intestinal bacteria. Carcinogenesis, 3, 1255-1260.

Chamberlain, A.C., 1983.   Fallout of lead and uptake by crops. Atmos. Environ., 17, 693-706.

Chamberlain, A.C., 1983.   Effect of airborne lead on blood lead. Atmos. Environ., 17, 677-692.

Chamberlain, A.C., Heard, M.J., Little, P., Newton, D., Wells, A.C. and Wiffen, R.D., 1978.   Investigations into lead from motor vehicles.   AERE Harwell, R9198.

Charbonneau, S.M.,   Hollins, J.G.,   Tam, G.K.H.,   Bryce, F., Ridgeway, J.M. and Wiles, R.F., 1980.   Whole body retention, excretion and metabolism of As-74 arsenic acid in the hamster. Toxicol. Lett., 5, 175-182.

Chmielnicka, J., Szymanska, J.A. and Tyfa, J., 1982.   Disturbances in the metabolism of endogenous metals (Zn and Cu) in nickel-exposed rats.   Environ. Res., 27, 216-221.

Chowdhury, P., Chang, L.W. and Rayford, P.L., 1983.   Catabolism and tissue distribution of Cd-109 in rats.   Bull. Environ. Contam. Toxicol., 31, 391-398.

Cikrt, M., 1972.   Biliary excretion of Hg-203, Cu-64, Mn-52 and Pb-210 in the rat.   Br. J. Ind. Med., 29, 74-80.

Cikrt, M. and Bencko, V., 1979.   Biliary excretion and distribution of Cr-51(III) and Cr-51(VI) in rats.   J. Hyg., Epidemiol. Microbiol. Immunol., 23, 241-246.

Clary, J.J., Bland, L.S. and Stokinger, H.E., 1975.   The effect of reproduction and lactation on the onset of latent chronic Be disease.   Toxicol. Appl. Pharmacol., 33, 214-221.

Cotes, J.E., Gilson, J.C., McKerrow, C.B. and Oldham, P.D., 1983.   A long term follow up of workers exposed to beryllium.   Brit. J. Indust. Med., 40, 13-21.

Coughtrey, P.J. and Thorne, M.C., 1983.   Radionuclide distribution and transport in terrestrial and aquatic ecosystems.   Vol. 2, A.A. Balkema, Rotterdam.

Cunningham, E.M., Ponteract, R.D. and O'Brien, R.C., 1976.   Quantitative relationships of faecal asbestos to asbestos exposure.   J. Toxicol. Environ. Health., 1, 377-379.

Dang, H.S., Jaiswal, D.D. and Somasundaram, S., 1983.   Distribution of arsenic in human tissues and milk.   Sci. Tot. Environ., 29, 171-175.

Decoufle, P., Blatner, W.A. and Blair, A., 1983.   Mortality among chemical workers exposed to benzene and other agents.   Environ. Res., 30, 16-25.

Dossing, M. and Paulev, P.E., 1983. Blood- and air-lead concentrations during five years of occupational exposure: the effectiveness of an occupational hygiene programme and problems due to welding operations. Ann. Occup. Hyg., 27, 367-372.

Drasch, G.A., 1983. An increase in cadmium body burden for this century - an investigation on human tissues. Sci. Tot. Environ., 26, 111-119.

Elinder, C.G., Kjellström, T., Lind, B., Linnman, L., Piscator, M. and Sundstedt, K., 1983. Cadmium exposure from smoking cigarettes: variations with time and country where purchased. Environ. Res., 32, 220-227.

Elinder, C.G., Kjellström, T., Lind, B., Molander, M.L. and Silander, T., 1978. Cadmium concentrations in human liver, blood and bile: comparisons with a metabolic model. Environ. Res., 17, 236-241.

Ellis, K.J., Morgan, W.D., Zonzi, I., Yasumura, S., Vartsky, D. and Cohn, S.H., 1980. In vivo measurement of critical level of kidney cadmium: dose effect studies in cadmium smelter workers. Am. J. Indust. Med., 1, 339-348.

Ellis, K.J., Yasumura, S., Vartsky, D. and Cohn, S.H., 1983. Evaluation of biological indicators of body burden of cadmium in humans. Fundam. Appl. Toxicol., 3, 169-174.

Ellis, K.J., Yuen, K., Yasumura, S. and Cohn, S.H., 1984. Dose-response analysis of cadmium in man: Body burden vs kidney dysfunction. Environ. Res. 33, 216-226.

Elwood, J.C., Nash, D.T. and Streeten, D.H.P., 1982. Effect of high-chromium brewer's yeast on human serum lipids. J. Am. Coll. Nutr., 1, 263-74.

Elwood, P.C., Gallacher, J.E.J., Phillips, K.N., Davies, B.E. and Tothill, C., 1984. Greater contribution to blood lead from water than from air. Nature (Lond.), 310, 138-140.

Engizek, T. 1981. Time dependent distribution accumulation and loss of lead-210 in various organs or rats. Turk. J. Nucl. Sci., 8, 48-52.

Falck, F.Y., Fine, L.J., Smith, R.G., McClaltchey, K.D., Annesley, T., England, B. and Schork, A.M., 1983. Occupational cadmium exposure and renal status. Am. J. Indust. Med., 4, 541-549.

Fischl, J. and Labi, M., 1966. Gas chromatographic determination of carbon tetrachloride in a case of accidental poisoning. Israel J. Med. Sci., 2, 84-85.

Fishbeck, W.A., Langner, R.R. and Kociba, R.J., 1975 Elevated urinary phenol levels not related to benzene exposure. Am. J. Ind. Hyg. Assoc. J., 36, 820-824.

Flanagan, P.R., Chamberlain, M.J. and Valberg, L.S., 1982   The relationship between iron and lead absorption in humans.   Am. J. Clin. Nutr., 36, 823-829.

Fletcher, J.G., Chettle, D.R., Al-Haddad, I.K., 1982.   Experience with the use of cadmium measurements of liver and kidney.   J. Radioanal. Chem. 71, 547-560.

Foa, V., Colombi, A., Moroni, M., Buratti, M. and Calzaferri, G., 1984.   The speciation of the chemical forms of arsenic in the biological monitoring of exposure to inorganic arsenic.   Sci. Tot. Environ., 34, 241-259.

Fowler, J.S.L., 1969.   Carbon tetrachloride metabolism in the rabbit. Br. J. Pharmacol., 37, 733-737.

Frank, H. and Durz, H., 1983.   Determination of alkanes in breath to monitor lipid peroxidation in the presence of volatile toxicants and metabolites.   An optimized, automatic method.   Arch. Toxicol., 53, 213-223.

Ganong, W.F., 1977.   Review of Medical Physiology 8th Edition.   Lange Medical Publications, Los Altos, California.

Garty, M., Wong, K.L. and Klaasen, C.D., 1981.   Redistribution of cadmium to blood of rats.   Toxicol. Appl. Pharmacol., 59, 548-554.

Gellert, J., Goldermann, L. and Teschke, R., 1983.   Effect of CO_2-induced hyperventilation on carbon tetrachloride (CCl_4) levels following acute CCl_4 poisoning.   Intensive Care Med., 9, 333-337.

Gerber, G.B., Maes, J. and Eyhens, B., 1982.   Transfer of antimony and arsenic to the developing organism.   Arch. Toxicol., 49, 159-168.

Ghafourian, H., Rahimi, H., Banisadr, A., Shakisavandi, K. and Bayat, I., 1983.   An investigation of the amount of lead in blood of Tehran citizens in 1980-1981.   Int. J. Environ. Studies, 21, 309-316.

Glende Jnr., E.A., 1972.   Carbon tetrachloride-induced protection against carbon tetrachloride toxicity.   Biochem. Pharmacol., 21, 1697-1702.

Goldermann, L., Gellert, J. and Teschke, R., 1983.   Quantitative assessment of carbon tetrachloride levels in human blood by headspace gas chromatography: application in a case of suicidal carbon tetrachloride intoxication.   Intensive Care Med., 9, 131-135.

Goldsmith, J.R. and Hexter, A.C., 1967.   Respiratory exposure to lead: epidemiological and experimental dose-response relationships.   Science, 158, 132-134.

Grandjean, P. and Kon, S.H., 1981.   Lead exposure of welders and by-
    standers in a ship repair yard.   Am. J. Indust. Med., 2, 65-70.

Grandjean, P., Selikoff, I.J., Shen, S.K. and Sunderman Jnr., F.W.,
    1980.   Nickel concentrations in plasma and urine of shipyard
    workers.   Am. J. Industr. Med., 1, 181-189.

Grandjean, P., Wulf, H.C. and Niebuhr, E. 1983.   Sister chromatid
    exchange in response to variations in occupational lead exposure.
    Environ. Res., 32, 199-204.

Gross, S.B., Yeager, D.W. and Middendorf, M.S., 1976.   Cadmium in
    liver, kidney, and hair of humans, foetal through old age.   J.
    Toxicol. Environ. Health, 2, 153-167.

Gruber, J.E. and Jennette, K.W., 1978.   Metabolism of the carcinogen
    chromate by rat liver microsomes.   Biochem. Biophys. Res.
    Commun., 82, 700-706.

Gruden, N., 1975.   Lead and active calcium transfer through the
    intestinal wall in rats.   Toxicology, 5, 163-166.

Gruden, N., 1982.   Transfer of cadmium through the rat's intestinal
    wall.   Environ. Res. 28, 340-343.

Gutenmann, W.H., Bache, C.A., Lisk, D.J., Hoffmann, D., Adams, J.D.
    and Elfving, D.C., 1982.   Cadmium and nickel in smoke of cigar-
    ettes prepared from tobacco cultured on municipal sludge-amended
    soil.   J. Toxicol. Environ. Health, 10, 423-431.

Haavikko, K., Anthilo, A., Helle, A., and Vuori, E., 1984.   Lead con-
    centrations of enamel and dentine of deciduous teeth of children
    from the Finnish Towns.   Arch. Environ. Health, 39, 78-84.

Haley, T.J., 1982.   Metabolism and pharmacokinetics of benzidine and
    its congeners in man and animals.   Drug Metab. Rev., 13,
    473-483.

Hartwell, T.D., Handy, R.W., Harris, B.S., Williams, S.R. and Gehl-
    bach, S.H., 1983.   Heavy metal exposure in populations living
    around zinc and copper smelters.   Arch. Environ. Health, 38,
    284-295.

Hassler, E., Lind, B., Nilsson, B. and Piscator M., 1983.   Urinary
    and faecal elimination of nickel in relation to air-borne nickel
    in a battery factory.   Ann. Clin. Lab. Sci., 13, 217-224.

Hatfield, T.R., Roberts, E.C., Bell, I.F., Clunie, J.C., Kalla, P.J.
    and McKay, P.G., 1982.   Urine monitoring of textile workers
    exposed to dichlorobenzidine-derived pigments.   J. occup. Med.,
    24, 656-658.

Heard, M.J., Chamberlain, A.C. and Sherlock, J.C., 1983.   Uptake of
    lead by humans and effects of minerals and food.   Sci. Tot. Env-
    iron., 30, 245 253.

Heck, J.D. and Costa, M., 1982.   Extracellular requirements for the endocytosis of carcinogenic crystalline nickel sulphide particles by facultative phagocytes.   Toxicol. Lett., 12, 243-250.

Hefner, R.E., Watanabe, P.G. and Gehring, P.J., 1975.   Preliminary studies of the fate of inhaled vinyl chloride monomer in rats. Ann. N.Y. Acad. Sci., 246, 135-149.

Herlant-Peers, M.C., Hildebrand, H.F. and Kerckaert, J.P., 1983.   In vitro and in vivo incorporation of [63]Ni [II] into lung and liver subcellular fractions of BALB/C mice.   Carcinogenesis, 4, 387-392.

Higgins, I., Welch, K, Oh, M., Bond, G. and Huowitz, P., 1981. Influence of arsenic exposure and smoking on lung cancer among smelter workers: a pilot study.   Am. J. Indust. Med., 2, 33-41.

Hogetveit, A.C. and Barton, R.H., 1977.   Monitoring Nickel Exposure in refinery workers.   In: Braun, S.S. (Ed.) Clinical Chemistry and Chemical Toxicology of metals.   Elsevier North - Holland Biomedical Press, Amsterdam, 265-268.

Holt, D. and Webb, M., 1982.   Intestinal and hepatic binding of cadmium in the neonatal rat.   Arch. Toxicol., 52, 291-301.

Holt, P.F., 1982.   Translocation of asbestos dust through the bronchiolar wall.   Environ. Res., 27, 255-260.

Hooper, W.F., 1981.   Acute beryllium lung disease.   NC Med. J., 42, 551-553.

Hsu, R.S. and Sikka, H.C., 1982. Disposition of 3,3' - dichlorobenzidine in the rat. Toxicol. Appl. Pharmacol., 64, 306-316.

Inamasu, T., 1983.   Arsenic metabolites in urine and faeces of hamsters pretreated with PCB. Toxicol. Appl. Pharmacalogy., 71, 142-152.

International Agency for Research on Cancer. 1979. Vinyl Chloride, polyvinyl chloride and vinyl chloride - vinyl acetate copolymers. IARC Monographs on the evaluation of the carcinogenic risk of chemicals to humans, 19, 377-438.

International Agency for Research on Cancer. 1982.   Benzene. IARC monographs on the evaluation of the carcinogenic risks of chemicals to humans, 29, 93-148.

International Commission on Radiological Protection, 1975.   ICRP Publication 23. Report of the Task Group on Reference Man. Pergamon Press, Oxford.

International Commission on Radiological Protection. 1981. Limits for Intake of Radionuclides by Workers. ICRP Publication 30, part 2. Annals of the ICRP, Vol 6, No. 2/3.

Iyengar, G.V. Kollmer, W.E. and Bowen, H.J.M. 1978. The Elemental composition of Human Tissues and Body Fluids. Verlag - Chemie, Weinheim.

Jaeger, R.J., Conolly, R.B., Reynolds, E.S. and Murphy, S.D. 1975. Biochemical toxicology of unsaturated halogenated monomers. Environ. Health Perspec., 11, 121-128.

Jarup, L., Rogerfelt, A., Elinder, C-G., Nogawa, K. and Kjellstrom, T. 1983. Biological half-time of cadmium in the blood of workers after cessation of exposure. Scand. J. Work. Environ. Health, 9, 327-331.

Johanisson, A., Camner, P., Jarstrand, C. and Wiernik, A. 1983. Rabbit alveolar macrophages after inhalation of soluble cadmium cobalt and copper: A comparison with the effects of soluble nickel. Environ. Res., 31, 340-354.

Josephy, P.D., Mason, R.P. and Eling, T. 1982. Chemical structure of the adducts formed by the oxidation of benzidine in the presence of phenols. Carcinogenesis, 3, 1227-1230.

Kalliomaki, P., Rahhonen, E., Vaaranen, V., Kalliomaki, K. and Aittorieni, K. 1981. Lung-retained contaminents, urinary chromium and nickel among stainless steel welders. Int. Arch. Occup. Environ Health, 49, 67-75.

Kang, H.K., Infante, P.F. and Carra, J.S. 1983. Determination of blood-lead elimination patterns of primary lead smelter workers. J. Toxicol. Environ. Health, 11, 199-210.

Kaul, B., Davidow, B., Yee, M. and Gewirtz, M.W. 1983. Lead, erythrocyte protoporphyrin and ferritin levels in cord blood. Arch. Environ. Health., 38, 296-300.

Kellner, H.M., Christ, O.E. and Latzch, K. 1973. Animal studies on the kinetics of benzidine and 3,3' - dichloro-benzidine. Arch. Toxicol., 31, 61-79.

Kiilunen, M., Kivicto, H., Ala-Lavrila, P., Tossavainen, A. and Aitio, A. Exceptional pharmacokinetics of trivalent chromium during occupational exposure to chromium lignosulfonate dust. Scand. J. Work Environ. Health, 9 265-271.

Kirkpatrick, D.C. and Coffin, D.E. 1974. The trace element content of representative Canadian diets in 1970 and 1971. J. Inst. Can. Sci. Technol. Alimentaire, 7, 56-58.

Kollmer, W.E. 1982. The significance of Cd in hair. Influence of the level of intake and the external contamination in the rat. Sci. Tot. Environ., 25, 41-51.

Kostial, K., Simonovic, I., Rabar, I., Blanusa, M. and Landeka, M., 1983. Age and intestinal retention of mercury and cadmium in rats. Environ. Res., 31, 111-115.

Kowal, N.E. and Zirkes, M. 1983. Urinary cadmium and Beta$_2$ - micro-globulin: normal values and concentration adjustment. J. Toxicol. Environ. Health., 11, 607-624.

Knuuttila, M., Lappalainen, R., Olkkonen, H., Lammi, S and Alhava, E.M., 1982. Cadmium content of human cancellous bone. Arch. Environ. Health., 37, 290-294.

Krajewski, J., Dobecki, M. and Gromiec, J. 1980. Retention of vinyl chloride in the human lung. Br. J. Industr. Med., 37, 373-374.

Kuehn, K. and Sunderman, F.W. 1982. Dissolution half-times of nickel compounds in water, rat serum and renal cytosol. J. Inorg. Biochem., 17, 29-39.

Kumpulainen, J., Lehto, J., Koivistoinen, P., Uusitupa, M. and Vuori, E., 1983. Determination of chromium in human milk, serum and urine by electrothermal atomic absorption spectrometry without preliminary ashing. Sci. Tot. Environ., 31, 71-80.

Kundomal, Y.R., Morgan, R.M. and Hupp, E.W. 1983. Metal content and testes weight in rats following cadmium and/or gamma radiation exposure. Environ. Pollut. Ser. A., 30, 161-172.

Labreche, F. and P'an, A. 1982. Relationships between three indica-tors of lead exposure in workers: blood lead, delta-aminolaevulinic acid and free erythrocyte protoporphyrin. Int. Arch. Occup. Environ. Health., 51, 35-44.

Leonard, A. 1984. Recent advances in arsenic mutagenesis and carcino-genesis. Toxicol. Environ. Chem. 7, 241-250.

Lilis, R., Fischbein, A., Valciukas, J.A., Blumberg, W. and Selikoff, I.J. 1980. Kidney function and lead: relationships in several occupational groups with different levels of exposure. Am. J. Indust. Med., 1, 405-12.

Lim, T.H., Sargent, T. and Kusubov, N. 1983. Kinetics of the trace element chromium III in the human body. Am. J. Physiol. 244, R445-454.

Lindgren, A., Vahter, M. and Dencker, L. 1982. Autoradiographic studies on the distribution of arsenic in mice and hamsters administered ^{74}As Arsenite (III) or arsenate (IV). Acta. Pharmacol. Toxicol., 51, 253-265.

Littlefield, N.A., Nelson, C.J. and Frith, C.H. 1983. Benzidine dihydrochloride: Toxicological assessment in mice during chronic exposures. J. Toxicol. Environ. Health., 12, 671-685.

Lowry, L.K. 1980. Chemical monitoring of urine from workers poten-tially exposed to benzidine-derived azo dyes. Toxicol. Lett., 7, 29-36.

Lu, C.C., Matsumoto, N. and Ijima, S. 1981. Placental transfer and body distribution of nickel chloride in pregnant mice. Toxicol. Appl. Pharmacol., 59, 409-413.

Lynch, G.P., Cornell, D.G. and Smith, D.F. 1974. Excretion of cadmium and lead into milk. In: Trace Element Metabolism in Animals. Ed. Hoekstra, W.G., Suttie, J.W., Ganther, H.E. and Mertz, W. University Park Press, Baltimore. 470-472.

Lynn, R.K., Garvie-Gould, C., Milam, D.F., Scott, K.F., Eastman, C.L. and Rodgers, R.M., 1983. Metabolism of the human carcinogen, benzidine, in the isolated perfused rat liver. Drug Metab. Dispos., 11, 109-114.

McCabe, L.J., Symons, J.M., Lees, R.D. and Roebuck, G.G., 1970. Survey of community water supply systems. J. Amer. Water Works Assoc., 62, 670-687.

McCabe, M., Maguire, D. and Nowak, M., 1983. The effects of arsenic compounds on human and bovine lymphocyte mitogenesis in vitro. Environ. Res., 31, 323-331.

McCollister, D.D., Beaver, W.H., Atchison, G.J. and Epeneer, H.C., 1951. The absorption, distribution and elimination of radioactive carbon tetrachloride by monkeys upon exposure to low vapour concentrations. J. Pharmacol. Exp. Ther., 102, 112-124.

McLellan, J.S., Flanagan, P.R., Chamberlain, M.J. and Valberg, L.S., 1978. Measurement of dietary cadmium absorption in humans. J. Toxicol. Environ. Health., 4, 131-138.

McNeill, K.G., McLellan, J.S., Amin, A.K., Mernagh, J.R., and Vohra, K. 1982. Measurement of cadmium in vivo in industrial workers. J. Radioanal. Chem., 71(2), 573-580.

Maibach, H.I. and Anjo, D.M. 1981. Percutaneous penetration of benzene and benzene contained in solvents used in the rubber industry. Arch. Environ. Health., 36, 256-260.

Maltoni, C., Conti, B. and Cotti, G. 1983. Benzene: A multipotential carcinogen. Results of long-term bio-assays performed at the Bologna Institute of Oncology. Am. J. Ind. Med., 4, 589-630.

Maltoni, C. and Lefemine, G. 1975. Carcinogenicity bioassays of vinyl chloride: current results. An. N.Y. Acad. Sci. 246, 195-218.

Manufacturing Chemists Association. 1978. Epidemiological study of vinyl chloride workers. Manufacturing Chemists Association, Washington.

Marafante, E., Vahter, M. and Dencker, L., 1984. Metabolism of arsenocholine in mice, rats and rabbits. Sci. Tot. Environ., 34, 223-240.

Marcus. A.H., 1979. The body burden of lead: comparison of mathematical models for accumulation. Environ. Res. 19, 79-90.

Marcus, A.H., 1982. Multicompartment kinetic models for cadmium. i) Effects of Zinc on cadmium retention in male mice. Environ. Res., 27, 46-51.

Martin, C.N. and Ehers, S.F., 1980. Studies on the macromolecular binding of benzidine. Carcinogenesis, 1, 101-109.

Marx, J.J.M., Beld, R.B. van den., Dongen, R. van. and Strackee, L.H., 1980. Simultaneous measurements of ^{59}Fe and ^{51}Cr in iron absorption studies using a whole-body scanner with mobile shielding. Nucl. Med., 19, 140-145.

Mealey, J., Brownell, G.L. and Sweet, W.H., 1959. Radioarsenic in plasma, urine, normal tissues and intracranial neoplasms. Arch. Neural. Psychiatry, 81, 310-320.

Meek, M.E. and Grasso, P. 1983. An investigation of the penetration of ingested asbestos into the normal and abnormal intestinal mucosa of the rat. Food. Chem. Toxicol., 21, 193-200.

Meigs, J.W., Brawn, R.M. and Sciarini, L.J., 1951. A study of exposure to benzidine and substituted benzidines in a chemical plant. Arch. Ind. Hyg., 4, 533-540.

Meigs, J.W., Sciarini, L.J. and Van Sandt, W.A., 1954. Skin penetration by diamines of the benzidine group. Arch. Ind. Hyg., 9, 122-132.

Merian, E., 1984. Introduction on environmental chemistry and global cycles of chromium, nickel, cobalt, beryllium, arsenic, cadmium and selenium, and their derivatives. Toxicol. Environ. Chem., 8, 9-38.

Mertz, W., 1974. Chromium as a dietary essential for man. Trace Element Metabolism in Animals III. Ed. Hoekstra, W.G., Suttie, J.W. and Ganther, H.F. University Park Press, Baltimore. 185-198.

Mico, B.A., Blanchflower, R.V. and Pohl, L.R., 1983. Formation of electrophilic chlorine from carbon tetrachloride - involvement of cytochrome P-450. Biochem. Pharmacol., 32, 2357-2359.

Moody, D.E., Clawson, G.A., Woo, C.H. and Smuckler, E.A., 1982. Cellular distribution of cytochrome P-450 loss in rats of different ages treated with alkyl halides. Toxicol. Appl. Pharmacol., 66, 278-289.

Moreau, T., Lellouch, J., Jughet, B., Festy, B., Urssaud, G. and Claude, J.R., 1983. Blood cadmium levels in a general male population with special reference to smoking. Arch. Environ. Health., 38, 163-167.

Morgan, A., Black, A. and Belcher, D.R., 1970. The excretion in breath of some aliphatic halogenated hydrocarbons following administration by inhalation. Ann. Occup. Hyg., 14, 219-233.

Morgan, A., Evans, J.C. and Holmes, A., 1977. Deposition and clearance of inhaled fibrous minerals in the rat. Studies using radioactive tracer techniques. In: Walton, W.H. (Ed). Inhaled particles IV. Pergamon Press, Oxford. 259-274.

Morinaga, K., Oshima, A. and Hara, I. 1982. Multiple primary cancers following exposure to benzidine and beta-naphthylamine. Am. J. Ind. Med., 3, 243-246.

Mukai, T., 1981. Experimental studies on the distribution, retention and excretion of lead with labeled lead nitrate in guinea pigs. Osaka-Shi Igakkai Zasshi., 30, 21-40.

Mykkäenen, H.M. and Wasserman, R.H., 1982. Effect of vitamin D on the intestinal absorption of Pb-203 and Ca-47 in chicks. J. Nutr., 112, 520-527.

Nomiyama, K. and Nomiyama, H., 1974. Respiratory retention, uptake and excretion of organic solvents in man. Benzene, toluene, n-hexane, trichloroethylene, acetone, ethyl acetate and ethyl alcohol. Int. Arch. Arbeitsmed., 32, 75-83.

Nomiyama, K., Yotoriyama, M. and Nomiyama, H., 1983. Urinary β_2-microglobulin and renal function in elderly people in an area with no known cadmium pollution. Arch. Environ. Toxicol., 12, 143-146.

Nomiyama, K., Yotoriyama, M. and Nomiyama, H., 1983b. Dose-effect relationship between cadmium and β_2-microglobulin in the urine of inhabitants of cadmium-polluted areas. Arch. Environ. Contam. Toxicol., 12, 147-150.

Nordberg, G.F. and Kjellstrom, T., 1979. Metabolic model for cadmium in man. Environ. Health Perspect., 28, 211-217.

Nordberg, G.F. and Nishiyama, K., 1972. Whole-body and hair retention of cadmium in mice, including an autoradiographic study on organ distribution. Arch. Environ. Health, 24, 209-214.

Norin, H. and Vahter, M., 1981. A rapid method for the selective analysis of total urinary metabolites of inorganic arsenic. Scand. J. Work. Environ. Health, 7, 38-44.

O'Flaherty, E.J., Hammond, P.B. and Lerner, S.I. 1982. Dependence of apparent blood lead half-life on the length of previous lead exposure in humans. Fundam. Appl. Toxicol., 2, 49-54.

Olguin, A., 1983. Arsenic levels in blood, urine, hair and nails from a chronically exposed human population. Proc. West. Pharmacol. Soc., 26, 175-177.

Olsen, I. and Jonsen, J., 1979. Whole-body autoradiography of ^{63}Ni in mice throughout gestation. Toxicol., 12, 165-172.

Ord, M.G. and Stocken, L.A. 1981. Enzyme induction in rat liver: the effects of Be^{2+} in vivo. Biosci. Rep. 1, 217-222.

Pallotti, G., Consolino, A., Bencivenga, B., Iacoponi, V., Morisi, G. and Taggi, F., 1983. Lead levels in whole blood of an adult population group from Rome. Sci. Tot. Environ., 31, 81-87.

Panholzer, M., Raptis, S.E. and Mueller, K., 1982. A simple method for determination of cadmium in urine. Microchim. Acta. 2, 189-198.

Payton, K.B., Flanagan, R.P., Stinson, E.A., Chodirker, D.P., Chamberlain, M.J. and Valberg, L.S., 1982. Technique for determination of human zinc absorption from measurement of radioactivity in a faecal sample or the body. Gastroenterol., 83, 1264-1270.

Perry, S.T., Kulkarn, S.B., Lee, K.L. and Kenney, F.T., 1982. Selective effects of the metallocarcinogen beryllium on hormonal regulation of gene expression in cultured cells. Cancer. Res., 42, 473-476.

Pershagen, G., Lind, B. and Bjorklund, N.E., 1982. Lung retention and toxicity of some inorganic arsenic compounds. Environ. Res. 29, 425-434.

Pershagen, G., Wall, S., Taube, A. and Linmann, L., 1981. On the interaction between occupational arsenic exposure and smoking, and its relationship to lung cancer. Scan. J. Work. Environ. Health 7, 302-309.

Picciano, D., 1979. Cytogenic study of workers exposed to benzene. Environ. Res., 19, 33-38.

Pirl, J.N., 1983. Death by arsenic: a comparative evaluation of exhumed body tissues in the presence of external contamination. J. Anal. Toxicol., 7, 216-219.

Post, C.T., Sqibb, K.S., Fowler, B.A., Gardner, D.E., Illini, J. and Hook, G.E.R. 1982. Production of low molecular weight cadmium - binding proteins in rabbit lung following exposure to cadmium chloride. Biochem. Pharmacol., 31, 2969-2975.

Post, G.B. and Snyder, R., 1983a. Fluoride stimulation of microcomal benzene metabolism. J. Toxicol. Environ. Health, 11, 799-810.

Post, G.B. and Snyder, R., 1983b. Effects of enzyme induction on microsomal benzene metabolism. J. Toxicol. Environ. Health, 11, 811-825.

Pounds, J.G., Wright, R. and Kodell, R.L., 1982. Cellular metabolism of lead: a kinetic analysis in the isolated rat hepatocyte. Toxicol. Appl. Pharmacol., 66, 88-101.

Rabinowitz, M.B., Wetherill, G.W. and Kopple, J.D., 1976. Kinetic analysis of lead metabolism in healthy humans. J. Clin. Invest., 58, 260-270.

Reeves, A.L., 1977. Beryllium carcinogenesis. In: Inorganic and Nutritional Aspects of Cancer, 13-27. (Ed. G.N. Schroeger), Plenum Press, New York.

Rehlund, S., Metall, B., Bergfors, P.G., Gustavson, K.H., Kollberg, H., 1979. Lead concentrations in the blood of children in the vicinity of a sulphide ore smelting plant. An evaluation of the influence of various sources of lead pollution in the children's environment. Ambio, 8, 118-120.

Reynolds, E.S., Moslew, M.T. and Treinen, R.J., 1982. Isoproponol enhancement of carbon tetrachloride metabolism in vivo. Life Sci., 31, 661-669.

Rickert, D.E., Baker, T.S., Bus, J.S., Barrow, C.S. and Irons, R.D. Benzene disposition in the rat after exposure by inhalation. Toxicol. Appl. Pharmacol., 49, 417-423.

Rinsky, R.A., Young, R.J. and Smith, A.B., 1981. Leukaemia in benzene workers. Am. J. Industr. Med., 2, 217-245.

Roels, H., Buchet, J-P., Croquet, F. and Lauwerys, R., 1982. The possible role of direct ingestion on the overall adsorption of cadmium or arsenic in workers exposed to CdO or As_2O_3 dust. Am. J. Indust. Med., 3, 53-65.

Roels, H.A., Lauwerys, R.R., Buchet, J.P., Bernard, A., Chettle, D.R., Harvey, T.C. and Al-Haddad, I.K., 1981. In vivo measurement of liver and kidney cadmium in workers exposed to this metal: its significance with respect to cadmium in blood and urine. Environ. Res., 26, 217-240.

Rogers, R.M., 1983. Metabolism, distribution and excretion of the carcinogenic aromatic amine, 3, 3'-dimethoxybenzidine in the rat. Formation of mutagenic urinary and biliary metabolites. Drug. Metab. Dispos., 11, 293-300.

Rom, W.N., Lockey, J.E., Bang, K.M., Dewitt, C. and Johns, R.E., 1983. Reversible beryllium sensitization in a prospective study of beryllium workers. Arch. Environ. Health, 38, 302-307.

Rosen, J.F., 1983. The metabolism of lead in isolated bone cell populations: interactions between lead and calcium. Toxicol. Appl. Pharmacol., 71, 101-112.

Ryu, J.E., Ziegler, E.E., Nelson, S.E. and Formon, S.J., 1983. Dietary intake of lead and blood lead concentration in early infancy. Am. J. Dis. Child, 137, 886-891.

Saito, F.U., Kocsis, J.J. and Snyder, R., 1973. Effect of benzene on hepatic drug metabolism and ultrastructure. Toxicol. Appl. Pharmacol, 26, 204-217.

Salmela, S.S., Vuori, E., Huunan-Seppala, Kilpio, J.O. and Sumuvuori, H., 1983. Body burden of cadmium in man at low level of exposure. Sci. Tot. Environ., 27, 89-95.

Salter, P.J., Currah, I.E. and Fellows, J.R., 1980. Further studies on the effects of plant density, spatial arrangement and time of harvest on yield and root size in carrots. J. Agric. Sci., Comb., 94, 465-478.

Sato, A., Nakajima, T., Fugiwara, Y. and Hirosawa, K., 1974. Pharmacokinetics of benzene and toluene. Int. Arch. Arbeitsmed., 33, 169-182.

Scheiner, D.M., Katz, S.A. and Samitz, M.H., 1976. Nickel levels in hair and nickel ingestion in guinea pigs. Environ. Res., 12, 355-357.

Schrenk, H.H. and Schreibeis, L., 1958. Urinary arsenic levels as an index of industrial exposure. J. Am. Ind. Hyg. Assoc., 19, 225-228.

Shah, P.V. and Guthrie, F.E., 1983. Dermal absorption of benzidine derivatives in rats. Bull. Environ. Contam. Toxicol., 31, 73-78.

Shaikh, Z.A. and Smith, J.C., 1980. Metabolism of orally ingested cadmium in humans. Dev. Toxicol. Environ. Sci., 8, 569-574.

Shank, K.E., Vetter, R.J. and Ziemer, P.L., 1977. A mathematical model of cadmium transport in a biological system. Environ. Res., 13, 209-214.

Sharma, R.P., Kjellstrom, T. and McKenzie, J.M., 1983. Cadmium in blood and urine among smokers and non-smokers with high cadmium intake via food. Toxicol., 29, 163-171.

Sherlock, J.C., Smart, G.A., Read, J.I., Brooke, P.J., Forbes, G., Patterson, W., Richards, W., Moore, M and Wilson, T., 1983. Intakes of copper, zinc, cadmium, tin, iron, nickel and arsenic in a population exposed to lead from water. Sci. Tot. Environ., 30, 255-260.

Sherwood, R.J., 1976. Comparative methods of biologic monitoring of benzene exposures. In: Proc. 17th, Int. Cong. Occup. health, 29-51.

Shimizu, T., Shijo, T. and Sakai, K., 1981. Determination of cadmium in human urine by graphite furnace atomic absoprtion spectrometry. Bunseki Kagaku., 30, 770-774.

Sjogern, B., Hedstrom, L. and Ulfvorsen, V., 1983. Urine chromium as an estimator of air exposure to stainless steel welding fumes. Int. Arch. Occup. Environ. Health., 51, 347-354.

Skilleter, D.N., 1984. Biochemical properties of beryllium potentially relevant to its carcinogenicity. Toxicol. Environ. Chem., 7, 213-228.

Smialawicz, R.J., Rogers, R.R., Riddle, M.M. and Statt, G.A., 1984. Immunologic effects of nickel: 1. Suppression of cellular and humoral immunity. Environ. Res., 33, 413-427.

Smith, T.J., Anderson, R.J. and Reading, J.C., 1980. Chronic cadmium exposures associated with kidney function effects. Am. J. Indust. Med., 1, 319-337.

Snee, R.D., 1982. Models for the relationship between blood lead and air lead. Int. Arch. Occup. Environ. Health, 50, 303-319.

Starich, G.H. and Blincoe, C., 1983. Dietary chromium - forms and availabilities. Sci. Tot. Environ., 28, 443-454.

Stern, R.M., 1983. Assessment of risk of lung cancer for welders. Arch. Environ. Health, 38, 148-155.

Stewart, R.D., 1960. Infra red analysis of carbon tetrachloride and ethanol in blood. J. Lab. Clin. Med., 56, 148-156.

Stewart, R.D., Boettrer, E.A., Southworth, R.R. and Lerny, J.C., 1963. Acute carbon tetrachloride intoxication. J. Am. Med. Assoc., 183, 994-997.

Stewart, R.D., Dodd, H.C., 1964. Absorption of carbon tetrachloride, trichloroethylene, tetrachloroethylane, methylene chloride, and 1, 1, 1 - trichloroethane through the human skin. Am. Ind. Hyg. Assoc. J., 25, 439-446.

Stewart, R.D., Gay, H.H., Erley, D.S., Hake, C.L. and Peterson, J.E., 1961. Human exposure to carbon tetrachloride vapour. Relationship of expired air concentration to exposure and toxicity. J. occup. Med., 3, 586-590.

Stowe, H.C., 1976. Biliary excretion of cadmium by rats. Effects of zinc, cadmium and selenium pretreatments. J. Toxicol. Environ. Health, 2, 45-53.

Subramanian, K.S. and Meranger, J.C., 1983. Blood levels of cadmium, copper, lead and zinc in children in a British Columbia community. Sci. Tot. Environ., 30, 231-244.

Suzuki, Y., 1981. Cadmium, copper and zinc distribution in blood of rats after long-term cadmium administration. J. Toxicol. Environ. Health, 7, 251-262.

Takahasi, W., Pfenninger, K. and Wong, L., 1983. Urinary arsenic, chromium and copper levels in workers exposed to arsenic based wood preservative. Arch. Environ. health, 38, 209-214.

Tam, G.K., Charbonneau, S.M., Bryce, F. and Sandi, E., 1982. Excretion of a single oral dose of fish-arsenic in man. Bull. Environ. Contam. Toxicol., 28, 669-673.

Tanaka, K., Nomura, H., Onosaka, S. and Min., K.S., 1981. Release of hepatic cadmium by carbon tetrachloride treatment. Toxicol. Appl. Pharmacol., 59, 535-539.

Tandon, S.K., 1982. Disposition of nickel-63 in the rat. Toxicol. Lett., 10, 71-73.

Tossavainen, A., Nurminea, M., Mutonen, P. and Tola, S., 1980. Application of mathematical modelling for assessing the biological half-times of chromium and nickel in field studies. Brit. J. Ind. Med., 37, 285-291.

Teisinger, J. and Fiserova-Bergerova, V., 1958. Valeur Comparee de la determination du phenol contenus dans l'urine. Arch. Malad. Prof., 16, 221-232.

Teschke, R., Vierke, W. and Goldermann, L., 1983. Carbon tetrachloride levels and serum activities of liver enzymes following acute CCl$_4$ intoxication. Toxicol. Lett., 17, 175-180.

Thorne, M.C. and Jackson, D., 1983. Models for the Metabolism of Chemical Carcinogens in Man. ANS Report No. 347.

Tipton, I.H. and Stewart, P.L., 1969. Patterns of elemental excretion in long-term balance studies. II. Health Physics Division Annual Progress Report (for period ending July 31, 1969). ORNL-4446, 303-305.

Tjälve, H. and Löfberg, B., 1983. Extrahepatic sites of metabolism of carbon tetrachloride in rats. Chem. Biol. Interact., 46, 299-316.

Tohyama, C., 1981. Elevated urinary excretion of metallothionein due to environmental cadmium exposure. Toxicology, 20, 289-297.

Tsukamoto, H., Parker, H.R., Gribble, D.H., Mariassy, A. and Peoples, S.A., 1983a. Nephrotoxicity of sodium arsenate in dogs. Am. J. Vet. Res., 44, 2310-2324.

Tsukamoto, H., Parker, H.R. and Peoples, S.A., 1983b. Metabolism and renal handling of sodium in dogs. Am. J. Vet. Res., 44, 2331-2335.

Tunek, A. and Oesch, F., 1981. Multi-step metabolic activation of benzene in rat liver microsomes. Adv. Exp. Med. Biol., 136A, 319-329.

Tyson, C.A., Hanu-Prather, K., Story, D.L. and Gould, D.H., 1983. Correlations of in vitro and in vivo hepatotoxicity for five haloalkanes. Toxicol. Appl. Pharmcol., 70, 289-302.

Vacher, J., Deraedt, R., Flahaut, M., 1975. Possible role of lysosomal enzymes in some pharmacological effects produced by Be. Toxic. Appl. Pharmacol., 33, 205-213.

Vacher, J. and Stoner, H.B., 1968. The removal of injected beryllium from the blood of the rat. The role of the reticulo-endothelial system. Br. J. Exp. Pathol., 49, 315-323.

Vahter, M. and Envall, J., 1983. In vivo reduction of arsenate in mice and rabbits. Environ. Res., 32, 14-24.

Vahter, M., Marafante, E., Lindgren, A. and Dencker, L., 1982. Tissue distribution and subcellular binding of arsenic in marmoset monkeys after injection of ^{74}As-arsenite. Arch. Toxicol. 51, 65-77.

Vahter, M. and Marafante, E., 1983. Intracellular interaction and metabolic fate of arsenite and arsenate in mice and rabbits. Chem. Biol. Interactions, 47, 29-44.

Vahter, M., Marafante, E. and Dencker, L., 1983. Metabolism of arsenobetaine in mice, rats and rabbits. Sci. Tot. Environ., 30, 197-211.

Versieck, J. and Cornelis, R., 1983. Normal levels of trace elements in human blood plasma or serum. Anal. Chim. Acta, 116, 217-254.

Van Stee, E.W., Boorman, G.A., Moorman, M.P. and Sloane, R.A., 1982. Time-varying concentration profile as a determinant of hepatotoxicity. J. Toxicol. Environ. Health, 10, 785-795.

Vincent, J.H., Johnston, W.B., Jones, A.D. and Johnston, A.M., 1981. Static electrification of airborne asbestos: a study of its causes, assessment and effects on deposition in the lungs of rats. Am. Ind. Hyg. Assoc. J., 42, 711-721.

Von Erlicher, H., 1958. Benzidine as an occupational hazard. Zbl. Arbeitsmed., 8, 201-207.

Wada, O., Wu, G.Y., Yamomoto, A., Manabe, S. and Ono, T., 1983. Purification and chromium-excretory function of low-molecular weight chromium-binding substance from dog liver. Environ. Res., 32, 228-239.

Walker, B. and Gerber, A., 1981. Occupational exposure to aromatic amine: benzidine and benzidine-based dyes. Natl. Cancer Inst. Monogr., 58, 11-13.

Wallach, S. and Verch, R.L., 1983. Radiochromium conservation and distribution in diuretic states. J. Am. Coll. Nutr. 2, 163-172.

Warren, H.V. and Horksy, S.J., 1983. Quantitative analysis of zinc, copper, lead, molybdenum, bismuth, mercury and arsenic in brain and other tissues from multiple sclerosis and non-multiple sclerosis cases. Sci. Tot. Environ., 29, 163-169.

Watanabe, T., Koizumi, A., Fujita, A., Fujita, H., Kumai, M. and Ikeda, M., 1983. Cadmium levels in the blood of inhabitants in non-polluted areas in Japan with special references to ageing and smoking. Environ. Res., 31, 472-483.

Watanage, P.G. and Gehring, P.J., 1976. Dose-dependent fate of vinyl chloride and its possible relationship to oncogenicity in rats. Env. Health Perspec., 17, 145-152.

Watanabe, P.G., Zempel, J.A. and Gehring, P.J., 1978. Comparison of the fate of vinyl chloride following single and repeated exposure in rats. Toxicol. Appl. Pharmacol., 44, 391-399.

Webb, M.A.H., Chettlet, D.R., Al-Haddad, I.K., Dawrey, S.P.M.J. and Morisey, T.C., 1982. Measurement of cadmium in liver and kidney using in vivo techniques. Ann. occup. Hyg., 25, 33-37.

Weber, H., 1983. Long-term study of the distribution of soluble chromate-51 in the rat after a single intratracheal administration. J. Toxicol. Environ. Health, 11, 749-764.

Weinzweig, M. and Richards, R.J., 1983. Quantitative assessment of chrysotile fibrils in the bloodstream of rats which have ingested the mineral under different dietary conditions. Environ. Res., 31, 245-259.

Welch, K., Higgins, I., Oh, M., Burchfield, C., 1982. Arsenic exposure, smoking and respiratory cancer in copper smelting workers. Arch. Environ. Health, 37, 325-335.

Wicks, M.J., Archer, V.E., Auerbach, O. and Kuschrer, M., 1981. Arsenic exposure in a copper smelter as related to histological type of lung cancer. Am. J. Indust. Med., 2, 25-31.

Williams, W.J. and Williams, W.R., 1983. Value of beryllium lymphocyte transformation tests in chronic beryllium disease and in potentially exposed workers. Thorax, 38, 41-44.

Withey, J.R., 1976. Pharmacodynamics and uptake of vinyl chloride monomer administered by various routes to rats. J. Toxicol. Environ. Health, 1, 381-394.

Yamaguchi, S., Jones, K. and Shimojo, N., 1983. On the biological half-time of hexavalent chromium in rats. Ind. Health, 21, 25-34.

Yamamoto, A., Wada, O. and Ono, T., 1981. A low-molecular weight, chromium-binding, substance in mammals. Toxicol. Appl. Pharmacol., 59, 515-523.

Yamauchi, H. and Yamamura, Y., 1983. Concentration and chemical species of arsenic in human tissue. Bull. Environ. Contam. Toxicol., 31, 267-277.

Zachariasen, H., Anderson, I., Kostal, C. and Barton, R. Techniques for determining nickel in blood by flameless atomic absorption spectrophotometry.

Zenser, T.V., Mattammal, M.B., Rapp, N.S. and Davies, R.B., 1982. Effect of aspirin on metabolism of acetaminophen and benzidine by renal inner medulla prostaglandins hydroperoxidase. J. Lab. Clin. Med., 101, 58-65.

Zenser, T.V., Mattammal, M.B., Wise, R.W., Rice, J.R. and Davis, B.B., 1983. Prostaglandin H synthase-catalysed activation of benzidine: a model to assess pharmacologic intervention of the initiation of chemical carcinogenesis. J. Pharmacol. Exp. Ther., 227, 545-530.

Zhdan, V.M., 1982. Benzidine content of the urine of rats after the administration of benzidine-based dyes. Gig. Tr. Prof. Zabol., 32-35.

Ziegler, E.E., Edwards, B.B., Jensen, R.L., Mahaffey, K.R. and Fomon, S.J., 1978. Absorption and retention of lead by infants. Pediat. Res., 12, 29-34.

5
Model of the GI tract

5.1   Introduction

With the respiratory system, the gastro-intestinal (GI) tract is an important organ of intake of potential carcinogens into the body. In the non-occupationally exposed person, it is probably the more important of the two, with the majority of the body burden being derived from dietary sources. Therefore, intakes via the GI tract must be taken into account when developing any model of systemic uptake and retention.

In occupationally exposed persons, carcinogenic substances present in the work environment can enter the GI tract by two routes:

- Accidental transfer of material from hand to mouth, possibly via food. This is normally due to poor industrial hygiene practices;

- transfer of inhaled material from the lung to the GI tract as a result of the swallowing of inhaled material cleared from the lung by the mucociliary escalator.

A model of the GI tract has been adopted by the International Commission for Radiological Protection (ICRP) (1979). This model, which is based on a paper by Eve (1966), is shown in Fig. 5.1. In the model, the GI tract is divided into 4 sections, the stomach, small intestine and the upper and lower large intestine. Any substance ingested is assumed to pass through each section in sequence in a well-defined manner. Absorption is assumed to take place only from the small intestine and the concept of a "f_1" value for a substance is used. This is the fraction of ingested material that is absorbed from the GI tract into the systemic circulation.

The ICRP model is used primarily in radiation protection calculations for workers occupationally exposed to radionuclides, though it is also employed in assessing the exposure of members of the public. The model serves several purposes:

- Estimation of the amount of radioactive material absorbed into the systemic circulation and hence transferred to other organs and tissues;

- estimation of the radiation dose delivered to the relevant region of the GI tract by the presence of radioactive material in the gut lumen;

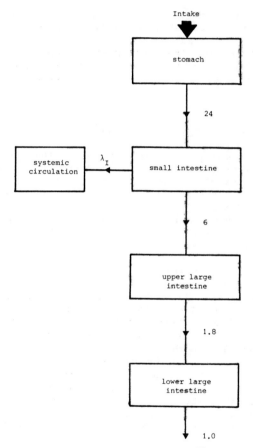

Notes: Rate constants given in units of d^{-1}
The value of λ_I can be calculated using

$$\lambda_I = 6f_1/(1-f_1)$$

where f_1 is the fractional absorbtion of the substance from the gastrointestinal tract. If f_1 is unity, the substance can be considered to go directly from the stomach to the systemic circulation with a rate coefficient of 24 d^{-1}.
From International Commission on Radiological Protection (1979).

FIGURE 5.1 THE GENERAL GASTROINTESTINAL TRACT MODEL FOR THE METALS AND METALLOIDS

- estimation of the radiation dose delivered to all organs and tissues as a result of the presence of γ-emitting radionuclides in the lumen.

However, for the purposes of this study, different considerations apply in the construction and implementation of a model of the GI tract. These are the requirements to estimate:

- Absorption of ingested material into the circulation;

- retention of certain compounds by the cells lining the lumen of the GI tract;

- modelling the transfer of ingested material through the GI tract and into the faeces, for possible monitoring purposes.

The long period since the ICRP model was formulated, together with the particular requirements of this study, indicated the need to review relevant literature on GI tract modelling. This topic is discussed below.

5.2   Physiology and anatomy of the GI tract

This Section contains a short review of the anatomy and physiology of the GI tract where relevant to construction of a model. For a more detailed review of the subject, the reader is directed to the standard text-books on the subject such as Gray's Anatomy (1981), Ham (1974) or Davenport (1971).

The GI tract consists of a long muscular tube, opening to the environment at the lips and the anus, together with certain large glands developed from the epithelial lining of this tube, and emptying their secretions into it. The parts of the tube and their general anatomical situation in the body are shown in Fig. 5.2.

The main functions of the gut are the breakdown and digestion of food, absorption of nutrients and essential substances and elimination of unabsorbed material. The length of the GI tract has been estimated as 8 m, but this value is based on measurements made in cadavers. In the live person, muscle tone in the gut wall will result in a smaller "physiological" length.

The structure of the wall of the tube is shown in Fig. 5.3. The muscle of the tube is all smooth muscle, except in the upper oesophagus and rectum, where voluntary (striated) muscle is present.

The nerve supply to the GI tract and its asociated glands is from both the sympathetic and parasympathetic nervous systems. The sympathetic supply is via the splanchnic nerves. The parasympathetic supply is via the vagus, which supplies all the glands (except salivary glands) and all of the gut up to and including the colon, and the sacral parasympathetics, which control the smooth muscle of the pelvic colon and rectum. There are several short reflexes also, involving local networks from the gut to the coeliac plexus, and back.

5.2.1   <u>Events in the mouth</u>

        Food and water pass very quickly through the mouth and
gullet, and so no consideration is usually made of residence time of
food in these locations when developing a model of the GI tract.
However, for the sake of completeness a brief account is given of the
digestive processes occurring in the mouth.
        Digestion of food is effected by two means:

-    Mechanical action of the parts of the GI tract;

-    digestion by enzymes, and acid, released by the glands of the
     tract.

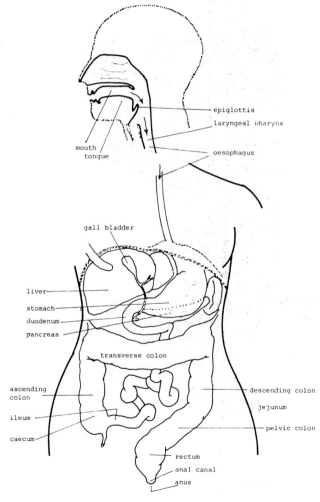

Note:
    Redrawn from Ham (1974)

FIGURE 5.2. ANATOMY OF THE GASTROINTESTINAL TRACT

When food enters the mouth, mechanical digestion begins with chewing. This breaks the food down into small pieces to facilitate the digestive action of the lower parts of the tract.

The presence of food and the chewing action both stimulate the salivary glands to increase their secretion. The functions of saliva are:

-    To lubricate the mouth and facilitate rapid articulation;

-    to initiate digestion of starch, by means of the enzyme amylase which is present in saliva;

-    to keep the mouth and teeth free from infection, by means of the bacteriocidal effect of the enzyme lysozyme.

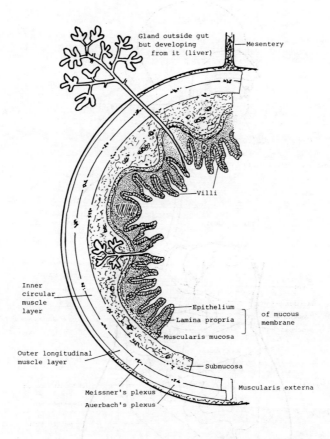

Note:
     Redrawn from Ham (1974)

FIGURE 5.3. A GENERALIZED CROSS-SECTION OF THE GASTROINTESTINAL TRACT

After several seconds chewing, the masticated food is passed into the oesophagus by swallowing.

The oesophagus is the first part of the GI tube. It is approximately 25 cm long and 2 cm in diameter. It connects the pharynx and the stomach. At each end of the oesophagus are two sphincters, controlling passage of food through the gut. The structure of the oesophagus wall is as described above.

Swallowing is a very complex process, which can be divided into three phases. The first phase is under voluntary control. The bolus of food is propelled into the oesophagus by a backward and upward movement of the tongue. At the same time, the soft palate rises and approaches the posterior pharyngeal wall which is brought forward to close off the nasopharynx. Respiration is reflexly inhibited and the larynx begins to rise as the bolus passes over the back of the tongue. From this point, the deglutition process is involuntary.

The next phase is designed to direct the food into the correct tube i.e. the oesophagus rather than the trachea, since both tubes connect with the pharynx. The tongue moves back towards the posterior pharyngeal wall and forces the bolus back against the epiglottis which arrests it for a short time and then becomes folded to form a cowl-like hood over the laryngeal orifice. The entrance to the larynx is closed by the sphincteric action of the girdle of muscles surrounding it. The bolus passes over the top of the larynx, and the upper oesophagal sphincter relaxes for approximately one second, allowing the bolus to enter the oesophagus. The reverse of the above procedure now occurs allowing resumption of breathing. The laryngeal sphincter then contracts.

The final phase involves the passage of the bolus down the oesophagus and into the stomach. The bolus is moved down the tube by peristalsis, a sequential and coordinated contraction of the muscle layers behind the bolus. A long reflex is activated by the presence of food in the oesophagus. This causes the lower oesophageal sphincter to relax, allowing the food to enter the stomach. Once the bolus has passed, the sphincter closes, preventing regurgitation. This lower sphincter has not been defined anatomically, although it must exist, since intragastric pressure is usually higher than intraoesophageal pressure.

5.2.2   The stomach

The stomach has 3 functions:

-      It acts as a food storage reservoir;

-      it liquidises and churns the food into chyme, as a result of its secretions and movements;

-      it delivers chyme to the duodenum at a controlled rate so that the digestive and absorptive processes are not overwhelmed by a large volume of chyme.

When food enters the stomach, the smooth muscle in the stomach wall relaxes. This is thought to be a long, vagally mediated reflex initiated by tension receptors in the oesophageal and stomach wall. The process is called receptive relaxation.

Once the food is in the stomach, digestion by locally produced secretions can begin. There are two main digestive secretions, pepsinogen and hydrochloric acid (HCl). The secretory glands of the stomach are the gastric pits, shown diagrammatically in Fig. 5.4. Parietal cells produce HCl and peptic cells produce pepsinogen. The large triangular cells shown in Fig. 5.4 are goblet cells. These release a secretion which forms a continuous layer over the whole surface of the stomach, approximately 100 μm thick. The functions of this barrier are:

-     To prevent autolysis of the stomach by pepsin and HCl;

-     to lubricate the stomach wall and to prevent mechanical damage by scraping of the contents against the wall.

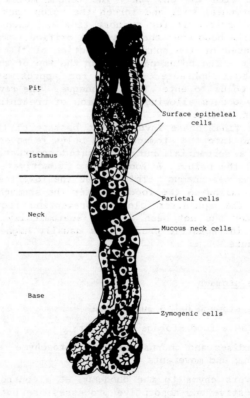

Pit

Surface epitheleal cells

Isthmus

Parietal cells

Neck

Mucous neck cells

Base

Zymogenic cells

Note:
    Redrawn from Ham (1974)

FIGURE 5.4.   THE CELLULAR ARRANGEMENT IN THE GASTRIC PITS

The stomach has two other secretions.

- Intrinsic factor, which is required for the absorption of vitamin B_{12} in the intestine. Its site of secretion is unknown.

- Gastrin, which is a hormone secreted by G cells in the gastric pits. It is released into the blood stream and controls the level of gastric secretion.

Pepsinogen is the inactive precursor of the protease pepsin. It is activated in an environment of pH 2 created by the HCl. Other functions of the HCl produced in the stomach are:

- To denature proteins by destroying their tertiary structure, thus aiding protease digestion;

- to kill bacteria;

- to hydrolyse sugars.

There is hardly any absorption from the stomach, since nothing has been completely digested. However, small molecules such as ethanol and aspirin (salicylic acid) are absorbed from the stomach. There is also a passive, bidirectional flux of water to maintain isosmolality of the chyme and plasma.

Controlled release of chyme into the duodenum is achieved by peristalsis. The stomach wall acts as a unit because the longitudinal

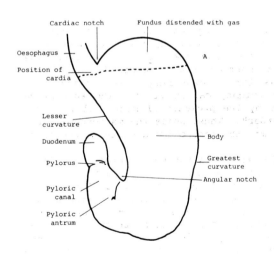
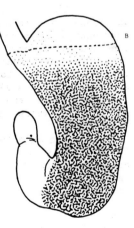

Note:
   Redrawn from Bell et al. (1976)

FIGURE 5.5.   A) THE ANATOMY OF THE STOMACH
              B) THE DISTRIBUTION OF ACID PRODUCING CELLS

and circular muscle are continuous sheets. There is an intrinsic rhythym at a frequency of 3 waves per minute. The waves initiate in an area high in the body of the stomach, called the pacemaker (see Fig. 5.5). The wave then progresses over the longitudinal muscle towards the pylorus and the excitation spreads from the longitudinal to the circular muscle. The wave moves over the body of the stomach at a velocity of 1 cm s^{-1} and as it passes over each region of muscle this area contracts, longitudinal first, circular shortly afterwards. As the wave approaches the antrum it accelerates to 3 or 4 cm s^{-1}.

The waves of contraction are no more than shallow ripples in the body, but as they approach the antrum they deepen, almost occluding the lumen, and force chyme past the pylorus into the duodenum. As the wave passes over the pylorus, its contraction stops the passage of chyme into the duodenum. The pylorus is normally relaxed, unlike the sphincters, so refluxing of duodenal contents can occur when suitable pressure gradients are present.

Control of gastric emptying can be exerted by changing the frequency on the force of contraction. In practice it is usually via the latter. Gastric motility is increased by the presence of food in the stomach. This is effected by distortion of recognised tension receptors in the stomach wall. Both short and long reflexes are involved. Inhibition of gastric motility is effected by four sets of receptors in the duodenum. These are sensitive to fat, hydrogen ions, osmolarity and tension. Thus, as chyme is squirted into the duodenum, these receptors are activated to varying degrees, depending on the composition of food and rate of emptying.

5.2.3   The small intestine

This is divided into three regions, the duodenum, jejunum and ileum. Its main function is digestion of chyme with absorption of nutrients and essential substances from the lumen. To fulfil the function of absorption, a large surface area is required. To achieve this, the intestinal mucosa is thrown into finger-like projections, varying from 0.5 to 1 mm in height, called villi. The absorptive surface is made still greater by the presence of micro-villi on the luminal surface, the "brush border". Thus, while the macroscopic area of the small intestine is ∿2.5 m^2, the absorptive area is in the range 200-500 m^2.

The main function of movement of the small intestine wall is to thoroughly mix the chyme with the digestive enzymes. This is achieved by localized contractions of concentric regions of the wall, resulting in a sausage-like appearance. This is called segmentation. There is no peristalsis in the small intestine, but movement of food along the tube is effected by different rates of contraction. In the duodenum, the rate is 18 contractions per minute, whereas in the ileum it is 7 per minute. This gradient in contraction rate moves food slowly along the intestine. Vagal stimulation and distension of the small intestine wall both increase the rate of contraction in the duodenum.

Digestion is effected by the enzymes and secretions of the pancreas which enter the duodenum together with the content of the bile duct, through the sphincter of Odi. Pancreatic secretion consists of a cocktail of enzymes. The enzymes all have an optimum pH of 7 to 8 and so the acidic chyme entering the duodenum has to be neutralised. This is achieved by the electrolyte present in the pancreatic secretion which neutralises the stomach-derived acid.

The enzymes of the pancreatic secretion are:

- An assortment of proteases;

- lipases, which break down fat;

- amylase, which breaks down carbohydrates;

- nucleases, which break down nucleic acids.

Pancreatic secretion is mainly controlled by the endocrine system. The two hormones secretin and cholecystokin pancreozymin (CCK-PZ) are produced by cells in the intestinal wall, in the presence of chyme in the lumen. The hormones are secreted into the blood stream and cause the pancreas to increase its rate of secretion. Secretin increases the electrolyte secretion and CCK-PZ increases the secretion of enzymes.

The secretion of the gall baldder is also controlled by these hormones. Secretin increases the electrolyte content of the bile, and CCK-PZ causes the walls of the gall-bladder to contract, expelling the contents into the duodenum. The functions of biliary secretions are as listed below.

- Neutralization of chyme as a result of its bicarbonate content.

- Emulsification of fats. Because fat is insoluble in the aqueous environment of chyme it would, in the absence of bile salts, be digested only very slowly. Bile salts aggregate in micelles which have a hydrophobic interior. Fat dissolves within this interior and an emulsion is formed which is more readily digested.

- Activation of pancreatic lipase.

5.2.4   The large intestine

There is a sphincter between the ileum and the colon. When the small intestine contracts this sphincter opens, allowing chyme to enter the colon. In the colon, the contents of the lumen are termed faeces. Most nutrients have already been absorbed from the contents which now consist mainly of water, salts and waste material. The function of the colon is to absorb water and electrolytes.

The longitudinal muscle of the colon is arranged into three bands, the taenia coli. These bands result in the colon being structured into discrete segments called haustrae. Movements are mainly concerned with mixing, but matter is also moved down the colon by haustral shunting.

In the lower region of the colon, there are mass propulsive movements to push the faeces into the rectum. There are usually three such movements per day and, in each, 20 cm of the colon contracts as a single entity.

The main function of the rectum is defaecation. The longitudinal and circular muscles in the rectum contract and the internal and external sphincters open. This is a reflex action, but can be controlled by higher centres of the central nervous sytem.

5.2.5   Digestion, absorption and excretion

5.2.5.1   Carbohydrates

About 60% of dietary carbohydrates are in the form of polysaccharides. These are macromolecules built up from several hexose sugars. These molecules are too large to be absorbed drectly and so must be digested into smaller molecules. This is achieved by the

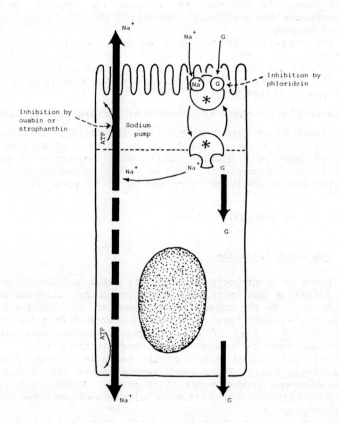

Note:
    Redrawn from Bell et al. (1976)

FIGURE 5.6.   SCHEMATIC DIAGRAM OF THE UPTAKE OF GLUCOSE BY THE INTESTINAL
    CELL

enzyme amylase and by HCl in the stomach. Both these agents have the effect of hydrolysing the 1-6 and 1-4 glycosidic linkages which join the hexose sub-units together.

The end products of the digestion are disaccharides. These are broken down by specific disaccharidases in the brush border of the villi to individual hexose units. Absorption of these has to take place against a concentration gradient. This is achieved by facilitated diffusion. On the luminal surface of the epithelial cells are hexose-specific co-transporter proteins (see Fig. 5.6). On the luminal side of the proteins are two specific binding sites, for a sodium ion and a specific hexose respectively. When both sites are occupied, the tertiary structure of the molecule becomes unstable, resulting in the translocation of the two sites to face the cell interior, where the two bound substances are released. This tranlocation requires no energy expenditure by the cell, since the sodium is moving down a concentration gradient. Thus, if the sodium were allowed to accumulate in the cell, the process would come to a halt. However, on the surface of cells, is the ubiquitous sodium-potassium ATPase. This protein acts to remove sodium ions from the cell and replace them with potassium ions from outside. This process requires the input of energy, which is supplied by ATP.

An exception to the above mechanism occurs for fructose which enters the cell by diffusion. In this case, a concentration gradient is maintained because fructose is metabolised in the cell to a glucose analogue.

5.2.5.2   Proteins

Proteins are macromolecules built of several hundred amino acids.   Their size is such that they are far too large to be absorbed, except by endocytosis. Because the endocytotic capacity for protein absorption is very small, such molecules have to be broken down into their constituent amino acids.

Digestion commences in the stomach, where the acid environment destroys the tertiary structure of the protein, enabling the endoprotease pepsin to attack peptide bonds along the length of the chain. When the chyme reaches the duodenum, pepsin is inactivated by the high pH environment and other endopeptidases, e.g. trypsin and chymotrypsin, continue digesting the protein. Endopeptidase cannot attack the terminal peptide bond and so the end result of digestion by this means are di- and tripeptides. These can be digested by exopeptidases, which are located in the brush border, and absorption of the resulting amino acids is by a facilitated sodium diffusion process similar to that which mediates carbohydrate absorption. Four specific co-tranporter molecules have been identified, for different types of amino acid.

5.2.5.3   Fat

Most dietary fat is in the form of tryglyceride, a glycerol ester comprising three fatty acid molecules. Because of the insolubility of fats, digestion is not initiated until entry into the duodenum. Here, fats are emulsified by bile salts and cholesterol into small stable droplets 0.5-1.0 μm in diameter, which present a large surface area for attack by pancreatic lipase. This enzyme de-esterifies the triglyceride, forming free fatty acids, mono- and diglycerides and glycerol. These products are still intrinsically very insoluble in aqueous media, but micelles are formed by aggrega-tion of bile salts and the digestion products. The micelles are separated from the microvilli by an aqueous phase and have a half-life in the order of milliseconds. On their breakdown, fatty acids are released, and diffuse the short distance to the cell membrane in which they are rapidly absorbed. Inside the cell, the fatty acids are reformed into triglycerides which are aggregated into chylomicra which are passed into the extracellular space and thence to plasma. These chylomicra are responsible for the milky appearance of plasma after a fatty meal has been eaten.

The central importance of bile salts in fatty acid digestion is evident. These salts are actively reabsorbed in the terminal ileum, and new bile salts are also synthesised by the terminal ileum to compensate for those which are lost in the faeces (∿10% of those secreted). It is noted that vitamin A and K are fat soluble and absorption of these vitamins is interlinked with that of fat.

Of interest in this study is that many of the organic car-cinogens considered are soluble in fat, and thus, any dietary intake will probably be absorbed with the lipid phase.

5.2.5.4   Water and ions

The major ions on which the body is dependent are sodium, potassium, calcium, iron and chloride. Sodium and potassium ions are very mobile, moving readily between the lumen of the GI tract and plasma, with net absorption being under the hormonal control of aldo-sterone. Chloride absorption is passive, but is related to sodium absorption because of the requirement to maintain electroneutrality of the plasma.

Iron and calcium are also absorbed into the intestinal cell by specific active transport mechanisms. They leave the cell by passive diffusion, but this process is much slower than the initial uptake so they tend to accumulate in intestinal cells. Calcium ab-sorption is increased by vitamin D. Several other non-essential diva-lent cations can also be absorbed by passive diffusion, which also mediates calcium and iron absorption to some extent. Of particular interest are cadmium and lead, since competetive effects lead to the apparent dependence on the absorption of these substances on the absorption of calcium and iron (see Section 5.3).

About 5 to 10 litres of water enter the small intestine each day via food, drink and secretions. In contrast only 0.7 l enters the colon. Thus, the small intestine has a large capacity to absorb water. The reabsorption of water can be studied by ingestion of a non-absorbable marker, and monitoring its concentration in various parts of the intestine. Thus, for example, after a meal of 0.65 l initial volume the concentration of previously administered marker in the duodenum decreased several-fold. The calculated volumes, on the basis of concentration of markers were mid-duodenum 1500 ml, jejunum

750 ml and ileum 250 ml. Throughout the gut, water movement across the ephithelial cells is such as to keep the gut contents similar to plasma, but in the stomach and duodenum, an additional volume of water in the form of secretions is added. As food is absorbed during its passage down the intestine, it tends to take water with it to maintain osmolarity e.g. absorption of 55 g glucose will cause 1 litre of water to be absorbed.

The net absorption of water is the small difference between the large fluxes from blood to lumen and vice versa. For example, when water labelled with deuterium oxide is placed in the upper intestine, 50% reaches the blood in 2-3 minutes, and 95% in 10 minutes. However, when 1 litre of water is drunk, only 50% is absorbed in 30 minutes. Therefore, the flux of water from lumen to blood is a factor of ten larger than the net absorption. Water movement is thought to occur via the paracellular pathway, the "tight" junctions. This movement may cause some solutes to be drawn with it,

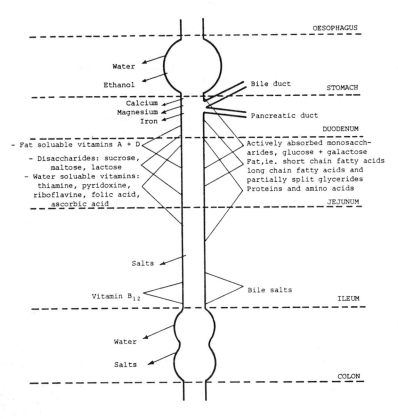

Note:
    Redrawn from Bell et al. (1976)

FIGURE 5.7. KNOWN SITES OF ABSORBTION IN THE ALIMENTARY CANAL

the process being termed "solvent drag", which could also be an important factor in the absorption of non-essential metalloids. A summary of the absorptive regions of the GI tract is given in Fig. 5.7.

5.2.5.5   The function of the colon

About 700 ml of faeces enter the colon per day, containing 85 m moles of sodium. The major function of the colon is to reabsorb this sodium (since severe salt depletion could otherwise occur). The reabsorption of sodium is an active process and as a side effect results in the passive reabsorption of chloride. Only 1-5 m moles of sodium are excreted in the faeces each day, i.e. less than 6% of that entering the colon. Water is passively reabsorbed, following the sodium and chloride , to maintain osmolarity. No potassium reabsorption occurs in the large intestine and 5 m moles are lost in the faeces each day. A total of 100-200 ml of faecal matter are passed each day by a subject eating a normal European diet. This consists of undigested matter, especially cellulose from plant cell walls, ions and water. The influence of diet should be noted. A group of African villagers consuming an unrefined diet passed an average of 400 g per day. The transit times of food through the gut are also much less for individuals on unrefined diet (see below).

Material absorbed from the intestine passes into the blood vessels of the mesentery which deliver their blood into the hepatic portal vein and thence to the liver, where processing of the nutrients continues.

5.3   Gastro-intestinal transit

The rate of transit of material through the gut determines both the amount of material that will be absorbed into the body and the rate of excretion of an unabsorbed ingested substance in the faeces.

These factors are both of interest when modelling the pharmacodynamics of ingested carcinogens, in relation to monitoring of exposure to these substances.

5.3.1   Gastric emptying

The rate of gastric emptying will determine the time delay between ingestion of a substance and the commencement of its absorption into the body from the small intestine (assuming that the stomach wall is impermeable to the substance).

Of the three regions of the human gut, most is known about the rate of transit of food through the stomach. This is because the stomach is more readily accessible to the techniques available for studying transit times and the rate of gastric emptying is a useful diagnostic tool, since it is affected by pathological conditions, especially in patients with gastro-duodenal ulcers.

There are several techniques used to measure the rate of gastric emptying. These include:

- Withdrawing the gastric contents through a tube;

- measuring the rate of efflux through the pylorus (by draining the duodenum through a fistula or an orally-introduced tube);

- measuring the volume of the stomach contents with an x-ray opaque material e.g. by the barium meal; or with a γ-ray emitting radio-nuclide marker, or by ultrasonic techniques).

Early work on the subject used the first technique and an excellent review of this work was published by Code and Carlsson (1968). The work can be represented by a paper by Hopkins (1966). He investigated the time-dependence of the volume of a standard liquid meal remaining in the stomach for meals of different volumes (Fig. 5.8). Despite wide variations in the initial volume of the meal a linear relation-

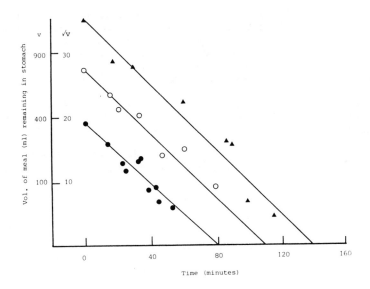

Note:
Redrawn from Hopkins (1966)

FIGURE 5.8. RELATIONSHIP BETWEEN THE VOLUME OF A STANDARD LIQUID MEAL REMAINING IN THE STOMACH AND TIME. THE INITIAL VOLUMES OF THE MEALS INTRODUCED INTO THE STOMACH WERE ▲ 1250 ml, ○ 750 ml AND ● 330 ml

ship was found between the square root of the volume remaining in the stomach and time. This was taken to imply the role of tension receptors in regulating gastric emptying (see Section 5.2.2) since the tension in the wall of the stomach is proportional to its radius (Laplace's law) and the radius of a cylinder is proportional to the square root of its volume.

Hunt and Spurvell (1951) observed that gastric emptying could be described by an exponential function. A model of this type was adopted by the ICRP based on a paper by Eve (1966). It was proposed that ingested food remained in the stomach with a half-time of one hour before being evacuated into the small intestine. This is an idealised situation, but is not unreasonable on the basis of gastric emptying data for different types of food (Eve, 1966).

The main problem with the intubation method of measuring gastric emptying is that it can only be used to study the emptying of liquid meals. Since it is known that liquids are emptied from the stomach far more quickly than solids, other techniques are required. In a study of subjects exhibiting similar gastric emptying patterns, Rinetti et al. (1982) showed that a barium meal and a similar volume (200 ml) of water labelled with Tc-99m showed identical emptying patterns. In a few seconds, both carriers fell from the cardia to the antrum, where a concentric contraction was initiated which began to discharge the stomach content into the duodenum. Quite different patterns were recorded when solid food labelled with Tc-99m, was used. The food remained in the fundus for several minutes, whilst passage to the antrum occurred after 25 minutes and to the duodenum after 35 minutes.

Gamma imaging techniques, such as that used in the above study have been used extensively in gastric emptying studies. In these techniques, gamma-ray emitting nuclides are tagged onto the food and emptying of food from the stomach is followed by imaging the activity in the stomach area, at various times after ingestion. Two nuclides have been particularly used, Tc-99m and Cr-51 (in the trivalent form). The advantage of using trivalent chromium is that only a small amount of this substance is absorbed by the body, and so the faecal excretion of this nuclide can be used as a measure of total gastrointestinal transit time. A number of groups have published data obtained in this way. Most of the results are expressed in terms of half-life for gastric emptying. The average value of this half-life is in the order of 60 minutes. However, examination of the individual emptying curves revealed a biphasic pattern so interpretation in terms of a single half-life should be regarded with caution (Claure, 1974; Jian, 1979).

The more rapid phase of clearance is probably associated with the liquid phase of the meal, with the slower phase being associated with clearance of the solid component. This subdivision of a solid meal into a liquid and a solid phase was investigated further by Malagelada (1977). He withdrew stomach contents via a gastric tube at various times after ingestion of a meal. In the stomach, the solid component of the meal was reduced in volume by a fifth, while endogenous secretion increased the volume of the liquid phase three-fold. Using Cr-51 bound to meat in the food, it was found that the Cr-51 gradually moved into the liquid phase during its time in the stomach, and that, in the duodenum, 95% of the Cr-51 was in the aqueous phase.

As has already been noted, liquid meals are emptied from the stomach far more quickly than are solid meals. Bateman (1982) studied the time dependence of gastric emptying of such meals, and concluded that after an initial rapid phase of emptying, an index of which is the volume remainig in the stomach after five minutes, emptying was mono-exponential, with a half-life of the order of 10 minutes.   This figure is similar to the value of 15 minutes obtained in normal subjects by Dugas et al. (1982).

In conclusion, there is a six-fold difference between the rate of emptying of liquid and solid meals. However, a solid meal has itself been shown to be composed of a solid and an aqueous phase. This implies that great care should be taken when interpreting data, concerned with gastric emptying, obtained after a radionuclide has been added to a solid meal.   The meal should be prepared in such a way that the nuclide becomes bound to the food consituents, rather than remaining in the aqueous phase, since, in the latter case, a misleadingly rapid gastric emptying pattern will be observed.   The effects of posture on emptying rates should also be noted (see Section 5.3.4).

5.3.2   Passage of food through the small intestine

A period of four hours was adopted by the ICRP for the transit of food through the small intestine.   This value was based mainly on studies of the passage of barium meals through the intestine.   Several new techniques have been developed to measure small-intestinal transit in animals, but as the majority of these necessitate killing the animal they are of little application in studies on man.

Transit times through the small intestine have not been widely investigated in man.   Apart from imaging techniques, either of radio-opaque materials or of γ-emitting radionuclides, the only methods available were complex invasive procedures involving the passage of tubes either from above into a specified section of the small intestine or from below into the ilio-caecal region.   Some information has also been obtained from patients subsequent to an ileostomy.   Here, the large intestine is removed, and the end of the small intestine is brought to the body surface and discharges waste material into a bag, which has to be periodically emptied.   A further technique has been developed which utilises the fact that in the large intestine are bacteria, which metabolise certain substances, providing volatile end-products, in particular, hydrogen.   This gas diffuses rapidly into the bloodstream, from where it is carried to the lungs and excreted in exhaled air.   If the hydrogen content of exhaled air is monitored, a reasonable indication of the passage of faecal matter into the large intestine can be obtained.

The relationship between the transit time of a meal through the small intestine, and the rate at which it leaves the stomach was first investigated by Lagerlof et al. (1974) who found that the rate at which a liquid meal passes the jejunum is proportional to the rate of gastric emptying.   Cobden et al. (1983) measured both gastric emptying and small intestinal transit time of a liquid meal in normal subjects.   Labelling with Tc-99m was used in conjunction with γ-imaging to monitor gastric emptying, and lactulose was added to the drink, as this sugar is poorly absorbed in the small intestine, and is fermented by the fauna of the large intestine, producing hydrogen. No significant correlation was found between gastric emptying half-times and intestinal transit time, but as the former represents a rate whereas the latter gives the time for the head of the bolus to reach the caecum, such a relationship should not be expected. The mean gastric emptying half-life was 62 minutes, larger than previous reported values for a liquid meal (see Section 5.3.1), but, as the meal was hypertonic, this is not unexpected (Section 5.2). Values for small intestinal transit time varied from 25 to 150 minutes (mean 72 minutes).

Read et al. (1982) used a variety of techniques to study the relationship between gastric clearance and transit time through the small intestine. They found that increasing the size of the meal by doubling the absorbable components delayed gastric emptying, but did not affect the time for the head of the meal to enter the caecum (lactose-H_2technique). The time for transfer of the majority of the meal into the caecum (measured by peak H_2 breath concentration) was increased by eating a larger meal. Incorporating fat in the meal affected all three parameters in the same way as increasing the size of the meal. A finding of interest was that lactulose did not affect gastric emptying times but significantly reduced intestinal transit times, placing in doubt its elligibility as a marker for intestinal transit under normal conditions. In control subjects, hydrogen breath concentration began to rise approximately 4 h after consuming the meal, and peak concentrations were observed after 7 h. This implies that the mean transit time of a solid meal through the intestine is somewhere between these values. (After subtracting the gastric emptying time, 1.5 h in this case).

Holgate and Read (1983) observed the effects of pharmacological agents on the small intestinal transit time and on absorption of dietary components in patients with terminal ileostomies. Lactulose, magnesium sulphate and the drug metaclopramide were used. All three agents significantly reduced the time taken for the meal to empty from the ileum. With lactulose and magnesium sulphate, this was associated with significant reductions in the absorption of fat, protein, carbohydrate and electrolytes, ascertained by analysing the contents of the ileal residues. Metaclopramide, although reducing transit time by a comparable amount to the other agents, had much less of an effect on absorption. Holgate and Read also attached a radioactive marker (Tc-99m) to the meal. Gastric emptying half-times exhibited a mean value of 67 minutes, a value similar to that obtained for normal subjects. The average time for the first appearance of the marker was 3.5 hr after eating the meal. This was almost identical to the mouth to caecum transit time of 3.4 h observed in normal subjects. In the patients, 50% of the marker had appeared by 6.9 hr.

The intestinal transit of solid and liquid meals was investigated by Kerlin and Phillips (1983). They used both dilution techniques involving a tube positioned in the terminal ileum, and the hydrogen in breath concentration method. Polyethylene glycol was used as an indicator for the liquid phase of a meal. Intestinal levels of polythylene glycol peaked 1.5 to 2 h post-prandially. Appreciable concentrations of hydrogen in breath were first detected 2 to 3 h

Subjects	Community	Race	Type of diet	No. of subjects	Time appearance of first pellet (hrs)		Transit time (hrs)		Weight of stools passed per day (gm)		Comments
					Range	Mean	Range	Mean	Range	Mean	
1. Naval ratings and wives.	UK	White	Refined	15	22-110	45.7	44-144	83.4	30-223	104	Shore based personnel.
2. Teenage boarding school pupils.	UK	White	Refined	9	19-103	57.4	35-120	76.1	71-142	110	Institutional diet together with cakes, sweets and so on from the school shop.
3. Students	South Africa	White	Refined	100	13-54	30.5	28-60	48.0	120-195	173	These ate more fruit than is usual in the UK.
4. Urban school children.	South Africa	African	Mixed	500	9-40	28.5	23-59	45.2	120-260	165	Partly European diet.
5. Manor House hospital patients	UK	White	Mixed	6	15-24	22.0	27-40	41.0	121-249	175	UK diet plus whole meal bread and added bran.
6. Senior boarding school pupils.	Uganda	African	Mixed	27	4-54	27.6	22-118	47.0	41-348	185	Traditional Ugandan diet plus refined sugar, white bread, jam and butter.
7. Vegetarians.	UK	White	Mixed	24	8-49	22.0	18-97	42.4	71-488	225	Similarity of values to those of Africans.
8. Nurses.	South	Indian (Vellore)	Mixed	13	9-34	27.6	23-64	44.0	-	155	Less refined diet than that of Western World.
9. Medical students (Present study)	India Assam	Indian	Mixed	30	7-42	20.40	19-126	46.65	17-420	126.82	Mixed institutional diet comprising of pulse, cereals, fish, meat, egg and vegetables.
10. Rural school children.	South Africa	Africa	Un-refined	500	5-28	12.8	20-48	35.5	150-350	175	
11. Rural villagers	Uganda	African	Un-refined	15	4-32	19.8	19-68	35.7	178-980	470	Villagers do not yet supplement their diet with processed food of western type.

Note: from Patowary et al. (1983)

TABLE 5.1

COMPARISON OF TRANSIT TIME ESTIMATED BY BINTON'S METHOD

after the meal represeting the passage of the first bolus of the solid
phase of the meal into the caecum. Peak concentrations were observed
5-6 hr post-prandially. Using indicator dilution techniques it was
calculated that approximately 1.8 l of chyme flows from the ileum into
the caecum per day, a value 50% higher than that assumed in the ICRP
model (see Eve, 1966).

        In conclusion, recent studies have shown that passage of
food through the small intestine taken from 2 to 6 h. The value of 4
h assumed by the ICRP as a half-time for transfer from the small
intestine to large intestine, corresponds to a mean residence time of
6 h and does not seem unreasonable.

5.3.3   Transit of food through the large intestine

        Measurement of the transit of matter through the large
intestine is very difficult and no references to such a study could be
identified. Information on this parameter may be obtained by studying
the passage of a barium meal through the entire intestine. Physiological measurements are usually made by measuring the total gastrointestinal transit time, and then subtracting the gastric and small
intestinal emptying time, to obtain the residence time in the large
intestine.

        Large intestine motility is studied by monitoring the change
in pressure in a balloon on a tube passed to different regions of the
large intestine. Loening-Baucke and Anuras (1983) showed that colonic
motility was increased during eating, this increase being due to an
increase in frequency of contraction, with the amplitude remaining
relatively constant. Motility returned to fasting levels when the
meal was completed. This finding was confirmed by Kerlin et al.
(1983).

        A review of published values of total gastrointestinal
transit time was presented by Petowary et al. (1972) (see Table 5.1).
These values were all obtained by measuring the transit of radio
-opaque pellets. A further study by Patoway et al. (1983) obtained a
transit time of 47 h for radio-opaque pellets in Indian medical stu-
dents. The major point of interest is the obvious correlation between
transit times and diet, in particular that a typical, refined, Western
diet gives longer transit times than does an unrefined diet. This is
thought to be related to the amount of undigested dietary fibre present in the diet, but further consideration of this topic is beyond
the scope of this review.

        Chromium sesquioxide (Cr_2O_3) has also been used as a marker
of gastrointestinal transit. Trivalent chromium ions are very poorly
absorbed from the intestine (Donaldson et al., 1966), and in a comparison with the radio-opaque pellet technique, Branch and Cummings
(1978), found very close agreement between the percentage faecal
contents of each marker as a function of time after ingestion.

        The faecal excretion of Cr-51 after a single oral dose of
tracer is shown in Fig. 5.9 (from Kerr et al., 1971). In a study by
Davignon et al. (1968) a transit time of 4 days was observed. Faecal
excretion of an oral dose of Cr-51 followed first order kinetics, and
had a half-time of 1.3 days (after correction for intestinal transit).

5.3.4   Effect of surgery, illness and pharmacological agents
         on gastrointestinal transit

         Gastric emptying rates can be markedly altered in patholo-
gical conditions. Of particular relevance to this review are studies
of gastric emptying in patients suffering from gastric and duodenal
ulcers, since these illnesses are common in the working population.
Harvey (1970) observed a doubling of the half-life of gastric emptying
in patients with gastric ulcers, whereas in patients with duodenal
ulcers the half-life of emptying was halved, compared with normal
subjects. Griffith (1966) also found a two-fold decrease in the
half-life of gastric emptying in duodenal ulcer sufferers.

         The operation of vagatomy is widely used in the treatment of
duodenal ulcers, but its long term effects on emptying are not clear.
Early investigators found that the operation was followed by a dis-
appointingly high incidence of recurrent ulceration and by troublesome
gastric stasis (Dragstedt et al., 1949). The recurrence could be

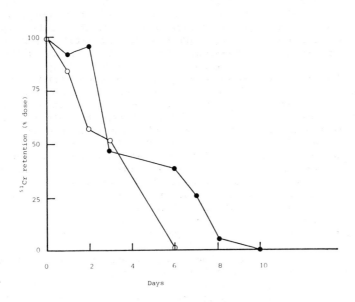

Note:
       Redrawn from Kerr et al. (1971)

FIGURE 5.9.   WHOLE BODY RETENTION OF ^{51}Cr FOLLOWING SINGLE ORAL DOSES
              OF TRACER IN TWO SUBJECTS; CASE A SHOWN WITH OPEN CIRCLES
              AND CASE B SHOWN WITH CLOSED CIRCLES

explained by an observation in rats by Poulsen et al. (1982). They found that cysteamine, a potent inducer of ulcers in rats, inhibited gastric motility, and this effect was even more marked after vagatomy, leading to stomach ulceration. If vagatomized patients are prescribed medication which inhibits gastric motility (as a side effect) the same effect may be observed in man. From a consideration of the physiological principles involved, it could be hypothesised that removing the vagal supply to the stomach would result in a slowing of gastric emptying (see Section 5.2). However, as the vagus also supplies the majority of the gastrointestinal tract, the net effect of sectioning the nerve may not be so predictable. This is reflected in the few studies that have ben performed on gastric emptying rates before and after vagatomy. Colmer et al. (1973) found that the rate of emptying as expressed by the half-life was not altered by the operation, but several patients suffering from gastric ulcers were also included in the study. Davies et al. (1974) observed an increase, no change, or a decrease in gastric emptying rate after such operations, but the interpretation of these results is not clear, since in some patients pyloroplasty was also performed. This involves restructuring the pylorus, and, thus, will obviously affect the emptying rate. Using a Cr-51 labelled meal, Faxen et al. (1978) showed that emptying of a solid meal was significantly slowed after parietal cell vagatomy (sectioning those nerve fibres supplying the parietal region of the stomach) in duodenal ulcer patients. This was in contrast to the rate of emptying of a liquid meal which was found to be unchanged.

The effect of posture on gastric emptying measurements is also noted. Hancock et al. (1974) could find no difference in emptying rates in normal volunteers when the subject was standing or lying down. However, in vagotomized patients, the rate of gastric emptying was significantly faster when standing than when the subject was supine. The same result was observed by Hulme-Muir et al. (1973) using liquid meals. It was also observed that vagotomy increased gastric emptying half-times by up to a factor of ten in the erect position. Using solid meals, the gastric emptying time was more rapid in the upright than in the supine position, and also after vagotomy.

These findings could be interpreted in terms of a gravitational assistance of gastric emptying, especially in the case of liquid meals, and also when partial gastric stasis has been induced by surgery.

Obese subjects were found to have abnormal gastric emptying (Wright et al., 1983). For solid meals, obese subjects had faster gastric emptying rates than did normal subjects. In obese subjects who lost weight to within 10% of their ideal body weight no reversal of this emptying pattern was observed. No difference was found in the emptying times of liquids for normal and obese individuals.

When considering the effects of pharmacological agents, it must be remembered that gastro-intestinal motility is controlled to a large extent by the central nervous sytem and so any agent which exerts its effect on the central nervous system can potentially affect the motility of the gut. This was demonstrated by Thompson et al. (1982) who found that caloric stimulation of the ear (inducing vertigo) caused a delay in gastric emptying.

Besides effects on the central nervous sytem, certain pharmaceuticals have direct effects on smooth muscle. For example, morphine reduces gastrointestinal motility in vitro and in vivo (Bianchi et al., 1983; Stewart, 1981; Weisbrodt et al, 1980).

Metaclopramide is sometimes given after vagatomy operations to overcome the gastric stasis usually induced by this operation. Justin-Besancon et al. (1964) and Connel and George (1969) both found that metaclopramide induced, or increased the rate of, gastric emptying of liquid meals. With solid meals, metaclopramide had no effect on gastric emptying in normal subjects or in vagatomized subjects with no gastric stasis (Hancock et al., 1974). However, in patients with abnormally delayed emptying ($T_{\frac{1}{2}}\sim350$ mins), metaclopromide produced a significant improvement ($T_{\frac{1}{2}}\sim200$ mins).

The construction of models for gastrointestinal transit and retention can be affected by common pathological states and by medications used by the individual. Notwithstanding their pathology and medication, such individuals are likely to be fit enough to continue their employment.

5.4 Absorption and retention of material by the intestinal wall

The ICRP model of the gastrointestinal tract assumes that all absorption occurs from the small intestine. As has been seen (Section 5.2), this may not be true for certain substances, for example, sodium and chloride ions are known to be absorbed in the large intestine. However, as the substances considered in this review are not known to have specific absorption sites, the assumption that all absorption is from the small intestine is likely to be a reasonable approximation.

5.4.1 Absorption of lipid soluble material

Several of the potential carcinogens studied in this work are lipid-soluble molecules. The normal route of exposure is by inhalation, but certain foodstuffs have significant concentrations of some of these substances. It is likely that the substances will be dissolved in the lipid phase and thus will be absorbed with this phase in the small intestine. Thus, they will be solubilized in the interior of the bile salt micelles (see Section 5.2) and absorbed with the fatty acids. Blood concentrations of the substances are, usually, so low that diffusion into the plasma is rapid. Transport in the plasma will probably be to the liver in chylomicra, where the substance will be metabolized.

5.4.2 Absorption of particulate matter and large molecules

Particulate matter reaches the gastrointestinal tract in ingested food and waste and from inhaled material that has been cleared from the lung and swallowed. Volkheimer and collaborators (Volkheimer, 1977) described the intestinal uptake of particles of diameter 5 to 150 µm in diameter, by a process called "persorption", and their appearance in portal and peripheal blood after ingestion. Le Fevre et al. (1980) demonstrated that 5.7 µm microspheres were absorbed by macrophages in Peyer's patches (lymphoid tissue in the intestinal wall).

Immunoglobulin and ferritin have both been demonstrated to cross the intestinal wall in the rat (Williams and Hemmings, 1978). However, it is unlikely that these molecules are taken up by macrophages.

5.4.3   Absorption of minerals

Fourteen elements are known to be essential to animal life in trace amounts. In addition to these, several elements are required in larger amounts. Of this latter group, the majority have to be absorbed from the lumen of the gastrointestinal tract against an electrochemical gradient. For net absorption to occur, active processes must exist, and specific pumps are required for these minerals. These pumps are under homeostatic control via the endocrine system. Chloride is an exception to this, since the absorption of cations leads to the development of a favourable electrochemical gradient for chloride absorption to occur.

The intestinal epithelium is a typical "tight" epithelium with closely packed cells linked by tight junctions. Passive ion diffusion can occur through these junctions. This process does not involve specific sites and so the potential for movement of a wide range of ions exists and competition between different ionic materials can occur. For example, lead absorption has been shown to be dependent on the amount of calcium present in the diet (Karhausen, 1972). In this context, it is noted that active calcium absorption occurs primarily in the jejunum and duodenum, but a facilitated diffusion pathway for calcium is known to be present throughout the gastrointestinal tract.

Once an ion has been absorbed into the cell, diffusion into plasma occurs down on electrochemical gradient. However, several minerals are known to be retained in the intestine bound to metallothionein. This protein binds several different metal ions and such competitive binding may result in interactions between the metabolism and absorption of different minerals.

The majority of work on the interaction of ions in absorption has used lead as the non-essential competitor, and the interaction of cadmium and zinc with respect to metallothionein binding is well known. These two aspects of absorption are discussed in detail below.

Gruden et al. (1974) showed that peroral application of lead significantly diminished the transfer of both calcium and strontium across the wall of the duodenum in vitro. Whereas more calcium is transferred by the active mechanism than by the passive, the latter mechanism is dominant for strontium. They suggest that lead affects the transport of both ions through a reduction of the passive transport pathway. In a further study, Gruden (1975) could not show any reduction in active calcium transport by lead.

With respect to intestinal uptake of lead, Gruden and Stantic (1975) could find no evidence for active transport.

In man, Blake and Mann (1983) demonstrated that calcium and phosphorus both reduced the gastrointestinal absorption of lead.

Consideration of these data suggests that calcium and lead compete for the same passive diffusion channel in the intestinal wall. It is also noted that Smith et al. (1978) showed that vitamin D stimulates lead absorption. Vitamin D is known to increase the transport rate of the active absorption pathway, and it was suggested that lead and calcium may also compete for this site. However, if the active mechanism is stimulated, less calcium will be available to the passive channel and so more lead will be absorbed.

The transfer of cadmium through the intestinal wall was found to be a passive process (Gruden, 1982). However, 20% of the initial mucosal cadmium was retained in the intestinal wall. Evans et al. (1970) isolated a metallothionein-like protein from the bovine duodenum. Copper, zinc and cadmium were all bound by this protein, explaining the known antagonism of these elements to the absorption of each other.

The storage of metals in the intestine leads to problems in the interpretation of absorption data. This is because the rate of turnover of cells in the intestinal epithelium is rapid and is probably faster than the absorption of metallothionein-bound cadmium from the intestinal cell. It is likely, therefore, that some cadmium will be lost in sloughed-off cells before complete absorption into the circulation can occur.

Holt and Webb (1983) found that cadmium administered intraperitoneally was also accumulated by the intestinal cells, showing that a bidirectional process of uptake and excretion is involved. Nickel has also been shown to affect the metabolism of metallothionein and its associated metals (Chmielnicka et al., 1982), but whether this element is bound in the cells of the small intestine was not stated.

5.5   Modelling retention in the gastrointestinal tract

Recent data concerning the transit of material through the gastrointestinal tract has been reviewed. Comparison of parameters obtained from the literature with parameter values used in the ICRP model of retention and transit by the gastrointestinal tract indicates adequate agreement. For this reason, it is not thought necessary to amend the model of transit of material through the gastrointestinal tract.

With respect to absorption, unless specific information is available, absorption of material is assumed to be from the small intestine. The retention of material within the cells of the intestinal wall has not been taken into account in the ICRP model. However, it has not been shown to occur for all substances, and also, there may be bidirectional transfer occurring, making this pathway one of excretion also. For this reason, where specific information exists, the retention and excretion of material by the intestinal cells has been incorporated into the specific model of systemic metabolism for that substance.

In conclusion, on the basis of the literature review, no changes in either model structure or parameter values from the ICRP model of gastrointestinal retention and transit are recommended. Specific information with regard to intestinal retention can be incorporated into the model of systemic metabolism.

Variation of transit times may be seen in various illnesses, but these subjects can be readily identified and appropriate changes to the model made, for specific modelling exercises are required.

5.6   References

Bateman, D.N., 1982.   Effects of meal temperature and volume on the emptying of liquid from the human stomach.   J. Physiol., 331, 461-467.

Bianchi, G., Ferretti, P., Recchia, M., Rocchetti, M., Tavani, A. and Manara, L., 1983. Morphine tissue levels and reduction of gastrointestinal transit in rats. Gastroenterology, 85, 852-858.

Blake, K.H.C. and Mann, M., 1983. Effect of calcium and phosphorous on the gastrointestinal absorption of Pb-203 in man. Environ. Res., 30, 188-194

Branch, W.J. and Cummings, J.H., 1978. Comparison of radio-opaque pellets and chromium sesquioxide as inert markers in studies requiring accurate faecal collections. Gut, 19, 371-376.

Burkitt, D.P., Walker, A.R.P. and Painter, N.S., 1972. Effect of dietary fibre on stools and transit time and its role in the causation of disease. Lancet, 2, 1408-1410.

Chmielnicka, J., Szymanska, J.A. and Tyfa, J., 1982. Disturbances in the metabolism of endogenous metals (Zn and Cu) in nickel-exposed rats. Environ. Res., 27, 216-221.

Claure, H., Calderon, C., Braunschweig, T. and Diaz, J., 1974. Gastric emptying time in normal subjects using Cr-51 and a gamma camera. Fev. Méd. Chile, 102, 936-938.

Cobden, I., Barker, M.C.J. and Axon, A.T.R., 1983. Gastrointestinal transit of liquids. Ann. Clin. Res., 15, 119-122.

Code, C.F. and Carlson, A.J., 1968. In: Handbook of Physiology, Section 6, Alimentary Canal, Vol.II, Secretion. Washington D.C., American Physiological Society.

Colmer, M.R., Owen, G.M. and Shields, R, 1973. Pattern of gastric emptying after vagotomy and pyloroplasty. Br. Med. J., 864, 448-450.

Connell, A.M. and George, J.D., 1969. Effect of metaclopramide on gastric function in man. Gut, 10, 678-680.

Davenport, H.W., 1971. Physiology of the Digestive Tract. 3rd Edition. Chicago, Medical Year Book publishers.

Davies, W.T., Griffith, G.H., Owen, G.M. and Shields, R., 1974. The effect of vagotomy and drainage operations on the rate of gastric emptying in duodenal ulcer patients. Br. J. Surg., 61, 509-515.

Davignon, J., Simmonds, W.J. and Ahrens, E.H., 1968. Usefulness of chromic oxide as an internal standard for balance studies in formula-fed patients and for assessment of colonic function. J. Clin. Invest. 47, 127-138.

Donaldson, R.M. and Barreras, R.F., 1966. Intestinal absorption of trace quantities of chromium. J. Lab. Clin. Med., 68, 484-493.

Dragstedt, L.R., Camp, E.H. and Fritz, J.M., 1949. Recurrence of gastric ulcer after complete vagatomy. Ann. Surg., 130, 843-854.

Dugas, M.L., Schade, R.R., Lhotsky, D. and Vanthiel, D., 1982. Comparison of methods for analysing gastric isotope emptying. Am. J. Physiol., 243, G237-242.

Evans, G.W., Majors, P.F. and Cornatzer, W.E., 1970. Mechanism for cadmium and zinc antagonism of copper metabolism. Biochem. Biophys. Res. Commun., 40, 1142-1148.

Eve, I.S., 1966. A review of the physiology of the gastrointestinal tract in relation to radiation doses from radioactive materials. Health Physics, 12, 131-161.

Faxen, A., Alpsten, M., Cederblad, A., Kewenter, J. and Rossander, L., 1978. The effect of parietal cell vagatomy and selective vagatomy with pyloroplasty on gastric emptying of a solid meal. Scan. J. Gastroenterol., 13, 727-733.

Gray, H. Anatomy, 36th Edit. (Eds. Warwick, R. and Williams, P.L.) London, Churchill Livingstone.

Griffith, G.H., Owen, G.M., Kirkman, S. and Shields, R., 1966. Measurement of rate of gastric emptying using chromium-51. Lancet 449, 1244-1245.

Gruden, N., 1982. Transfer of cadmium through the rat's intestinal wall. Environ. Res., 28, 340-343.

Gruden, N., 1975. Lead and active calcium transfer through the intestinal wall in rats. Toxicology, 5, 163-166.

Gruden, N. and Stantic, M., 1975. Transfer of lead through the rat's intestinal wall. Sci. Tot. Environ. 3, 288-292.

Gruden, N., Stantic, M., and Buben, M., 1974. The effect of lead on the absorption of calcium and strontium in the rat. Environ. Res. 8, 203-209.

Ham, A.W. Hisology, 7th Edit. Philadelphia, J.B. Lippincott Company.

Hancock, B.D., Bowen-Jones, E., Dixon, R., Dymock, I.W. and Cowley, D.J., 1974. The effect of metaclopramide on gastric emptying of solid meals. Gut, 15, 462-467.

Hancock, B.D., Bowen-Jones, E., Dixon, R., Testa, T., Dymock, I.W. and Cowley, J., 1974. The effect of posture on the gastric emptying of solid meals in normal subjects and patients after vagatomy. Br. J. Surg., 61, 326.

Harvey, R.F., Mackie, D.B., Brown, N.J.G., Keeling, D.H. and Davies, W.T., 1970. Measurement of gastric emptying time with a gamma camera. Lancet, 636, 16-18.

Holgate, A.M. and Read, N.W., 1983. Relationship between small bowel transit time and absorption of a solid meal. Influence of meta-clopramide magnesium sulphate and lactulose. Dig. Dis. Sci. 28, 812-819.

Holt, D. and Webb, M., 1983. Intestinal and hepatic binding of cadmium in the neonatal rat. Arch. Toxicol. 52, 291-301.

Hopkins, A., 1966. Gastric emptying of a liquid meal in human subjects. J. Physiol. 182, 144-149.

Hulme-Moir, I., Donnan, S.P., McAlister, J. and McColl, I., 1973. The effect of surgery and posture on the pattern and rate of gastric emptying. Aust. N.Z., J. Surg., 43, 80-84.

Hunt, J.N. and Spurvell, W.R., 1951. The pattern for emptying of the human stomach. J. Physiol. 113, 157-168.

International Commission on Radiological Protection, 1979. Limits for intakes of radionuclides by workers. Part 1, Annals of the ICRP, Vol.2, Nos.3/4.

Jian, R., Pecking, A., Najean, Y. and Bernier, J.J., 1979. Gastric emptying of an ordinary meal in man. Nouv. Presse Méd, 8, 667-671.

Justin-Besancon, L., Grivaux, M. and Wattez, E., 1964. L'épreuve au metaclopramide en radiologie digestive. Bull. Soc. Med. Hop. 115, 721-726.

Karhausen, L., 1972. Intestinal lead absorption. International symposium of environmental health. Aspects of lead (Amsterdam), 427-440.

Kerlin, P. and Phillips, S., 1983. Differential transit of liquids and solid residue through the human ileum. Am. J. Physiol. 245(1), G38-43.

Kerlin, P., Zinsmeister, A. and Phillips, S., 1983. Motor responses to food of the ileum, proximal colon and distal colon of healthy humans. Gastroenterology, 84, 762-770.

Kerr, M.K., Hitchman, A., Hudson, H., Rapoport, A. and Harrison, J.E., 1971. The value of carrier-free ^{51}Cr as a stool marker. Clin. Biochem. 4, 233-240.

Lagerlof, O.H., Johansson, C. and Ekelund, K., 1974. Studies of gastrointestinal interactions. VI Intestinal flow, mean transit time and mixing after composite meals in man. Scan. J. Gastroenterol, 9, 261-270.

Le Fevre, M.E., Hancock, D.C. and Joel., D.D. 1980. Intestinal barrier to large particulate in mice. J. Toxicol. Environ. Health, 6, 691-704.

Loening - Baucke, V. and Anuras, S. 1983. Effects of a meal on the motility of the sigmoid colon and rectum in healthy adults. AM. J. Gastroenterol. 78, 393-£)7.

Malagoela, J.R. 1977. Quantification of gastric solid-liquid discrimination during digestion of ordinary meals. Gastroenterology 72, 1264-1267.

Martin, J.L., Beck, W.J., McDonald, A.P., Carlson, G.M., and Mathias, J.R., 1983. Tc-99m - labelled solid-phase meal: A quantitative clinical measurement of human gastric emptying. J. Clin. Gastroenterol., 5, 315-319.

Meves, V.M. and Beger, H.G. 1979. Gastric emptying in patients with ulcers ventriuli. Z. Gastroenterol. 17(4), 215-221.

Patowary, A.G., Patowary, S. and Ahmed, G., 1983. A study on intestinal transit time on healthy volunteers in Assam. Trop. Gastroenterol. 4, 104-108.

Poulsen, s.s., Kirkegaard, P., Olsen, P.S., Jensen, K.K. and Christiansen, J. 1982. Rate of delayed gastric emptying in the pathogenesis of cysteamine - induced duodenal ulcer in the rat. Scan. J. Gastroenterol. 17, 325-330.

Read, N.W., Cammack, J., Edwards, C., Holgate, A.M., Cann, P.A. and Brown, C. 1982. Is the transit time of a meal through the small intestine related to the rate at which it leaves the stomach? Gut. 23, 824-828.

Rinetti, M., Ugolotti, G., Zinelli, L.C., Calbiani, B. and Frigeri, S., 1982. A study of gastric kinetics (comparison between different isotope carriers). Ric. Clin. Lab. 12, 607-612.

Smith, C.M., DeLuca, H.F., Tanaka, Y. and Mahaffey, K.A. 1978. Stimulation of lead absorption by vitamid D administration. J. Nutr. 108, 843-847.

Stewart., J.J., 1981. Interactions of reserpine and morphine on rat intestinal transit. J. Pharmacol. Exp. Ther. 216(3), 521-5.

Thompson, D.G., Richelson, E. and Malagelada, J.R. 1982. Perturbation of gastric emptying and duodenal motility through the central nervous system. Gastroenterology. 83, 1200-1206.

Volkheimer, G. 1977. Persorption of particles: Physiology and pharmacology. Adv. Pharmacol. Chemother., 14, 163-187.

Weisbrodt, N.W., Sussman, S.E., Stewart, J.J. and Burks, T.F. 1980. Effect of morphine sulphate on intestinal transit and myaelectric activity of the small intestine of the rat. J. Pharmacol. Exp. Therap. 214, 333-338.

Williams, E.W. and Hemmings, W.A., 1978. Intestinal uptake and transport of proteins in the adult rat. Proc. R. Soc. Lond. (B). 203, 177-189.

Wright, R.A., Krinsky, S., Fleeman, C., Trujilo, J. and Teague, E., 1983. Gastric empty and obesity. Gastroenterology. 84, 747-751.

6
Modelling the deposition and retention of particulate materials in the lung

6.1   Introduction

            In a previous study (Thorne and Jackson, 1983) metabolic
models for several metals and semi-metals were developed under the
assumption that the ICRP model for deposition and retention of radioactive particulates in the lungs (ICRP, 1979) was applicable. Because
the ICRP model is based on that recommended by the ICRP Task Group on
Lung Dynamics nearly twenty years ago (ICRP, 1966), it was thought
appropriate to reconsider the lung model to be used in conjunction
with the systemic retention models proposed for the metals and semi-
metals under consideration. Particular areas which required review
are discussed in detail below. They include:

-    the effects of exposure conditions, aerosol characteristics and
     respiratory parameters on the amount of inhaled particulate
     material deposited in the respiratory tract and on the distribu-
     tion of that material between the different regions of the tract;

-    the clearance of deposited material in the first few days after
     deposition, taking account of the effects of disease, smoking
     habits and other modifying factors;

-    the dissolution of particulate material in the lung, together
     with the fate of the material liberated by dissolution, whether
     retained in the lung and associated tissues or transferred to the
     systemic circulation;

-    the translocation of particulate material within and from the
     deep lung, including clearance via the mucociliary escalator as
     well as movement via the lymphatic system and within tissues.

            While particular consideration is given to the materials for
which systemic models have been developed, i.e. arsenic, beryllium,
cadmium, chromium, nickel and lead, data and models for other materials are reviewed in so far as they help to give an understanding of
the relevant processes occurring in the respiratory system.

6.2   The anatomy and physiology of the respiratory tract

6.2.1   Gross anatomy

Schematically, the respiratory tract is as shown in Fig. 6.1. Air normally passes through the following regions: nasal cavity, pharynx, larynx, trachea, bronchi and gas exchange (pulmonary) region. For descriptive purposes the respiratory tract is sometimes divided into an upper respiratory tract, comprising the nasal cavity and related sinuses, pharynx and larynx, and a lower respiratory tract, comprising all levels below the larynx (Ballantyne and Schwabe, 1981). With respect to clearance of particles, it is often convenient to distinguish the lower respiratory tract into the air passages of the tracheo-bronchial region and the gas exchange, or pulmonary, region (ICRP, 1966). A brief anatomical description of these various regions was given by Ballantyne and Schwabe (1981) and is summarised below.

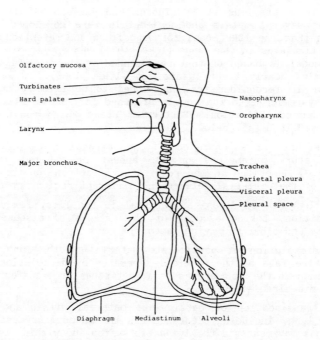

FIGURE 6.1.   DIAGRAMMATIC REPRESENTATION OF THE HUMAN RESPIRATORY TRACT.   From Ballantyne and Schwabe (1981).

6.2.1.1 Nasal cavity and pharynx

The cavity of the nose lies above the hard palate and is divided into left and right halves by a vertical midline nasal septum. Each separate nasal cavity opens in front to the atmosphere through a naris, or nostril, and is in free communication posteriorly with the nasopharynx. The free margin of the soft palate, lying behind, and attached to, the hard palate, can be moved up to the wall of the pharynx, isolating the nasopharynx from the oropharynx. This action prevents materials from passing into the nasopharynx during swallowing or vomiting.

A widened part of the nasal cavity, lying just behind the nares, is referred to as the vestibule and in its anterior part has many coarse hairs which filter large particles from inspired air. The posterior part of the vestibule and the remainder of the nasal cavity are lined with a highly vascular ciliated mucosa. Cilia-driven movement of the mucus is responsible for the transport of deposited foreign material to the nasopharynx where it is either swallowed or coughed out.

Arising from the side walls of each nasal cavity are the superior middle and inferior turbinates (conchae) which are also covered with a highly vascular mucosal layer.

The nasal cavity acts to transmit, warm and humidify inspired air; remove larger inhaled particles; and generate impulses responsible for the sensation of smell. When the nasal mucosa is congested, as in upper respiratory tract infection or some allergic reactions, the nasal passage may present considerable resistance to air flow.

6.2.1.2 Larynx

The larynx is a complex structure interposed between the pharynx and the trachea. It consists, essentially, of a series of articulating cartilages, muscles and lining mucosa. Two pairs of folds pass anteroposteriorly. Movement of the vocal folds forms part of the mechanism isolating the respiratory tract during swallowing and plays a major role in voice production.

6.2.1.3 Trachea, bronchi and alveolar region morphometry

The trachea is a cylindrical structure 10 to 12 cm in length and 1.5 to 2.0 cm in diameter. It extends from the lower border of the larynx into the upper part of the thoracic cavity where it divides into left and right major bronchi, which pass to the corresponding lungs. The structure of the tracheo-bronchial tree has been described by Horsfield (1981). The main bronchi have the same shape on section as the trachea, and are situated outside the lung. The right bronchus is much shorter and wider than the left, and the total cross-sectional area of the two may be less than that of the trachea, in marked contradistinction to what occurs further down the airways. Within the lung, the airways divide dichotomously, though an occasional apparent trichotomy occurs, which can be interpreted both mathematically and embryologically as two successive dichotomies with a suppressed, or very short, branch between them. On the right, the main bronchus divides into the upper lobe bronchus and the first part of the lower lobe bronchus, which in turn divides into the middle lobe bronchus and second part of the lower lobe bronchus. On the left, the main bronchus divides into upper and lower lobe bronchi. The five lobar bronchi give rise, by further division, to 19 named bronchopulmonary segment branches. The bronchopulmonary segments are units of bronchial and blood supply, and can be separately removed without dividing major vessels or bronchi below those supplying the segment itself. From this level downward, the summed cross-sectional area of the airways increases at each dichotomy, while the individual diameters progressively decrease.

After a varying number of dichotomies the bronchi become bronchioles, the most peripheral of which are the terminal bronchioles. These are the most 'peripheral' structures not to bear an alveolus and number about 25,000. Many airways angle back upon their parent branches so that their peripheral bronchi are situated deep within the lung substance.

The geometry of the conducting airways is of considerable importance in determing the deposition of inhaled particles in the micron size range. Weibel (1963) described early work on this topic and reported in detail on his own morphometric studies. He distinguished two types of dichotomy, i.e. 'regular' and 'irregular'. In a regular dichotomy, the conjugate elements are of equal dimensions and branch off their parent at equal angles. As Weibel noted, "in a strict sense this situation is quite improbable in nature". Nevertheless, Weibel proposed a lung model, his lung model A, which incorporated such a regular dichotomy. This model has been used widely in theoretical studies of tracheo-bronchial deposition (see below), and, therefore, requires some discussion.

The basic assumptions of the Weibel's model 'A' are as follows:

-    the airways multiply by regular dichotomy so that all elements (branches) in a given generation, z, have identical dimensions;

-    all generations are complete.

The airways of the model branch over 23 generations which can be grouped into three zones. These are:

-    the conductive zone comprising generations 0 to 16;

-    the respiratory bronchioles comprising generations 17 to 19;

-    the alveolar ducts and sacs comprising generations 20 to 23.

The number of airways in each generation, n(z) is given by:

$$n(z) = 2^z$$

Airway diameters, D(z), lengths, L(z), total airway cross-section at any generation, A(z), and overall volume of airways in each generation, V(z), are given by the following formulae:

$D(z) = 1.8e^{-0.388z}$ cm for $z \leq 3$

$D(z) = 1.3e^{-(0.2929-0.00624z)z}$ cm for $z > 3$

$L(z) = 12e^{-0.92z}$ cm for $z \leq 3$

$L(z) = 2.5e^{-0.17z}$ cm for $z > 3$

$A(z) = 2.54e^{-0.083z}$ cm^2 for $z \leq 3$

$A(z) = 1.32e^{(0.1074+0.0125z)z}$ cm^2 for $z > 3$

$V(z) = 30.5e^{-1.003z}$ cm^3 for $z \leq 3$

$V(z) = 3.3e^{(0.0125z-0.0626)z}$ cm^3 for $z > 3$

The constants used refer to an average sized adult human lung at 75% maximal inflation. It has a total air volume of about 4.8 l, of which 66% is contained in the alveoli.

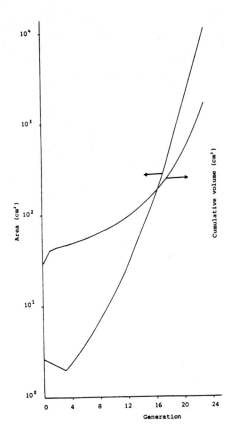

FIGURE 6.2.   AIRWAY AREA AND CUMULATIVE VOLUME AS A FUNCTION
OF GENERATION NUMBER IN THE WEIBEL 'A' LUNG MODEL.

TABLE 6.1

MORPHOMETRIC PARAMETERS OF THE LUNGS AS CALCULATED
FROM THE WEIBEL 'A' MODEL

Generation	Number	D(cm)	L(cm)	A(cm^2)	V(cm^3)	ΣL(cm)	ΣV(cm^3)
0	1	1.80E+0	1.20E+1	2.54E+0	3.05E+1	1.20E+1	3.05E+1
1	2	1.22E+0	4.78E+0	2.34E+0	1.12E+1	1.68E+1	4.17E+1
2	4	8.28E-1	1.91E+0	2.15E+0	4.10E+0	1.87E+1	4.58E+1
3	8	5.62E-1	7.60E-1	1.98E+0	1.50E+0	1.95E+1	4.73E+1
4	16	4.45E-1	1.27E+0	2.48E+0	3.14E+0	2.07E+1	5.04E+1
5	32	3.51E-1	1.07E+0	3.09E+0	3.30E+0	2.18E+1	5.37E+1
6	64	2.81E-1	9.01E-1	3.94E+0	3.55E+0	2.27E+1	5.73E+1
7	128	2.27E-1	7.61E-1	5.17E+0	3.93E+0	2.35E+1	6.12E+1
8	256	1.86E-1	6.42E-1	6.94E+0	4.45E+0	2.41E+1	6.57E+1
9	512	1.54E-1	5.41E-1	9.55E+0	5.17E+0	2.46E+1	7.08E+1
10	1024	1.30E-1	4.57E-1	1.35E+1	6.16E+0	2.51E+1	7.70E+1
11	2048	1.10E-1	3.85E-1	1.95E+1	7.52E+0	2.55E+1	8.45E+1
12	4096	9.50E-2	3.25E-1	2.90E+1	9.42E+0	2.58E+1	9.39E+1
13	8192	8.28E-2	2.74E-1	4.41E+1	1.21E+1	2.61E+1	1.06E+2
14	16384	7.32E-2	2.31E-1	6.88E+1	1.59E+1	2.63E+1	1.22E+2
15	32768	6.54E-2	1.95E-1	1.10E+2	2.15E+1	2.65E+1	1.43E+2
16	65536	5.92E-2	1.65E-1	1.81E+2	2.97E+1	2.67E+1	1.73E+2
17	131072	5.43E-2	1.39E-1	3.04E+2	4.22E+1	2.68E+1	2.15E+2
18	262144	5.04E-2	1.17E-1	5.24E+2	6.14E+1	2.69E+1	2.77E+2
19	524288	4.74E-2	9.89E-2	9.26E+2	9.16E+1	2.70E+1	3.68E+2
20	1048576	4.51E-2	8.34E-2	1.68E+3	1.40E+2	2.71E+1	5.08E+2
21	2097152	4.34E-2	7.04E-2	3.12E+3	2.20E+2	2.72E+1	7.28E+2
22	4194304	4.24E-2	5.94E-2	5.95E+3	3.53E+2	2.72E+1	1.08E+3
23	8388608	4.19E-2	5.01E-2	1.16E+4	5.82E+2	2.73E+1	1.66E+3

Note: Based on Weibel (1963); D = tube diameter: L = tube length:
       A = total cross-sectional area: V = volume of generation:
       ΣL and ΣV = cumulative values of L and V.

Results from the model are listed in Table 6.1. For comparison, total airway cross-section and cumulative lung volume are
plotted as a function of airway generation and as a function of depth
of penetration, i.e. total length of airway traversed, in Figs. 6.2
and 6.3 respectively.

A particular feature of the lung which is well illustrated
in Figs. 6.2 and 6.3 is the very considerable increase in airway area
with generation number. The implications of this in respect to deposition are discussed below, here it is sufficient to note that it
implies much higher air velocities centrally than peripherally during
inspiration and expiration.

Weibel (1963) also proposed a lung model based on irregular
dichotomy. In this model, the lung was supposed to be divided into η_u
units, each one being supplied by an entrance bronchus of diameter D^*.
Each of these units was assumed to have an equivalent volume v_u and to
contain an equivalent number of alveoli. Weibel took, as a point of
departure, $D^* = 2$ mm and found that $\eta_u = 400$ and $v_u = 12$ ml. He
reported that bronchi of diameter 2mm were found in generations 4 to
13 and that their density in each generation, z, could be well approximated by a binomial distribution:

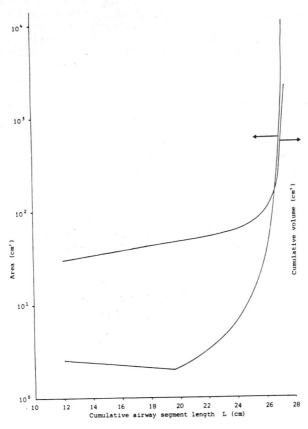

FIGURE 6.3.   AIRWAY AREA AND CUMULATIVE VOLUME AS A FUNCTION OF
CUMULATIVE AIRWAY SEGMENT LENGTH IN THE WEIBEL 'A'
LUNG MODEL.

$$f_2(z) = 10!p^{z-4}(1-p)^{14-z}/(14-z)!(z-4)!$$

Furthermore, the density of branches with $D^*=2mm$ found at a distance Δ from the root of the trachea was well represented by a normal distribution:

$$F_2(\Delta) = 0.157e^{-0.078(\Delta-24.5)^2}$$

The functions $f_2(z)$ and $F_2(\Delta)$ fix the locations of the entrance bronchi. Beyond these, 14 generations of regular dichotomy can be assumed taking dimensions from the Weibel 'A' model for generations 9 to 23. Weibel (1963) also gave more complex formulations for smaller airways, but did not attempt to justify these by reference to his observations.

More recent studies of lung morphometry have concentrated on asymmetries of the tracheo-bronchial tree and have included additional morphometric parameters, such as airway branching angles. Thus, Phalen et al. (1978) presented morphometric data for several mammalian species in terms of an idealised model comprising three connected tubular segments. This morphometric model uniquely defines an identification number for each branch segment, a branching angle, an airway segment length and diameter, an inclination of each segment and the degree of alveolarisation of each segment. Phalen et al. (1978) presented illustrative data for branching angles, diameter ratios and length: diameter ratios as a function of diameter of the parent bronchus, but did not apply their model to deposition calculations. However, Yeh and Schum (1980) extended the work of Phalen et al. (1978) using a silicone rubber replica cast of the tracheo-bronchial airways of a 60 year old male subject who died of a myocardial infarction. No abnormalities in the lung were observed in lung sections. Every airway segment with a diameter of 3mm or more and about 20% of the rest, randomly selected, were measured to the nearest 0.1 mm for length and diameter and 5° for angles. On the basis of these data, Yeh and Schum (1980) developed the concept of a "typical path lung model". A computer program was written to trace all available pathways from the trachea down to each terminal bronchiole. Taking the trachea as generation 1 (generation 0 in the Weibel 'A' model) the number of pathways terminating at various generations was counted to form a frequency distribution. From this distribution, the median generation number was obtained. The median values and observed ranges were as follows:

Lobe	Generation number between trachea and terminal bronchioles	
	Range	Median
Right Upper	9-20	15
Right Middle	10-20	15
Right Lower	12-22	17
Left Upper	11-22	15
Left Lower	13-22	16
Whole lung	9-22	16

The limited inter-lobe variation in median values contrasts strongly with the wide intralobe variation in individual values and suggests that morphometric distinctions in lobar structure may be of limited significance.

Having determined median generation numbers, mean or median geometric parameters were determined by tracing all pathways terminating at the median generation number. These parameters included airway segment diameters, lengths, branching angles and gravity angles. The number of segments in each generation, N_n, was calculated using:

$$N_n = X^{n-I}$$

where

n   is the generation number; and

I   is the generation number of the main stem segment.

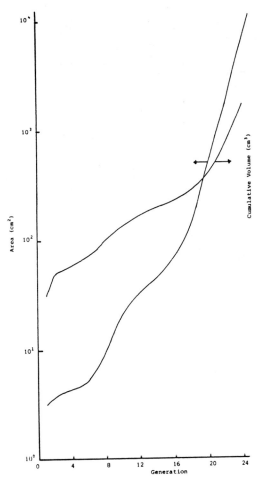

FIGURE 6.4. AIRWAY AREA AND CUMULATIVE VOLUME AS A FUNCTION OF GENERATION NUMBER IN THE YEH AND SCHUM MODEL.

TABLE 6.2

MORPHOMETRIC PARAMETERS OF THE LUNGS AS CALCULATED
FROM THE MODEL OF YEH AND SCHUM

Generation	No. of tubes	D(cm)	L(cm)	Θ^0	Φ^0	A(cm^2)	V(cm^3)	ΣL(cm)	ΣV(cm^3)
1	1	2.01	10.0	0	0	3.17	31.73	10.0	31.73
2	2	1.56	4.36	33	20	3.82	16.67	14.36	48.40
3	4	1.13	1.78	34	31	4.01	7.14	16.14	55.54
4	8	0.827	0.965	22	43	4.30	4.15	17.11	59.69
5	16	0.651	0.995	20	39	5.33	5.30	18.10	64.98
6	32	0.574	1.01	18	39	8.28	8.36	19.11	73.35
7	64	0.435	0.890	19	40	9.51	8.47	20.00	81.81
8	128	0.373	0.962	22	36	13.99	13.46	20.96	95.27
9	256	0.322	0.867	28	39	20.85	18.07	21.83	113.34
10	512	0.257	0.667	22	45	26.56	17.72	22.50	131.06
11	1024	0.198	0.556	33	43	31.53	17.53	23.05	148.59
12	2048	0.156	0.446	34	45	39.14	17.46	23.50	166.05
13	4096	0.118	0.359	37	45	44.79	16.08	23.86	182.13
14	8192	0.092	0.275	39	60	54.46	14.98	24.13	197.10
15	16384	0.073	0.212	39	60	68.57	14.54	24.34	211.64
16	32768	0.060	0.168	51	60	92.65	15.57	24.51	227.21
17	65536	0.054	0.134	45	60	150.09	20.11	24.65	247.32
18	131072	0.050	0.120	45	60	257.36	30.88	24.77	278.20
19	262144	0.047	0.092	45	60	454.81	41.84	24.86	320.04
20	524288	0.045	0.080	45	60	833.84	66.71	24.94	386.75
21	1048576	0.044	0.070	45	60	1594.39	111.61	25.01	498.36
22	2097152	0.044	0.063	45	60	3188.78	200.89	25.07	699.25
23	4194304	0.043	0.057	45	60	6090.97	347.19	25.13	1046.44
24	8388608	0.043	0.053	45	60	12181.95	645.64	25.18	1692.08
25	3×10^8	0.030	0.025	45	60	–	3871.80	25.21	5563.88

Note: Derived from Yeh and Schum (1980); Θ = branching angle; Φ = gravity angle, with 90^0 corresponding to a horizontal tube; other quantities as Table 6.1.

Experimentally, X was determined as 1.99, but a value of 2, corresponding to dichotomous branching, was used for simplicity. The model was extended to include several generations of respiratory bronchioles, alveolar ducts, sacs and alveoli, assuming a total of 3×10^8 alveoli (Weibel, 1963) and a total lung capacity of 5600 cm^3 for a Reference Man (ICRP, 1974). Results for the whole lung are summarised in Table 6.2, while total areas and cumulative lengths are plotted against generation number and total path length in Figs. 6.4 and 6.5 respectively.

A third detailed analysis of human lung morphometry was that carried out by Horsfield and his co-workers (Horsfield and Cumming, 1968; Horsfield et al., 1971; Cumming, 1974; Horsfield et al., 1976). These data were discussed by Horsfield (1981) and used in a model for mucus transport by Yeates and Aspin (1978). The ordering system used by Horsfield (1981) differs from that employed in the simple symmetric dichotomous or pseudo-symmetric dichotomous systems described above.

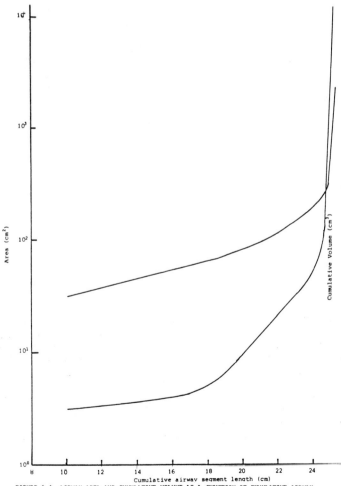

FIGURE 6.5. AIRWAY AREA AND CUMULATIVE VOLUME AS A FUNCTION OF CUMULATIVE AIRWAY
SEGMENT LENGTH IN THE YEH AND SCHUM MODEL.

In the Horsfield system, end branches are of order 1 and the rules are:

- two order n branches meet to form a branch of order n+1;
- where two branches of differing order meet the parent branch is one order more than the order of the higher of the two daughter branches.

On this basis, Horsfield (1981) gave the following summary of the number and dimensions of the conducting airways.

Horsfield order	Number	Diameter (cm)	Length (cm)
28	1	1.60	10.00
27	1	1.11	2.20
26	2	1.05	3.80
25	2	0.70	1.20
24	2	0.70	0.97
23	3	0.67	1.13
22	6	0.59	1.13
21	8	0.54	0.97
20	12	0.43	1.08
19	14	0.35	0.95
18	20	0.35	0.86
17	30	0.31	0.99
16	37	0.29	0.80
15	46	0.28	0.92
14	64	0.27	0.82
13	85	0.25	0.81
12	114	0.24	0.77
11	158	0.22	0.64
10	221	0.20	0.63
9	241	0.18	0.52
8	499	0.16	0.48
7	760	0.14	0.42
6	1104	0.11	0.36
5	1675	0.095	0.31
4	2843	0.076	0.25
3	5651	0.064	0.11
2	11300	0.056	0.13
1	25000	0.051	0.11

In this nomenclature, orders 28 to 25 include the trachea, main bronchi and lower lobe bronchi; orders 24 to 20 include other lobar and broncho-pulmonary segment bronchi; orders 19 to 5 include intrasegmental bronchi; orders 4 to 2 are bronchioles; and order 1 represents the terminal bronchioles. It is noted that only a fraction of paths traverse all orders in this model. For this reason, cross-sectional areas and cumulative volumes cannot be computed straight-forwardly as in the geometrically less complex models. However, it is noted that Horsfield (1981) has interpreted the data of Hansen and Ampaya (1975) as indicating an initial increase and subsequent de-crease in total cross-sectional area with total path-length from the trachea. While superficially this appears to be in contradiction with

results from the simpler models, this is primarily a result of including real variations in path length from trachea to alveolar sacs,
or terminal bronchioles.

The above discussion has related exclusively to the morphometric characteristics of a small number of adult human lungs. It is
recognised that intersubject variations in these characteristics will
exist.   The significance of these is discussed in the context of
calculations of aerosol deposition. It is also important to note that
the lungs are not fully developed at birth and that there is a considerable period of postnatal development.   An account of early
studies on this topic was given by Dunnill (1962) who also reported
data on twenty lungs from ten children aged from birth to eight years,
in addition to several adult lungs.   The total number of alveoli
increased from 2.4×10^7 at birth to $\sim 8 \times 10^7$ at 3 months, $\sim 1.6 \times 10^8$ at 2
years and $\sim 2.8 \times 10^8$ at 8 years. The number of alveoli present in the
8-year-old was comparable with the value of 2.96×10^8 given for the
adult. The total number of respiratory airways increased to a similar
extent; from 1.5×10^6 at birth to $\sim 7 \times 10^6$ at age 2 years and $\sim 1.4 \times 10^7$ at
8 years or more.   Dunnill (1962) particularly noted that the fraction
of lung volume occupied by tissue in the infant was considerably
larger than that recorded for the adult. A mathematical model for
post-natal growth of the human lung has recently been described by
Hofmann (1982). In this model, the Weibel 'A' structure was taken as a
basis, since theoretical deposition data obtained using this model
were stated to be in fair agreement with experimental results.   However, Hofmann noted that the methodology proposed can be applied to
the more detailed anatomical models of Horsfield and Cumming (1968)
and Yeh and Schum (1980).   The basis of the model is summarised as
follows.

-   Morphometric studies have shown that the non-respiratory air
    passages, down to the level of the terminal bronchioles, are
    complete at birth.   Therefore, in generations 0 to 16 the number
    of airways was assumed to remain constant during post-natal
    growth.

-   With progressing age, each individual branch of the non-respira-
    tory airways was taken to grow in a symmetrical way both in
    length and diameter and in constant relationship to the whole
    organ.

-   Most of the post-natal increase in size of the lung comes from
    the respiratory structures which grow not only by increasing in
    size, but also by increases in the total number of alveoli and
    respiratory airways.

-   Growth in number of respiratory airways and alveoli is largely
    completed by eight years of age.

On the basis of these assumptions, and by fitting a variety
of anatomical data, Hofmann (1982) proposed the following analytical
functions:

Diameter of trachea (mm)
$$d(t) = (1-e^{-0.07t})12.71 + 5.5$$

Length of trachea (cm)

$$l(t) = (1-e^{-0.1t})8.72 + 4$$

Diameter of main bronchi (mm)

$$d(t) = (1-e^{-0.12t})8.63 + 4.2$$

Length of main bronchi (mm)

$$l(t) = (1-e^{-0.1t})29.31 + 15$$

Diameter of terminal bronchioles (mm)

$$d(t) = (1-e^{-0.1t})0.57 + 0.08$$

Number of 'respiratory airways'

$$N(t) = \{[1.13(t-6)-(1.13(t-6)^2+2)^{0.5}]0.92 +14.04\}10^6$$

Diameter of alveoli (μm)

$$d_{alv}(t) = (1-e^{-0.2t})172.76 + 100$$

Number of alveoli

$$N_{alv}(t) = [(1-e^{-0.4t})286.21 + 37.6]\ 10^6$$

Total lung volume (l)

$$V_{tot}(t) = [0.23(t-22)-(0.23(t-22)^2 + 0.5)^{0.5}]0.53-5.6$$

Hofmann (1982) commented that experimental data on diameters and lengths of trachea, main bronchi and terminal bronchioles lead to the supposition that their growth can be described by very similar functions. For this reason, it was assumed that the increase in airway dimensions for generations 2 to 16 could be represented by the functions for the main bronchi.

Hofmann (1982) also considered respiratory standards as a function of age. These are discussed in detail in Section 6.2.3.

It is noted that Hughes et al. (1972) studied the effects of lung inflation on airway dimensions in excised lungs of dogs and reported that changes in bronchial length and also in many cases diameter, were proportional to the cube root of the absolute lung volume. No difference was found in the percentage changes for airways of different sizes. It was also noted that changes in length and diameter were in many cases greater than would have been predicted from the behaviour of airways dissected free of lung tissue, suggesting that bronchi in situ are exposed to distending forces in excess of transpulmonary pressure. Further discussion of the morphometric structure of the human lung, in the context of particle deposition is given by Raabe (1982).

The structure of the respiratory region of the lung has been summarised by Ballantyne and Schwabe (1981) and is illustrated in Fig 6.6. Each terminal bronchiole gives rise to a series of respiratory bronchioles. These in turn open into alveolar ducts which divide into several alveolar sacs. The alveolar sacs and ducts, and the respiratory bronchioles, communicate with numerous surrounding alveoli. About 200 alveoli are supplied per respiratory bronchiole. The diameter of the alveoli varies with the stage of breathing, but averages about 0.25 mm. It has been estimated that there are $\sim 3 \times 10^8$ alveoli per lung and that, in healthy adult subjects, the internal surface area of the lung varies from 40 to 80 m^2.

6.2.2   Detailed structure

In order to appreciate mechanisms of clearance of particulate material from the lungs some information on the cellular architecture of the respiratory system is required. Recent reviews on this topic include those of Corrin (1981) and Gil (1982) from which the following brief summary is taken.

6.2.2.1   Conductive zone

The respiratory epithelium, which lines the trachea and bronchi, is traditionally described as consisting of pseudo-stratified ciliated cells interspersed with occasional goblet cells. This type of epithelium is found from the trachea to the bronchioles, with only a gradual reduction in cell height and pseudo-stratification signifying a more peripheral location. In the small bronchioles, goblet cells are scanty and ciliated cells are outnumbered by Clara cells. In addition to these three main cell types, there are also found basal, intermediate, serous, brush and endocrine cells. The cells are bound to each other by desmosomal attachments and, near the surface of the

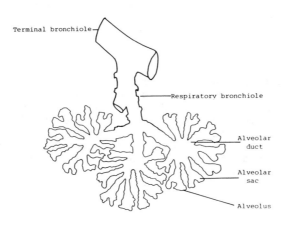

FIGURE 6.6. SCHEMATIC REPRESENTATION OF THE RELATIONSHIPS OF THE
TERMINAL AND RESPIRATORY BRONCHIOLES, AND THE ALVEOLAR
COMPLEX. From Ballantyne and Schwabe (1981).

lumen, by tight junctions. Within the epithelium there may also be migrating leucocytes without desmosomal attachments and deep in the surface epithelium are bronchial glands of mixed sero-mucous type (Corrin, 1981). The extraordinary complexity of the airway epithelium has only recently been recognised. It acts as an epithelial lining, a mechanical and immunological defence organ, and a secretory tissue (Gil, 1982).

The two cell types of particular interest in respect of lung clearance are the ciliated and goblet cells. The ciliated cells, which account for the bulk of the cell population, are responsible for moving mucous secretions. They are columnar, with abundant mito-chondria, secondary lysosomes, rough endoplasmic reticulum, multi-vesicular bodies, smooth vesicles and well-developed Golgi. Their lumenal surface is covered with long slender microvilli and approx-imately 250 cilia per cell, each 6 μm long and 0.3 μm wide (Gil, 1982). The cilia beat in an aqueous lining layer and mucus is thought to be found as discrete particles on the surface of this film (Corrin, 1981). Ciliary action and the movement of mucus is discussed in detail in Section 6.4.1.

Goblet cells vary in appearance with a cycle of activity which culminates in discharge of mucus into the lumen of the airways. Devoid of mucus, they are slender and exhibit abundant endoplasmic reticulum as well as a well-developed Golgi. Toward the lumen are found mucus granules of fibrillary, granular or homogeneous structure. As these accumulate they fuse to produce a large secretion vacuole which distends the apical cell cytoplasm to give the cell its charac-teristic wine-glass, or goblet, shape. Discharge takes place by further fusion involving the secretion vacuole and apical cell mem-branes, and mucus is often seen extending from the discharging secre-tory vacuole some distance into the lumen (Corrin, 1981).

Clara cells require a brief mention because of their import-ance in the bronchiolar region. These smooth-surfaced cells are most numerous in the peripheral airways where they tower above the more cuboidal ciliated cells, which they equal or exceed in number. Clara cells have been proposed as a source of bronchiolar surfactant inde-pendent of the alveoli, both in respect of the lipidic surface layer and in respect of the aqueous hypophase (Corrin, 1981).

The submucosal seromucous glands are thought to be the main source of tracheo-bronchial secretions. They consist of a ciliated duct continuous with the surface epithelium, a collecting duct lined with tall nonciliated cells and of mucous and secretory end-pieces (Gil, 1982). Mucous secretion appears to be a discontinuous process, whereas serous secretion is continuous (Corrin, 1981). The precise nature of the serous secretions is not known, but they may include enzymes used to modulate the final composition of the mucus produced by the mucous cells of the glands.

6.2.2.2 Respiratory zone

The gas exchanging parenchyma consists, at minimum, of an endothelium and a thin epithelium. A diagrammatic representation of alveolar fine structure is shown in Fig. 6.7. The type I alveolar epithelial cell covers almost all the interalveolar septum; it is a cell with few organelles, but remarkable for its very thin cytoplasmic extensions. Cytoplasmic processes of this cell may even spread through the interalveolar septum to line the opposite side. On one side of a septum alone, a type I cell may cover over 2000 μm^2 yet measure as little as 0.2 μm in thickness. Type I cells are connected to each other and to type II cells by tight junctions and this epithe-lium forms the major barrier to fluid movement into, and out of, an alveolus. However, pinocytotic fluid transport does occur, as does macromolecular transport to the interstitium. Furthermore, although the phagocytic potential of type I cells is very limited, extremely small particles may gain entry to the alveolar interstitium by a pinocytotic transport mechanism similar to that for fluids (Corrin, 1981).

Type II alveolar epithelial cells are slightly more numerous than are type I cells. However, they cover little of the surface of the alveolar septum, being generally cuboidal, or low columnar, in profile. They are generally found occupying a niche in a corner of an alveolus and often all but the apical pole is covered by neighbouring type I cells. The free surface bears blunt microvilli and the cyto-plasm contains many mitochondria, a plentiful rough endoplasmic reti-culum, Golgi apparatus and distinctive osmiophilic lamellar vacuoles. Type II cells are regarded as the source of pulmonary surfactant. This surfactant consists of an aqueous hypophase and surface-active lipid layer. The surfactant layer is reported to be relatively thick

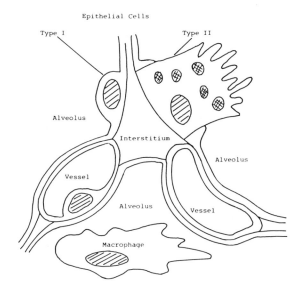

FIGURE 6.7. DIAGRAMMATIC REPRESENTATION OF ALVEOLAR FINE
STRUCTURE. From Corrin (1981).

in the corners of the alveoli and thin over lateral extensions of the
type I cells. It is continuous with the mucus lining of the airways
and may thereby contribute to sputum (Corrin,1981).

The alveolar capillaries form a mesh with quite small
(∿10 µm) inter-capillary gaps filled with interstitial tissue. The
capillary wall consists of endothelium resting on a basement membrane
and, on one side or other of the interalveolar septum, the capillary
is closely applied to the alveolar epithelium. In this region, the
endothelial and epithelial basement membranes fuse to form a single
lamina giving an air/blood barrier thickness of 0.15 µm. Elsewhere,
interstitial tissue separates endothelium from epithelium, so that the
arithmetic mean thickness of the air/blood barrier is 1.25 µm and the
harmonic mean thickness is 0.57 µm. In contrast to the alveolar
epithelium, the endothelial cell junctions readily permit the passage
of small molecular weight proteins. Larger molecules, e.g. albumin,
are retained, but small amounts can cross the endothelium into the
interstitium by pinocytotic transport (Corrin, 1981).

The interstitial space contains collagen and elastin fibre
bundles, an occasional elongated interstitial cell, unmyelinated axons
attended by Schwann cells and two types of nerve endings. While some
interstitial cells resemble fibroblasts, others represent a cell form
intermediate between blood monocytes and alveolar macrophages. Kinetic studies indicate that the interstitium is the immediate source of
alveolar macrophages, though the ultimate source is the bone marrow.
It appears that the number of intra-alveolar macrophages may be increased in response to challenge by both enhanced migration of marrow-
derived interstitial cells and division of pre-existing intra-alveolar
cells (Corrin, 1981).

Migration of intra-alveolar macrophages is discussed in
detail in the context of translocation of inhaled particulate material
from the respiratory region (Section 6.4.4.1).

6.2.3   Mechanisms of breathing

In this Section, concern is solely with the flow of air
into, and out of, the lungs. A discussion of gas exchange is outside
the scope of this review and considerations of particle transport in
the airflow, and deposition from it, are dealt with in later sections.

Movement of air into and out of the lungs is effected by
sinusoidal alterations in the volume of the thoracic cavity, with the
lungs following these volume changes as a result of fluid mediated
adhesion between the visceral and parietal pleura. Due to the elastic
properties of the lungs and thoracic wall, work is necessary to increase the volume of the lungs on inspiration. This work is performed
by contraction of the intercostal muscles, which increases the trans-
verse and anteroposterior dimensions of the thoracic cavity, and by
contraction of the musculature of the diaphragm, which increases the
vertical dimensions of the cavity. During resting breathing, movements of the diaphragm contribute about 75% to ventilation (Ballantyne
and Schwabe, 1981). In contrast, expiration is essentially a passive
process governed by controlled muscular relaxation.

When there are increased breathing requirements, accessory
muscles are invoked to raise the sternum and increase the anteropost-

erior dimensions of the thorax. Also, expiration is facilitated by contraction of the abdominal muscles to force the viscera against the diaphragm and displace it upward into the thoracic cavity (Ballantyne and Schwabe, 1981).

In discussing breathing, particularly with respect to particle inhalation and deposition, several quantities are conventionally defined. Most of these are illustrated in Fig. 6.8, which is taken from Raabe (1982). Definitions of the various quantities of interest are given below.

Tidal Volume (TV) - the volume of air inhaled or exhaled in a single breath.

Inspiratory Capacity (IC) - the maximum volume of air that can be inspired at the end of a normal tidal expiration.

Inspiratory Reserve Volume (IRV) - the maximum volume of air that can be voluntarily inhaled after a normal tidal inspiration; i.e. the difference between the inspiratory capacity and the tidal volume.

Expiratory Reserve Volume (ERV) - the maximum volume of air that can be voluntarily exhaled at the end of a normal tidal expiration.

Residual Volume (RV) - the volume of air remaining in the respiratory tract following a maximum possible expiration.

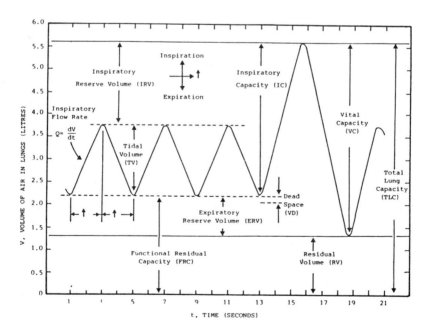

FIGURE 6.8. PARAMETERS USED IN RESPIRATORY PHYSIOLOGY ILLUSTRATED USING A HYPOTHETICAL SPIROMETRIC RECORD OF BREATHING PATTERNS. From Raabe (1982).

Functional Residual Capacity (FRC) - the volume of air remaining in the respiratory tract at the end of a normal tidal expiration, i.e. the sum of the expiratory reserve volume and residual volume.

Dead Space Air (VD) - the volume of air in those parts of the respiratory tract which are not involved in gas exchange. The anatomical dead space, i.e. the volume of air in the respiratory system above the respiratory bronchioles, is distinguished from the physiological dead space which may include some nonfunctioning alveoli. The existence of nonfunctioning alveoli or alveoli with reduced function occurs both in pathological conditions and in the normal individual in the erect position, since, for the latter, blood flow, and hence gas exchange, is reduced at the apices of the lungs.

Vital Capacity (VC) - the maximum volume of air that can be exhaled following a maximum inspiration, i.e. the sum of inspiratory reserve volume, tidal volume and expiratory reserve volume.

Forced Expiratory Volume (FEV_t) - the proportion of the vital capacity that can be exhaled in a fixed period of time t (seconds). Typically, $FEV_{0.75}$ or FEV_1 values are used as indices of airway resistance.

Total Lung Capacity (TLC) - the sum of the vital capacity and the residual volume.

Inspiratory Flow Rate (Q) - the rate of change of lung volume on inspiration.

Respiratory Frequency (F) - the number of cycles of inspiration plus expiration in unit time.

Other derived quantities include the respiratory minute volume, (the volume of air breathed per minute), the maximum voluntary ventilation (the largest volume of air that can be breathed in a given period) and the alveolar ventilation.

The concept of alveolar ventilation requires some further description. When the tidal air is inspired it is carried down the bronchial tree to the respiratory portion of the lungs. However, only a proportion of the tidal air reaches the alveoli, the remainder occupying the volume of displaced air in the nasal cavity, pharynx, trachea, bronchi and nonrespiratory bronchioles. This is the anatomical dead space air and is typically ~140 ml. Thus, the alveolar ventilation is defined as the difference between the tidal and dead space volumes multiplied by the breathing rate. It is important to note that the presence of dead space air means that variations in breathing rate and tidal volume will produce differing alveolar ventilations for a given respiratory minute volume.

For reference, some typical values of respiratory parameters were given by Ballantyne and Schwabe (1981) and are listed below.

Parameter	Volume (ml)	
	Men	Women
Tidal Volume	500	500
Inspiratory Capacity	3800	2400
Inspiratory Reserve Volume	3300	1900
Expiratory Reserve Volume	1000	700
Residual Volume	1200	1100
Vital Capacity	4800	3100
Functional Residual Capacity	2200	1800

It is noted that tidal volume and respiratory frequency vary considerably with degree of exertion and that, in addition, resting values vary considerably with age. From an analysis of available data, Hofmann (1982) has proposed the following functions for tidal volume (ml) and respiratory frequency (min.$^{-1}$) at rest as functions of age, t (years):

$$TV(t) = 21.7 + 35.13t - 0.64t^2$$

$$F(t) = 15.17/(0.25t + 0.5) + 11.75$$

Data for varying levels of activity at different ages were given by the ICRP (1974) and are summarised below:

Individual	Activity level	F (min^{-1})	TV (ml)	Minute volume (l)
Adult	Rest	12-15	500-750	6-7.5
Man	Light activity	~16	~1500	20-29
	Heavy work	21	2000	43
	Maximal work	40	3000	110
Adult	Rest	12-16	340-650	4.5-10
Woman	Light activity	~20	~900	16-19
	Heavy work	30	880	25
	Maximal work	46	2100	90
Adolescent	Rest	~15	~300	~5
	Maximal work	~50	1900-2500	90-110
Child	Rest	16	300	4.8
	Light activity	24	600	14
	Maximal work	60-70	500-1300	34-71
Infant (1y)	Rest	30	48	1.4
Newborn	Rest	34	15	0.5

With respect to average inspiratory flow rate, Raabe (1982) gave a value of 43.5 l min^{-1}, corresponding to a tidal volume of 1450 ml and a respiratory frequency of 15 min^{-1}, for conditions of light activity.

Finally, in respect of breathing patterns, it is noted that particle deposition in the lungs can be very different following mouth, as opposed to nose, breathing. The degree to which individuals breath through the nose is very variable, depending on personal habits, activity and state of health. Some quantitative data on this subject were given by Camner and Bakke (1980) who reported that, in healthy subjects, the volume of air breathed through the nose during casual conversation is less than 50% of the volume breathed through the nose during quiet reading. Camner (1981) later interpreted these results as indicating that 80% of air is inhaled via the nose during reading and that ~40% is inhaled via the nose during quiet conversation.

6.3   Deposition

6.3.1   Introduction

Five major processes of particle deposition in the respiratory tract are commonly identified (Raabe, 1982). These are:

- interception;

- impaction;

- gravitational settling;

- electrostatic attraction;

- brownian diffusion.

When, as a result of any of these processes, a particle contacts the walls of the airways it is irreversibly removed from the airstream. The contact process can occur during inspiration or expiration of a single breath, or subsequently, if the particle has been transferred to unexhaled lung air. Deposition increases with duration of breath holding and depth of breathing (Raabe, 1982).

The five major processes of particle deposition are illus-

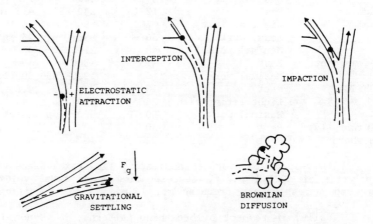

FIGURE 6.9.   REPRESENTATION OF FIVE MAJOR MECHANISMS OF DEPOSITION
OF INHALED AIRBORNE PARTICLES IN THE RESPIRATORY TRACT.
From Raabe (1982).

trated schematically in Fig. 6.9. Interception consists of non-inertial incidental meeting of a particle and a surface and, therefore, depends on the physical size of the particle. The probability of this process would be zero for pointlike particles and is of importance primarily for particles with large aspect ratio, e.g. asbestos fibres.

Impaction is of major importance for deposition in the nasopharyngeal and tracheo-bronchial regions. In this process, changes in direction or magnitude of air velocity streamline or eddy components are not duplicated by airborne particles because of their inertia and, as a result, the particles impact upon surfaces.

Gravitational settling occurs because of modification of particle velocities relative to the airflow by the acceleration due to gravity and deposition due to diffusion is the result of velocity modifications induced by random collisions of small particles with air molecules.

Electrostatic attraction, due to the induction of image charges in the airway walls, is probably a minor mechanism of deposition in most cases, but may have to be included as a deposition enhancing factor for some aerosols and is relevant in interpreting the results of some experimental studies on deposition.

A more detailed discussion of the various deposition processes is given later in this section. However, as a basis for this discussion, it is convenient first to define the relevant physical characteristics of the depositing aerosols.

6.3.2   Aerosol characteristics

An aerosol is a relatively stable suspension in a gas of very small liquid drops or solid particles. If the particles are smooth and spherical, or near spherical, their respective sizes can be conveniently described in terms of their respective geometric diameters. However, aerosols of solids rarely contain smooth spherical particles and various conventions are employed to represent the physical characteristics of the individual particles by single numerical values. In the present context, the most useful parameters are those relating to aerodynamic properties and in particular to diffusive and inertial characteristics.

The diffusive diameter of a particle is equal to the geometric diameter of an ideal spherical particle with the same diffusivity as the actual particle under identical conditions. This quantity is primarily of interest for particles with a physical diameter of less than 0.5 µm.

An aerodynamic diameter has customarily been used to describe the aerodynamic properties of a particle. The most common definition is the diameter of a unit density sphere having the same settling speed under gravity as the particle in question. Based on Stoke's Law, the terminal settling speed of a spherical particle for viscous settling conditions is given by:

$$V_t = g\rho C(D) \; D^2/18\eta$$

TABLE 6.3

SLIP CORRECTION FACTORS AS A
FUNCTION OF PARTICLE DIAMETER

Diameter (μm)	Slip correction factor $[C(D)]$	$C(D)D^2$
0.01	24.199	0.00242
0.02	12.383	0.00495
0.04	6.499	0.01040
0.06	4.556	0.01640
0.08	3.597	0.02302
0.1	3.029	0.03029
0.2	1.937	0.07748
0.3	1.601	0.1441
0.4	1.443	0.2309
0.5	1.351	0.3378
0.6	1.292	0.4651
0.8	1.218	0.7795
1.0	1.174	1.174
1.5	1.116	2.511
2.0	1.087	4.348
3.0	1.058	9.522
4.0	1.044	16.704
6.0	1.029	37.044
8.0	1.022	65.408
10.0	1.017	101.700

where

g   is the acceleration due to gravity (9.8 m s^{-2} at sea level);

ρ   is the difference in density between the particle and the gas;

D   is the physical diameter of the particle;

η   is the viscosity of the gas (1.85x10^{-4} P for air at 25°C); and

C(D) is a slip correction factor, which is a semi-empirical correction required when the aerosol particles are almost as small, or smaller, than the mean free path of air molecules.

Raabe (1982) gave the following formulae for the slip correction factor for spherical particles:

$$C(D) = 1 + 2A(\lambda/D)$$

$$A = \alpha + \beta \exp(-\gamma D/2\lambda)$$

where

λ   is the mean free path of the gas molecules,

α   = 1.26,

β   = 0.45,

γ   = 1.08, and

λ   is 0.0646 μm at 21°C or 0.0692 μm at 37°C for air at sea level.

Using λ = 0.0692 μm, appropriate for air in the respiratory tract, the slip correction factor as a function of D is as listed in Table 6.3. It is emphasised that the aerodynamic diameter is mainly of relevance for particles with diameters of greater than 0.5 μm. Thus, the slip correction factor is usually less than 1.35 in practical applications.

      Using the above equations, the aerodynamic diameter of a particle is given by:

$$C(D_{ad})D_{ad}^{2} = \rho C(D)D^{2}$$

where

D_{ad} is the aerodynamic diameter.

For convenience of comparison values of the function $C(D)D^{2}$ are given in Table 6.3.

      Because aerosols rarely consist of particles of a single size they must necessarily be characterised by a distribution, which is conveniently expressed mathematically as a probability density function in aerodynamic or physical dimensions. The function most usually used is the log-normal distribution, which, for diameter is given by:

$$f(D) = \exp \{-(\ln D - \ln D_0)^2 / 2(\ln \sigma_g)^2\} / \sqrt{(2\pi)}(\ln \sigma_g)D$$

where

   D_0 is the count median diameter; and

   σ_g is the geometric standard deviation of the distribution.

Alternatively, distributions are often expressed in terms of the mass of the particles, i.e. $f(M)$ rather than $f(D)$. It is noted that a log-normal distribution in D implies a log-normal distribution in M for which:

$$M_0 = \pi \rho D_0^3 / 6$$

$$\ln \sigma_g^M = 3\ln \sigma_g^d$$

where

   ρ is the density of the particles; and

   σ_g^m, σ_g^d relate to the mass and diameter distributions respectively.

In the literature, distinction is often made between poly-disperse and monodisperse aerosols. It is emphasised that monodisperse aerosols are not composed of particles of a single size, but are characterised by small values of σ_g, typically less than 1.22. Further discussions on the topic of aerosol characteristics are given by Raabe (1982) and Morrow (1981).

6.3.3   Deposition mechanisms

There have been a large number of accounts of mechanisms governing deposition in the respiratory system (e.g. Raabe, 1982; Morrow, 1974; Stuart, 1973; Yeh et al., 1976; Taulbee and Yu, 1975). These reviews should be consulted as a supplement to the brief comments given below. In addition, attention is directed to a review of the mechanics of aerosols by Fuchs (1964).

6.3.3.1   Inertial impaction

In inertial impaction, the inertia of an airborne particle tends to cause it to travel in its initial path when the supporting airstream is suddenly deflected, e.g. at the turbinates or bifurcations in the bronchial tree. The probability of inertial deposition, has been stated (Stuart, 1973) to exhibit the following functional dependence.

$$P_I \ \alpha \ U_t U \sin\theta / R$$

where

U_t is the terminal settling velocity of the entrained particle;

U is the velocity of the airstream;

θ is the angle of the bend; and

R is the radius of the airway.

Raabe (1982) quoted a formula developed by Yeh for impaction at a bend, as relevant, and appropriately simple, for calculating impaction at an airway branch. This formula is:

$$P_I = 1-(2/\pi)\cos^{-1}(\theta.Sk/2) + (1/\pi)\sin[2\cos^{-1}(\theta.Sk)]$$

where

Sk   is Stoke's number;

θ is the bending angle; and

the expression applies for $\theta.Sk/2<1$.

Values of Sk are given by:

$$Sk = 2L_s/d$$

where

L_s is the stopping distance; and

d   is the tube diameter.

Yeh et al. (1976) gave an expression for Stoke's number of the following form:

$$Sk = C\rho_p r_p^2 \bar{v}/9\mu R$$

where

C   is the slip correction factor;

ρ_p is the particle density;

r_p is the particle radius;

$\bar{v}$ is the mean flow velocity;

μ is the fluid viscosity; and

R   is the tube radius.

It will be noted that the term $C\rho_p r_p^2$ in the above formulation can be replaced by $C(D_{ad})$ $D_{ad}^2/4$ where D_{ad} is the aerodynamic diameter discussed above (Section 6.3.2). Also, $\bar{v}$ for a given respiratory system will be almost exactly proportional to the inspiratory or expiratory flow rate. For these reasons, it is generally convenient to plot deposition efficiencies against $\bar{Q}D_{ad}^2$, where $\bar{Q}$ is the mean inspiratory flow rate.

6.3.3.2   Gravitational settling

The probability of deposition by gravitational settling is usually estimated with equations describing gravitational settling of particles in an inclined cylindrical tube under laminar flow conditions (Raabe, 1982);

$$P_s = (2/\pi)[2K(1-K^{0.667})^{0.5} - K^{0.333}(1-K^{0.667})^{0.5}\sin^{-1}(K^{0.333})]$$

with K, the characteristic parameter, given by:

$$K = t\rho_p C(D)D^2 g.\cos\beta/48\eta R$$

where

t   is the residence time in the tube;

g   is the acceleration due to gravity;

β   is the inclination angle relative to the horizontal; and

all other quantities are as defined previously.

As with impaction, settling probabilities are determined by D_{ad}^2. However, in contrast to impaction, K decreases as $\bar{Q}$ increases. Thus, a relevant parameter for plotting deposition in the gravitational settling regime is $D_{ad}^2/\bar{Q}$.

6.3.3.3   Diffusion

For diffusion it is appropriate to consider airways separately from the respiratory region of the lung. In the airways, Raabe (1982) has argued that diffusive deposition, P_D, can be calculated using the Thomas modification of the Gormley-Kennedy equation, i.e.

$$P_D = 1-0.819\exp(-1.828u) + 0.097\exp(-11.15u)+0.032\exp(-28.5u)$$

$$+0.027\exp(-61.5u)+0.025\exp(-375u)$$

with

$$u = 2\pi\Delta L/Q.$$

In this expression, Q is the volumetric flow rate, L is the length of the tube and Δ is the particle diffusion coefficient. The above expression assumes that the aerosol is well mixed at the entrance of the cylinder and may, therefore, over-estimate deposition in conditions where there is limited mixing from one generation of airways to the next.

The degree of diffusion of a particle is dependent upon its physical, rather than its aerodynamic, size. Diffusive deposition in the lung is mainly of important for particles with diameters of less than 0.5 μm, whereas impaction and sedimentation are more important for larger particles. For this reason, it is conventional to report data in terms of physical size for particles of less than 0.5 μm diameter and in terms of aerodynamic size for larger particles (Raabe, 1982).

For alveolar deposition by diffusion, Stuart (1973) cited the formulation of Landahl (1950):

$$D = 1-\exp(-0.58\Lambda/r)$$

where

D   is the fractional deposition;

r   is the dimension ('radius') of the confining space; and

Λ is the average Brownian displacement after time t.

Stuart (1973) gave the following formula for calculating Λ for particles in air:

$$\Lambda = \left(\frac{RT}{N} \cdot \frac{Ct}{3\pi\gamma D}\right)$$

where

R   is the gas constant;

T   is the absolute temperature;

N   is Avogadro's number;

C   is the slip correction factor;

t   is the time of residence;

δ is the viscosity of the gas; and

D   is the diameter of the particle.

6.3.4   Total deposition

In discussing total deposition of aerosols in the human respiratory system, reliance can be placed, almost exclusively, on direct measurements made on human subjects. In such studies particle densities are measured in the inhaled and exhaled air and differences are attributed to deposition (Davies et al., 1972). By studying the time course of exhaled air concentrations in such experiments, it is possible to obtain some information on the depth of penetration of the aerosol into the respiratory system and on the mixing phenomena which occur. Thus, Davies (1972) reported that mixing between tidal and reserve air takes place in the dead space above the respiratory bronchioles. In contrast, in the alveolated regions there is no mixing, so that the tidal air penetrates and retreats axially and is surrounded by a sheath of reserve air which is itself separated from the walls by the residual air. On the basis of exhaled air concentrations, Davies (1972) calculated that 0.5 µm particles are airborne for a mean time of 14.8s in the reserve air and 6.8s in the residual air.

On the basis of experimental data for 0.5 µm aerosols, Heyder and Davies (1971) developed a compartmental model for dispersion of aerosols in the lungs which gave the possibility of predicting

TABLE 6.4

CONSTANTS USED FOR CALCULATION OF THE
DEPOSITION OF PARTICLES IN THE LUNGS
DURING STEADY BREATHING THROUGH THE MOUTH

Particle aerodynamic diameter (μm)	B	C	D	E
0.5	400	50	0.5	3.5
0.7	400	67	0.61	2.7
0.9	370	85	0.68	2.7
1.0	300	92	0.70	3.0
1.1	240	93.5	0.69	3.3
1.2	200	94.8	0.66	3.75
1.3	170	96	0.62	4.4
1.4	140	97	0.52	5.6
1.5	120	98	0.45	6.6
1.75	86	99.5	0.36	9.6
2.0	65	100	0.30	13.3
2.25	50	100	0.24	17.6
2.5	42	100	0.20	22.0
3.0	35	100	0.14	28.0
4.0	30	100	0.07	36.0
5.0	28	100	0.03	39.5
6.0	28	100	0.01	40.4
7.0	28	100	0	38.8
10.0	28	100	0	29.5

Note: from Davies (1981).

the behavious of aerosols in different breathing manoeuvres. However, the transfer coefficients were evaluated only for a single individual breathing according to a single respiratory pattern (see also Davies, 1972a; Davies, 1980).

More recent work of Davies and co-workers has concentrated on predictions of total deposition for different respiratory patterns of mouth breathing and for different subjects (Davies et al., 1977); Davies, 1981). Davies et al. (1977) reported data from 424 experiments on 12 subjects and on the basis of these data proposed the following formula for calculating total deposition in the respiratory system:

$$D_e = V_t/B + C/F^D - E - (V_r - V_{ro})/A$$

where

D_e is the percentage deposition;

V_t is the tidal volume (ml);

F is the frequency of breathing (min^{-1}); and

V_r is the expiratory reserve volume (ml).

The constants A and V_{ro} are taken to be dependent upon subject, but not upon particle size. In contrast, the constants B, C, D and E are taken to be dependent on particle size, but not on subject. The value of A is typically $\sim$300, whereas values of V_{ro} are found to vary over the range 600 to 3500 ml. Values of B, C, D and E as functions of particle size are given in Table 6.4 and deposition fractions for different values of F, V_t and V_r are shown in Fig. 6.10.

Heyder et al. (1980) also considered the effects of particle diameter, particle density, inspiration time and flow rate on total deposition. They proposed a deposition parameter, X_m, defined by:

$$X_m = [\log_{10}(Q/Q_o) - 1.43]\ \log_{10}[(\rho/\rho_o)(d/d_o)^2(\tau/\tau_o)^{24/\sqrt{(Q/Q_o)}}]$$

where

Q is the mean flow rate;

ρ is the particle density;

d is the particle diameter, and

τ is the half-period of the breathing cycle.

The values of the constants were given as $\rho_o = 1\ g\ cm^{-3}$, $d_o = 1\ \mu m$, $Q_o = 1\ cm^3\ s^{-1}$, and $\tau_o = 1\ s$.

Heyder et al. (1980) also gave a physiological representation for X_m as follows:

$$X_m = [\log_{10}(V/30V_o) - 1.43]\log_{10}[(\rho/\rho_o)(d/d_o)^2(30F_o/F)^{24/\sqrt{(V/30V_o)}}]$$

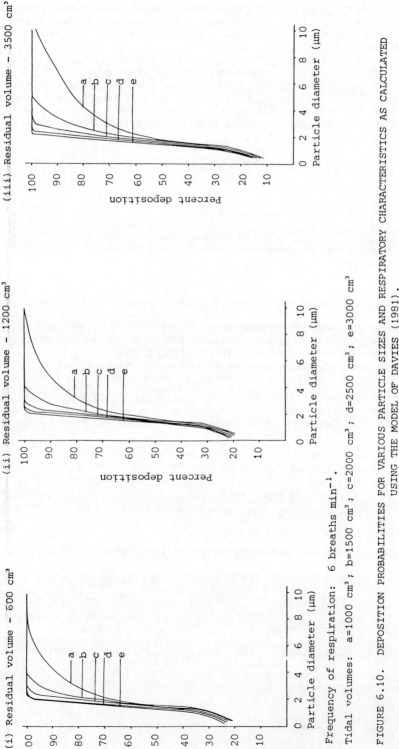

Frequency of respiration: 6 breaths min⁻¹.

Tidal volumes: a=1000 cm³; b=1500 cm³; c=2000 cm³; d=2500 cm³; e=3000 cm³.

FIGURE 6.10. DEPOSITION PROBABILITIES FOR VARIOUS PARTICLE SIZES AND RESPIRATORY CHARACTERISTICS AS CALCULATED
USING THE MODEL OF DAVIES (1981).

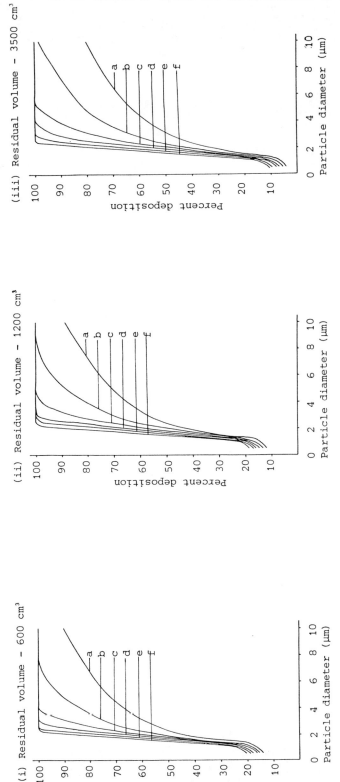

(i) Residual volume – 600 cm³

(ii) Residual volume – 1200 cm³

(iii) Residual volume – 3500 cm³

Frequency of respiration: 12 breaths min⁻¹.

Tidal volumes: a=500 cm³ ; b=1000 cm³ ; c=1500 cm³ ; d=2000 cm³ ; e=2500 cm³ ; f=3000 cm³ .

FIGURE 6.10   Contd.

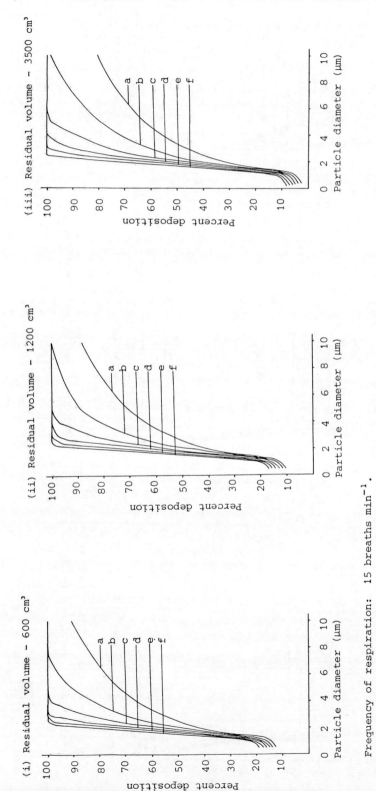

(i) Residual volume – 600 cm³

(ii) Residual volume – 1200 cm³

(iii) Residual volume – 3500 cm³

Frequency of respiration: 15 breaths min⁻¹

Tidal volumes: a=500 cm³; b=1000 cm³; c=1500 cm³; d=2000 cm³; e=2500 cm³; f=3000 cm³.

FIGURE 6.10 Contd.

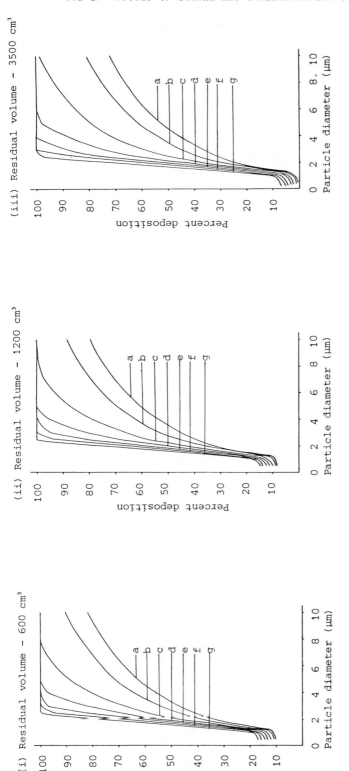

FIGURE 6.10   Contd.

Frequency of respiration: 20 breaths min⁻¹.

Tidal volumes: a=250 cm³ ; b=500 cm³ ; c=1000 cm³ ; d=1500 cm³ ; e=2000 cm³ ; f=2500 cm³ ; g=3000 cm³ .

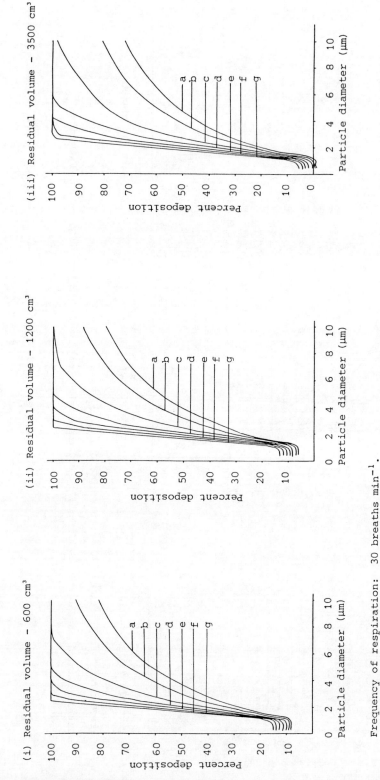

(i) Residual volume – 600 cm³

(ii) Residual volume – 1200 cm³

(iii) Residual volume – 3500 cm³

Frequency of respiration: 30 breaths min⁻¹.

Tidal volumes: a=250 cm³; b=500 cm³; c=1000 cm³; d=1500 cm³; e=2000 cm³; f=2500 cm³; g=3000 cm³.

FIGURE 6.10   Contd.

Breathing rate (min⁻¹)	Tidal Volume (ml)	Minute Volume (ml)	Aerodynamic diameter (μm)	X_M	Deposition (%) Davies (1)	Deposition (%) Heyder et al (2)
6	1000	6000	0.5	0.51	0.19	0.15
			2.5	1.73	0.72	0.68
			7.5	2.56	0.97	0.90
	2000	12000	0.5	0.28	0.22	0.12
			2.5	1.92	0.96	0.75
			7.5	3.03	1.00	0.94
15	500	7500	0.5	-0.14	0.11	0.08
			2.5	1.21	0.48	0.35
			7.5	2.14	0.80	0.82
	1000	15000	0.5	-0.35	0.12	0.07
			2.5	1.42	0.60	0.50
			7.5	2.63	0.97	0.90
	2000	30000	0.5	-0.59	0.14	0.05
			2.5	1.61	0.84	0.60
			7.5	3.11	1.00	0.94
30	250	7500	0.5	-0.58	0.06	0.05
			2.5	0.77	0.35	0.20
			7.5	1.69	0.72	0.66
	500	15000	0.5	-0.76	0.07	0.05
			2.5	1.01	0.41	0.28
			7.5	2.22	0.81	0.85
	1000	30000	0.5	-0.95	0.08	0.04
			2.5	1.25	0.52	0.40
			7.5	2.75	0.97	0.92
	2000	60000	0.5	-0.11	0.11	0.09
			2.5	1.49	0.76	0.54
			7.5	3.27	1.00	0.95

Notes: 1. based on A=300, $V_r = V_{ro} = 1200$ ml.
      2. estimated from Fig.6.11.

TABLE 6.5

COMPARISON OF DAVIES AND HEYDER ET AL MODELS OF TOTAL DEPOSITION IN MOUTH BREATHING

where

   V   is the minute volume;

   F   is the breathing rate;

   V_o is 1 cm³ min⁻¹; and

   F_o is 1 min⁻¹.

   The dependence of total deposition for controlled mouth breathing on the parameter X_m is shown in Fig. 6.11.

   In view of these two different analyses of total deposition based on distinct data sets, it is appropriate to compare the two methods of calculation for a range of values of F and V_t. This is done in Table 6.5. Taking into account the substantial intersubject variability that is known to occur in total deposition, the two models can be stated to give very similar results.

   A recent theoretical analysis of total, and regional, deposition is that presented by Yu and Diu (1983). This model included contributions from impaction, sedimentation and diffusion and gave results which were reasonably satisfactory representations of total

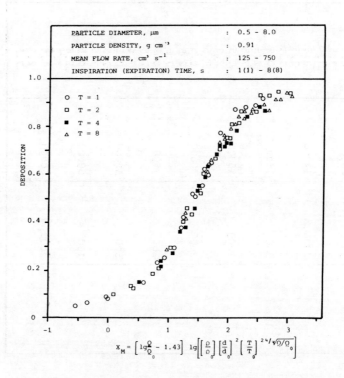

FIGURE 6.11.   DEPENDENCE OF TOTAL DEPOSITION FOR CONTROLLED MOUTH-
BREATHING ON THE DEPOSITION PARAMETER X_M. From
Heyder et al. (1980).

TABLE 6.6

REGIONAL DEPOSITION OF AEROSOLS AS MEASURED BY LIPPMANN AND ALBERT (1969)

Subject	d_m	Minute vol.(l)	Average inspiratory flow(l min^{-1})	Total deposition (%)	Regional deposition (%)			
					Mouth	P-L	T-B	Alv.
DA	3.02	10.8	22.8	90.9	0.77	51.49	32.89	14.85
	5.33	8.7	18.4	91.0	16.15	56.70	23.85	3.30
RA	4.45	7.1	14.2	[41.2]	–	–	52.91	47.09
	4.65	21.5	35.6	97.1	39.65		33.16	27.19
	4.77	16.2	61.3	88.6	53.50		42.78	3.72
	3.56	19.0	–	87.7	9.12	5.70	34.09	51.08
	3.43	9.8	–	86.9	3.22	2.53	26.35	67.89
	5.03	15.1	–	95.9	22.52	45.26	19.29	12.93
RB	3.68	17.5	36.7	95.7	16.30	33.65	43.57	6.48
	4.96	16.2	33.9	90.7	26.35	31.64	37.82	4.19
	2.46	15.2	30.2	[69.9]	1.57	–	64.95	33.48
	3.16	17.0	32.5	[7.6]	3.68	–	79.87	16.45
	5.76	16.1	36.5	97.2	16.98	56.28	>24.90	<1.85
	7.25	17.3	36.3	98.7	29.08	46.61	>23.30	<1.01
	1.34	11.1	25.7	81.3	1.85	10.95	24.48	62.73
	2.04	10.0	22.1	77.6	1.42	14.18	28.74	55.67
RJB	3.90	19.1	34.4	92.3	1.95	29.47	65.11	3.47
	5.04	19.1	35.5	95.6	2.41	40.69	54.08	2.82
VB	3.94	15.7	28.1	95.3	4.41	38.72	44.39	12.49
	5.19	16.2	26.6	97.9	11.13	34.73	49.85	4.29
WB	3.77	14.1	32.8	97.7	40.33		47.70	11.98
	2.59	6.3	20.2	70.9	4.09	21.30	29.90	44.71
	5.14	12.7	23.6	96.9	21.88	48.92	26.63	2.58
	6.80	13.3	22.2	97.9	29.62	53.52	>16.64	<0.20
	5.00	12.0	–	96.2	20.79	10.40	66.74	2.08
	5.10	16.3	–	97.9	45.97	15.73	32.89	5.41
CC	3.68	21.0	40.4	69.7	2.58	17.07	63.41	16.93
	3.90	17.0	38.5	92.1	19.22	50.49	20.30	9.99
	5.19	20.3	39.5	93.3	60.34	5.79	27.12	6.75
	4.05	15.2	28.0	93.5	73.26		13.37	13.37
	5.33	16.0	32.2	99.3	85.10		14.90	–
FC	3.41	20.4	41.7	95.4	12.37	21.28	46.44	19.92
	4.65	26.2	45.6	92.4	13.10	22.84	58.98	5.09
NC	3.41	19.7	42.8	92.5	11.57	32.65	45.73	10.05
	∿4.7	22.1	43.4	93.6	14.21	42.20	38.35	5.24
	4.05	23.2	45.5	97.3	38.34	40.70	16.75	4.21
	5.10	23.7	47.7	96.1	32.99	46.72	16.65	3.64
RD	3.62	13.9	30.8	[84.1]	13.08	–	78.24	8.68
	4.98	17.2	34.7	[75.4]	28.25	–	70.29	1.46
MH	3.59	21.4	42.5	92.8	10.45	42.67	32.76	14.12
	4.93	23.2	44.4	97.2	13.37	60.80	23.25	2.57
EK	3.74	15.5	29.9	82.2	9.25	22.63	31.39	36.74
	5.12	17.4	34.5	83.5	16.29	35.93	31.02	16.77

TABLE 6.6 (Contd.)

Subject	d_m	Minute vol.(l)	Average inspiratory flow(l min^{-1})	Total deposition (%)	Regional deposition (%)			
					Mouth	P-L	T-B	Alv.
KK	3.60	11.3	21.3	100.0	10.40	25.40	55.90	8.30
	4.90	12.8	23.6	99.9	18.12	30.23	47.05	4.60
	2.10	18.0	35.3	88.3	1.25	2.94	39.30	56.51
	2.84	17.4	33.3	93.7	2.88	13.87	54.11	29.14
GL	3.78	18.2	36.6	83.5	24.67	13.65	28.38	33.29
	5.89	13.9	26.7	84.2	15.44	31.47	44.06	9.03
	7.90	13.8	29.4	93.0	30.22	38.60	>30.86	<0.32
	4.79	17.1	36.9	92.3	13.33	37.38	37.49	11.81
	7.16	16.2	35.2	96.0	19.27	42.92	36.67	1.15
ML	4.64	16.0	36.0	89.2	61.66		27.58	10.76
	4.82	19.4	63.8	99.2	85.38		11.69	2.92
	2.36	23.8	48.6	89.4	4.25	15.88	31.99	47.87
	3.77	18.9	37.5	92.2	6.83	20.07	55.53	17.57
	6.76	21.5	43.7	97.3	30.11	49.95	17.99	1.95
	2.91	12.4	–	96.1	11.76	2.81	34.13	51.30
	5.05	17.8	–	97.6	41.80	41.80	11.48	4.92
SL	4.05	12.1	29.3	94.4	23.73	37.71	31.99	6.57
	5.15	14.2	31.8	Error in original publication				
FN	3.80	11.0	23.8	96.7	3.93	51.60	34.23	10.24
	5.04	12.7	26.2	96.6	9.83	66.77	21.53	1.86
AO	3.76	7.2	20.7	75.7	27.48		61.69	10.83
HTP	3.56	12.6	34.4	99.1	4.14	71.75	21.49	2.62
	4.86	10.6	30.0	98.0	6.84	75.20	17.45	0.51
	1.82	11.2	27.3	85.0	1.29	23.41	37.65	37.65
	2.42	13.8	30.5	90.7	0.99	32.52	45.20	21.28
JR	4.12	15.9	32.6	95.1	24.08	43.53	25.24	7.15
	5.08	17.7	36.2	96.6	53.93	25.57	17.81	2.69
LR	5.48	13.9	26.9	100.0	6.20	44.90	46.90	2.00
CS	3.76	14.6	30.1	88.0	12.50	53.07	26.25	8.18
	5.02	12.9	30.4	94.3	15.38	51.01	29.90	3.71
CQS	3.63	20.4	37.2	87.7	11.40	32.73	33.52	22.35
	4.95	25.1	48.0	99.5	11.86	39.10	43.12	5.93
DS	3.66	15.6	34.0	94.0	4.47	43.30	41.81	10.43
	4.99	19.6	42.6	97.3	31.96	44.50	20.55	2.98
	2.34	16.8	32.9	74.2	1.08	0.67	22.64	75.61
	3.22	15.9	30.4	79.1	4.42	36.92	35.78	22.89
	7.08	16.2	30.0	92.7	45.09	36.03	17.91	0.97
GVS	3.52	21.7	39.4	92.8	20.15	38.47	31.03	10.34
	4.85	20.3	40.8	96.4	34.65	41.70	21.27	2.39
IS	4.04	18.8	40.9	96.7	10.55	54.60	26.47	8.38
	5.30	14.1	28.4	97.1	14.42	67.25	15.96	2.37
BA	5.20	15.0	–	94.3	19.72	38.81	37.33	4.14
DB	4.80	17.5	–	96.3	58.98	23.57	16.61	0.83
FB	5.20	13.5	–	94.5	31.32	16.19	44.66	7.83

TABLE 6.6 (Contd.)

Subject	d_m	Minute vol.(1)	Average inspiratory flow(1 min^{-1})	Total deposition (%)	Regional deposition (%)			
					Mouth	P-L	T-B	Alv.
HB	5.30	14.0	−	91.7	29.77	39.48	27.70	3.05
DH	5.30	13.5	−	95.5	34.87	44.19	19.90	1.05
HGP	5.10	19.8	−	96.8	45.04	19.01	29.55	6.40
LP	4.90	11.7	−	93.3	45.02	8.36	39.66	6.97
JS	4.80	16.3	−	94.8	34.39	2.11	60.34	3.16
	5.20	16.0	−	97.2	53.50	20.68	25.82	0.00

Notes: from Lippmann and Albert (1969); d_m is mass median diameter (μm); regional deposition values are relative to total deposition; P-L = pharynx plus larynx; T-B = tracheobronchial region; Alv. = alveolar region.

and regional deposition under various breathing regimes.

There have been a large number of experimental studies on total deposition in the human respiratory system in addition to those on which the models of Davies and Heyder et al. are based. In addition some animal studies are relevant to this topic.

Thus, Stokinger et al. (1951) demonstrated distinctions in lobar deposition in rats, with higher concentrations being found in the upper right lobe for 0.45 and 2.6 μm particles. This result was confirmed by Sneddon and Brain (1981) who also demonstrated that apex to base gradients occurred irrespective of the orientation of the animal relative to gravity for aerosols with an Activity Median Aerodynamic Diameter (AMAD) of 0.7 to 0.8 μm. Use of different carrier gases (He and SF_6) gave contradictory results for animals in different orientations. The authors were not able to offer an adequate explanation of the apex to base gradients, but noted the combined effects of gravity, aerodynamics, lung density and breathing patterns as potential contributory factors.

Also in rats, Ferin et al. (1983) demonstrated that charged particles of titanium oxide exhibited higher fractional values of deposition than did near-neutral particles. Similar effects have been reported in man. Thus, Melandri et al. (1977) reported on experiments in which volunteers, breathing through the mouth at 12 respirations min^{-1}, inspired monodisperse carnuba wax particles of 0.3 to 1.1 μm diameter. These particles were unipolarly charged with 30 to 110 elementary charges per particle. For 0.75 μm particles, deposition efficiencies increased from ∿25% for neutral particles to ∿38% for particles carrying more than 100 elementary charges (Fig. 6.12). Further work on this topic has recently been reported by this group (Melandri, 1983; 1983a).

Early studies of total deposition in man included those of Landahl et al. (1951), Altshuler et al. (1957), Morrow et al. (1958) for sub-micronic NaCl and Dautrebande et al. (1959) for sub-micron dusts. In addition, attention is drawn to the studies of Lippmann and Albert (1969) which gave detailed data on the partition of inhaled material between different regions of the lung for mouth breathing. Deposition in the mouth was defined as that part of the head deposit recoverable, within the first few minutes after inhalation, by garg-

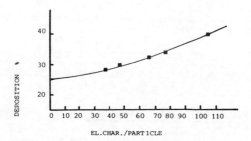

FIGURE 6.12. DEPOSITION EFFICIENCY VS. ELEMENTARY CHARGES CARRIED BY 0.75μm AEROSOL. From Melandri et al. (1977).

ling and mouthwashing. Residual head deposition was designated the pharyngeal and laryngeal (P-L) component. Alveolar deposition was estimated by thoracic counting at 24 h after exposure and tracheo-bronchial deposition was estimated by difference. Results are listed in Table 6.6 and indicate the variability of regional deposition at high values of total deposition, i.e. large X_m values. This can be attributed to the variable filtration efficiency of the mouth in mouth breathing and differences in penetration reflecting differences in airway geometry and breathing pattern.

Lippmann and Albert (1969) demonstrated correlation of deposition with $\rho d^2 Q$, in the cases of head and tracheo-bronchial deposition, and correlation with aerodynamic diameter, in the case of alveolar deposition (Fig. 6.13). However, in each case the range of reported values was large.

Kimura (1971) studied the deposition of monodisperse aerosols of different sizes in the upper, median and pulmonary regions of the respiratory space of a single individual and recorded the following results.

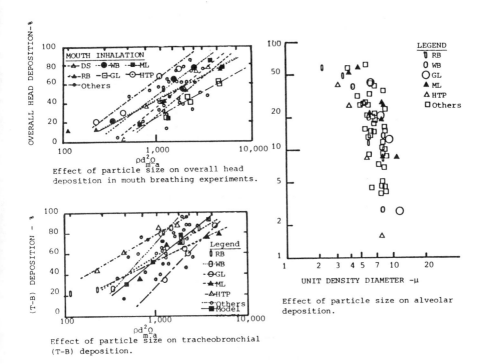

Effect of particle size on overall head deposition in mouth breathing experiments.

Effect of particle size on tracheobronchial (T-B) deposition.

Effect of particle size on alveolar deposition.

FIGURE 6.13. REGIONAL DEPOSITION IN THE HUMAN RESPIRATORY SYSTEM DURING MOUTH BREATHING. From Lippmann and Albert (1969).

Particle diameter (μm)	Condition	Resp. Rate (min⁻¹)	Tidal Vol. (cm³)	Deposition (%)			
				Upper tract	Median tract	Pulmon. space	Total
0.109	rest	20	554	5.5	17.5	18.6	32.0
	exercise	20	821	6.5	12.4	22.5	35.0
	rest	10	751	4.4	15.4	38.7	39.3
	exercise	10	1811	7.2	12.4	51.7	55.5
0.500	rest	20	532	3.3	16.4	21.5	28.2
	exercise	20	983	5.5	12.7	22.4	36.7
	rest	10	850	3.4	13.8	34.8	37.8
	exercise	10	1694	6.0	12.8	47.3	51.8
1.090	rest	20	527	14.0	22.2	36.5	48.5
	exercise	20	798	16.7	25.5	32.3	56.8
	rest	10	789	12.0	26.5	52.4	58.7
	exercise	10	1483	21.0	22.7	69.3	74.2
1.857	rest	20	561	22.8	23.7	34.7	57.2
	exercise	20	910	21.3	32.0	45.0	69.0
	rest	10	995	18.8	36.1	70.0	82.0
	exercise	10	1693	30.5	26.6	76.9	87.6

These data demonstrate that deposition probabilities in the upper respiratory tract decrease rapidly with decreasing particle size, whereas deposition probabilities in the median and pulmonary regions of the tract decrease much less substantially.

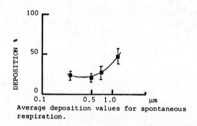

Average deposition values for spontaneous respiration.

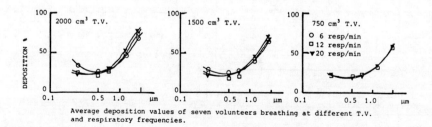

Average deposition values of seven volunteers breathing at different T.V. and respiratory frequencies.

FIGURE 6.14. DEPOSITION EFFICIENCIES FOR NOSE-IN-MOUTH-OUT BREATHING. From Giacomelli-Maltoni et al. (1972).

Giacomelli-Maltoni et al. (1972) studied the deposition of aerosols of carnuba wax during nose-in-mouth-out respiration. These studies concentrated on sub-micron aerosols. Results from these studies (Fig. 6.14) indicate limited effects of tidal volume and respiratory frequence in this size range, with a minimum deposition probability ∿20% for 0.5 µm diameter particles.

Giacomelli-Maltoni et al. (1972) also computed particle deposition efficiencies in the nose by comparing nose-in-mouth-out and mouth-in-mouth-out modes of breathing. Total deposition data and nasal deposition efficiencies from these studies are shown in Fig. 6.15. This illustrates that nasal trapping of particulate material is almost completely ineffective in the sub-micron size range.

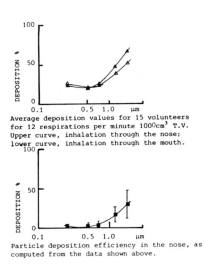

Average deposition values for 15 volunteers for 12 respirations per minute 1000cm³ T.V. Upper curve, inhalation through the nose; lower curve, inhalation through the mouth.

Particle deposition efficiency in the nose, as computed from the data shown above.

FIGURE 6.15. DEPOSITION VALUES AND NASAL DEPOSITION EFFICIENCIES.
From Giacomelli-Maltoni et al. (1972).

Other studies on the total deposition of micron and sub-micron particles of carnuba wax during mouth breathing were reported by Tarroni et al. (1980). Results, shown in Fig. 6.16, indicate a minimum at a particle diameter ∿0.6 µm, but with considerable inter-subject variation in the magnitude of deposition.

Tarroni et al. (1980) also investigated deposition efficiency (DE) as a function of expiratory reserve volume (ERV) for the individuals studied. They demonstrated a unique relationship between DE/DE_N and ERV/ERV_N where DE_N and ERV_N were values appropriate to normal breathing by the individual (Fig. 6.17). As Tarroni et al. (1980) noted the inverse correlation between DE and ERV is in contrast to the positive correlation predicted by Davies model.

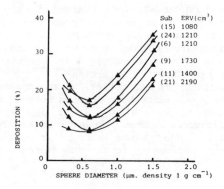

FIGURE 6.16. TOTAL DEPOSITION CURVES AS A FUNCTION
OF PARTICLE SIZE FOR SIX SUBJECTS
From Tarroni et al. (1980).

In respect of the effects of respiratory parameters, Love
and Muir (1978) reported a relationship between total deposition and
respiratory characteristics in coal miners inhaling 1 μm particles of
octyl sebacate. However, the effect was not very marked and was
generally much less than intrinsic inter-subject variability.

Foord and co-workers studied the regional deposition of
monodisperse polystyrene particles in mouth breathing subjects, using
retention at 24 h after inhalation as a measure of pulmonary (respiratory region) retention. A preliminary account of these experiments was given by Foord et al. (1978). Total deposition for 2.5 to
7.5 μm particles was closely related to D^2F where F was the average
inspired airflow and the results were consistent with the model of
Davies (discussed above).

Foord et al. (1978) also demonstrated that the ratio of
pulmonary to pulmonary plus tracheo-bronchial deposition was related

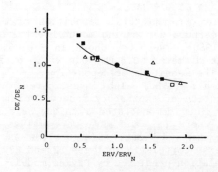

FIGURE 6.17. RELATIVE DEPOSITION DE/DE_N VS RELATIVE
EXPIRATORY RESERVE VOLUME ERV/ERV_N.
From Tarroni et al. (1980).

to D^2F and was consistent with the predictions of the ICRP (1966). The relevant results and comparision are shown in Fig. 6.18.   This comparison factors out mouth deposition, which is somewhat variable, but can be approximated by:

$$M = 20\log_{10}D^2F - 40.7$$

where D^2F, in units of μm^2 l min^{-1}, has a value of more than 108.4.

More recently, Pritchard et al. (1980) compared the deposition of 2.5 to 7.5 μm particles between mouth-breathing smokers and non-smokers.   Results are summarised below:

		Non-Smokers			Smokers	
		Total deposition	P/(P+TB)		Total deposition	P/(P+TB)
D^2F	No.	(% ± s.e.)	(% ± s.e.)	No.	(% ± s.e.)	(% ± s.e.)
125	5	70.0±2.3*	90.6±2.1	5	78.8±2.5*	80.2±6.5
368	6	81.2±2.0	82.5±4.8	6	82.0±2.6	77.3±2.6
500	7	91.1±3.0	72.0±3.1*	6	91.8±1.6	60.5±3.4*
1125	5	95.4±1.3	38.3±7.2	5	95.0±2.3	32.6±7.2
1268	7	93.7±0.8	50.3±8.2	6	94.7±0.5	41.5±8.5

Pairs of results marked with * are significant at $p<0.05$.

These data indicate limited differences in deposition in smokers relative to non-smokers during mouth breathing.

A number of recent studies on deposition are also of note. Thus, Garrard et al. (1981) noted that the pattern of aerosol deposition in healthy humans is influenced by mild degrees of obstruction to airflow and that measurements of initial distribution may be a better clinical measure than is obtained from clearance studies.

Emmett et al. (1982) measured the regional deposition of monodisperse polystyrene particles of between 3.5 and 10 μm diameter in subjects breathing via a mouthpiece (see also Emmett et al., 1979).

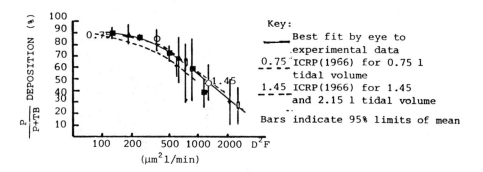

FIGURE 6.18.   AVERAGE PULMONARY DEPOSITION RELATIVE TO THE DEPOSITION IN THE LOWER RESPIRATORY TRACT. From Foord et al. (1978).

Four regional deposits were distinguished, these being:

- an oral deposit, f_o;
- a throat deposit, f_t;
- a tracheo-bronchial deposit, f_{tb}; and
- an alveolar deposit, f_a.

The oral deposit was obtained by repeated mouthwashings within a few moments after aerosol administration. The throat deposit was measured by external gamma scanning. The total tracheo-bronchial plus alveolar deposit was also determined by scanning soon after inhalation and the alveolar deposit was determined by scanning one day after inhalation. Results from these studies are summarised below:

		Deposition (% inhaled)				
Subject	Particle size (μm)	f_o	f_t	f_{tb}	f_a	f_{total}
DCFM	3.5	0.01	0.00	0.26	0.44	0.70
AM	3.5	0.01	0.03	0.23	0.53	0.79
AR	3.5	0.01	0.25	0.22	0.39	0.88
Average		0.01	0.09	0.24	0.45	0.79
HG	5.2	0.01	0.14	0.35	0.29	0.79
RB	5.2	0.02	0.15	0.35	0.38	0.89
PCE	5.2	0.00	0.00	0.37	0.37	0.75
Average		0.01	0.10	0.36	0.35	0.81
PT	8.0	0.04	0.45	0.36	0.06	0.91
PH	8.0	0.04	0.36	0.44	0.10	0.93
KD	8.0	0.10	0.46	0.31	0.09	0.96
Average		0.06	0.42	0.37	0.08	0.93
TDW	10.0	0.06	0.44	0.40	0.04	0.94
JH	10.0	0.17	0.29	0.33	0.08	0.86
AD	10.0	0.05	0.36	0.36	0.07	0.84
Average		0.09	0.36	0.36	0.06	0.88

It is of interest to note that there is significant alveolar deposition even with 10 μm particles and that the magnitude of this deposition is consistent with that predicted by the ICRP (1966).

Stahlhofen and his co-workers have reported several studies on the total and regional deposition of particles in the human respiratory tract using aerosols of di-(2-ethyl-hexyl) sebacate and iron oxide (Heyder et al., 1973; 1980; Rudolf et al., 1983; Stahlhofen et al., 1980; 1983). Heyder et al. (1973) found a total deposition of 10% of an inhaled aerosol of sebacate for all subjects at all particle sizes between 0.2 and 1 μm. For larger particles, deposition increased, reaching ~20% at 1.6 μm diameter. The more extensive data of Heyder et al. (1980) are discussed above, in the context of development of the parameter X_m.

Of particular note is the work of Stahlhofen et al. (1980) who used a special breathing manoevre to deposit 0.6 μm particles of

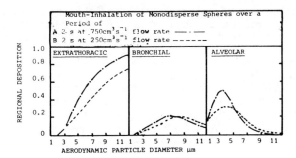

FIGURE 6.19. EFFECT OF PARTICLE SIZE AND FLOW RATE ON
REGIONAL DEPOSITION FOR MOUTH-BREATHING.
From Stahlhofen et al. (1983).

iron oxide exclusively in the alveolar region of the lungs. The
particles were radioactively tagged and their retention in the lungs
was followed, for up to 200 h, by external gamma counting. This study
demonstrated that there is little, or no, early clearance of material
deposited in the respiratory region of the lung and validated the use
of 24h post-inhalation assays in the estimation of such deposition.
Having established the validity of this assay, Stahlhofen et al.
(1980; 1983) produced a variety of results on regional deposition
under various respiratory regimes (see also Rudolf et al., 1983).
These results are illustrated in Figs. 6.19 and 6.20.

Much of the work which has been undertaken on total, or
regional, deposition has involved the use of monodisperse aerosols or
of polydisperse aerosols without any assay of particle size distributions in the inspired and expired air. Recently, Hiller et al. (1982)
have described the use of a single particle aerodynamic relaxation
time (SPART) analyser to provide a detailed real time analysis of
deposition with size for multi-modal or heterodisperse aerosols.

There is also the possibility of using excised human lungs
to study total or regional deposition in vitro (Mitchell, 1977).

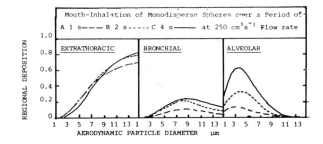

FIGURE 6.20. EFFECT OF PARTICLE SIZE AND INSPIRATION TIME
ON REGIONAL DEPOSITION FOR MOUTH-BREATHING.
From Stahlhofen et al. (1983).

While such studies are of interest, the availability of in vivo data, and observed differences of deposition in the lungs of dogs under in vivo and in vitro conditions (Swift et al., 1977), make data obtained from such studies of secondary importance.

In conclusion, with respect to regional and total deposition studies, attention is drawn to the work and reviews of Davies (1974), Mercer (1975), Yeh et al. (1976) and Chan and Lippmann (1980). The data included in these reviews is discussed in more detail in subsequent sections, but, for comparison, a compilation of deposition data and calculations derived from Chan and Lippmann (1980) is shown in Fig. 6.21.

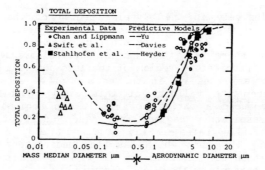

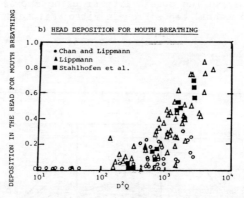

FIGURE 6.21. REGIONAL DEPOSITION DATA AND THEORIES.

6.3.5   Nasal, oral and pharyngeal deposition

Several early studies considered the nasal deposition of inhaled particulate material.   Thus, Boyland et al. (1947) demonstrated that nasal penetration decreased with increasing particle size and flow rate, as did Landahl and Black (1947).   For a particular flow rate, Landahl and Tracewell (1949) demonstrated that nasal penetration was a unique function of an 'equivalent impaction diameter' defined operationally by cascade impactor results.   Asset (1957) emphasised the importance of wind speed on nasal sampling efficiency.   Detailed studies by Vincent and Mark (1982) and by Armbruster and Breuer (1982) have revealed the importance of considering wind speed and direction, together with the shape of the human head and torso, in determining the inhalability of large particles (see also Ogden and Birkett, 1977).   While a full discussion of this subject is outside the scope of this review, it is relevant to note that Vincent and Mark (1982)

c) TRACHEOBRONCHIAL DEPOSITION

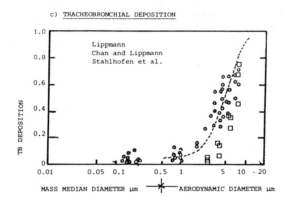

d) ALVELOLAR DEPOSITION

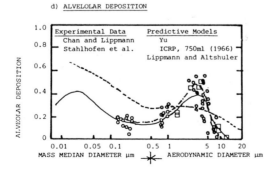

FIGURE 6.21 Contd.

recorded inhalabilities (sampling efficiencies) of 0.6 to 1.6 for individuals facing winds of 1 to 4 m s[-1] over a particle size range of 10 to 130 μm. For slow continuous rotation relative to the wind direction, Vincent and Mark (1982) recorded inhalabilities dropping from ∿0.9 for 10 μm particles to ∿0.5 for 40 μm particles and then maintaining a constant value up to ∿100 μm. Average sampling efficiencies for nose and mouth breathing, as presented by Ambruster and Breuer (1982) are consistent with this general trend (see Fig. 6.22). These data indicate that while sampling efficiencies may be very dependent upon orientation and windspeed, average efficiencies are likely to be between 0.5 and 2.0. It is noted that, in calm air, efficiencies may appear reduced for particles with diameters of >40 μm (Swift, 1981). However, this problem may be overcome by sampling suitably close to the respiratory zone.

With respect to head deposition of inhaled particulate material distinctions have to be made between nose and mouth breathing. Wolfsdorf et al. (1969) noted this distinction in mist aerosols produced by jet and ultrasonic nebulisers, but included only limited quantitative data. In respect of mouth breathing, Wilson et al. (1973) reported that 25 μm diameter pollen particles were deposited entirely in the oropharyngeal region and did not penetrate distal to the trachea. However, more recently, Michel et al. (1977) have shown that the methods used by Wilson et al. (1973) were insufficiently sensitive and that a small fraction of inhaled pollen grains do pene-

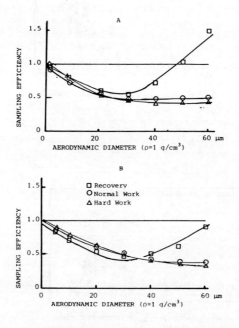

FIGURE 6.22. AVERAGED SAMPLING EFFICIENCIES FOR (A) FOR MOUTH BREATHING (B) FOR NOSE BREATHING. From Armbruster and Breuer (1982).

trate into the pulmonary region of the lung.

Early work on nasal deposition was reviewed by Lippmann (1972), Albert and Lippmann (1972) and Morrow (1974). Head deposition data, during mouth-in-mouth-out and nose-in-mouth-out breathing, are shown in Figs. 6.23 and 6.24 respectively. Morrow (1974) noted that nasal deposition had been represented by Pattle using the formulation:

$$N = -0.62 + 0.475 \log_{10} D_{ad}^2 F$$

where

    N   is the fractional nasal deposition;

    D_{ad} is the aerodynamic diameter (μm); and

    F   is the mean airflow rate (1 min^{-1}).

Heyder and Rudolf (1977) performed some 2000 experiments involving four breathing manoeuvres, four volunteers, a wide range of particle diameters and various breathing patterns. The particles used were bis (2-ethyl-hexyl) sebacate ($\rho = 0.93$ g cm^{-3}) and deposition in the nose was calculated from total deposition in the respiratory tract for mouth, nose, mouth-nose and nose-mouth breathing. This allowed

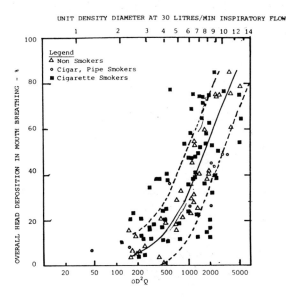

Note: Eye-fit median and upper and lower limit lines are drawn through the nonsmoker data, for whom the intersubject and intrasubject variability were similar.

FIGURE 6.23. HEAD DEPOSITION DURING MOUTH INHALATIONS OF MONODISPERSE TAGGED AEROSOLS OF VARIOUS SIZES. From Albert and Lippmann (1972).

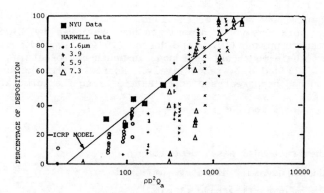

Notes: The ICRP model, (Pattle's data), and the Harwell data were based
on constant flows drawn in through the nose and out of the mouth.
The NYU data were obtained during normal nasal inhalations, with
exhalations via the mouth.

FIGURE 6.24. HEAD DEPOSITION DURING NASAL INHALATIONS FOR MONODISPERSED
TAGGED AEROSOLS. From Albert and Lippmann (1972).

determination of total nasal deposition and nasal efficiencies for
inspiration and expiration. For inspiration, the data from all four
subjects (Fig. 6.25) were well fitted by a function of the form:

$$N_i = 3.04 + 0.39 \log_{10} (\rho D^2 p^{0.667})$$

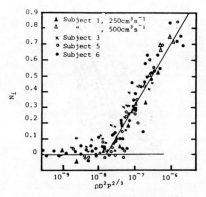

Notes: See text for a discussion of the fit to the data.

FIGURE 6.25. INSPIRATORY EFFICIENCY OF THE NASAL PASSAGES OF FOUR
SUBJECTS AS A FUNCTION OF THE PARAMETER $\rho D^2 p^{2/3}$.
From Heyder and Rudolf (1977).

where

  N_i is the fractional efficiency on inspiration;

  ρ is the particle density;

  D is the particle diameter; and

  P is the pressure drop across the nose.

Units of $\rho D^2 P^{0.667}$ are kg m^{-1} Pa$^{0.667}$.

It is noted that the requirement to invoke the pressure drop across the nose was due to the otherwise anomalous results reported for subject 1. Excluding this subject the data could be fitted by:

  $$N_i = -1.15 + 0.47 \log_{10}(\rho D^2 Q)$$

where

  Q (cm^3 s^{-1}) is the respiratory flow rate;

  D (μm) is the particle diameter; and

  ρ (g cm^{-3}) is the particle density.

On expiration, the data for three of the subjects were well fitted by:

  $$N_e = -1.01 + 0.43 \log_{10}(\rho D^2 Q)$$

where the various symbols are defined as for inspiration.

Results for subject 1 were again anomalous, exhibiting a similar functional dependence, but at lower values of $\rho D^2 Q$.

With respect to small particles, Giacomelli-Maltoni et al (1972) compared nose-in-mouth-out and nose-in-nose-out breathing patterns to calculate nasal deposition efficiencies. Results (Fig. 6.15) indicate significant nasal trapping of 1 to 2 μm particles of carnuba wax as would be expected at the $\rho D^2 Q$ values of 370 to 1500 g μm^2 s^{-1} associated with these particle sizes.

Possibly the most extensive series of studies of nasal deposition have been those undertaken at Harwell (Hounam et al. 1969; Fry, 1970; Hounam et al., 1971; Fry and Black, 1973; Foord et al. 1977; 1978). Hounam et al. (1969; 1971) reported on the results of studies using monodisperse aerosols of polystyrene of 1.6 to 7.3 μm diameter. Nasal deposition was found to be more closely related to $D^2 R$ than to $D^2 F$, where R is the resistance drop across the nose. Fry (1970) also used polystyrene particles and demonstrated that naso-pharyngeal deposition probabilities were not significantly affected by unipolar charging of the particles up to $\sim$40 elementary charges per particle. Thus, the relationship proposed by Hounam et al. (1971) may be taken to be appropriate for both charged and uncharged aerosols. This relationship is:

  $$N = -0.975 + 0.66 \log_{10} D_a^2 P_{nm}$$

where

N   is the fractional deposition in the nasopharynx;

D_a (μm) is the aerodynamic diameter of the particles; and

P_{nm} (mm water gauge) is the pressure drop across the nose and mouth.

P_{nm} is related to flow rate, F, for each individual, but the relationships differ between individuals and for the same individual for different environmental conditions and states of health. Data presented by Hounam et al. (1971) indicate a group averaged relationship of the form:

$$\log_{10} P_{nm} = -1.035 + 1.51 \log_{10} F$$

where

F   is in litres min^{-1}.

Combining the two expressions given above yields a group-averaged nasopharyngeal deposition function:

$$N = -1.658 + 0.66 \log_{10} D_{ad}^2 F^{1.5}$$

This suggests that an explanation for the scatter on results plotted against $D_{ad}^2 F$ may be largely due to the use of an inappropriate aerodynamic parameter. While $D_{ad}^2 F$ is appropriate for laminar flow regimes in tubes, it is not necessarily appropriate for mixed laminar and turbulent flow in the upper respiratory tract. In these expressions, flow rate, F, is the steady flow rate through the nose in the artificial nose-in-mouth-out breathing regime employed.

With respect to the distribution of deposits in the nasopharyngeal region, Fry and Black (1973) reported that, for 2 to 10 μm diameter particles of polystyrene, at least 45% of the retained material was deposited in the anterior region of the nasal passages. Because this region is partly non-ciliated, clearance was very variable and a component of long-term retention, with a half-life of more than 3 h, was always observed.

Data for mouth breathing were given by Foord et al (1977) for polystyrene particles. Results were as listed below.

Particle Diameter (μm)	Mouth Deposition (%)	Range (%)
2.5	4.8	0.8-14.9
5.0	17.0	1.0-52.4
7.5	39.8	5.9-76.8

More extensive data on this topic were presented by Foord et al. (1978). Three studies were conducted relating to variable

TABLE 6.7

REGIONAL AND TOTAL FILTRATION EFFICIENCIES OF THE
NOSE FOR DIFFERENT PARTICLE SIZES

Particle diameter (μm)	ε_I	ε_{II}	ε_{III}	ε_{IV}	ε_V	ε_n
A. Flow = 10 L/min						
0.2	0.00	0.00	0.00	0.00	0.00	0.00
0.4	0.00	0.00	0.01	0.00	0.00	0.01
0.6	0.00	0.00	0.01	0.00	0.00	0.01
0.8	0.00	0.00	0.02	0.00	0.00	0.02
1.0	0.00	0.00	0.03	0.00	0.00	0.03
2.0	0.01	0.00	0.09	0.00	0.01	0.11
3.0	0.02	0.00	0.18	0.01	0.01	0.21
4.0	0.03	0.00	0.28	0.02	0.02	0.32
5.0	0.04	0.00	0.37	0.03	0.03	0.43
6.0	0.06	0.00	0.46	0.04	0.04	0.53
7.0	0.07	0.01	0.54	0.05	0.06	0.62
8.0	0.10	0.02	0.60	0.07	0.08	0.69
9.0	0.12	0.03	0.66	0.08	0.10	0.76
10.0	0.14	0.04	0.70	0.10	0.12	0.82
B. Flow = 20 L/min						
0.2	0.00	0.00	0.00	0.00	0.00	0.00
0.4	0.00	0.00	0.01	0.00	0.00	0.01
0.6	0.00	0.00	0.02	0.00	0.00	0.02
0.8	0.00	0.00	0.03	0.00	0.00	0.04
1.0	0.00	0.00	0.05	0.00	0.00	0.06
2.0	0.01	0.00	0.17	0.01	0.01	0.19
3.0	0.03	0.00	0.30	0.02	0.02	0.35
4.0	0.05	0.00	0.43	0.03	0.04	0.50
5.0	0.07	0.01	0.54	0.05	0.06	0.63
6.0	0.10	0.02	0.63	0.07	0.09	0.73
7.0	0.14	0.04	0.70	0.10	0.12	0.80
8.0	0.17	0.06	0.75	0.13	0.15	0.86
9.0	0.21	0.08	0.79	0.16	0.19	0.90
10.0	0.24	0.10	0.82	0.20	0.23	0.93
C. Flow = 30 L/min						
0.2	0.00	0.00	0.00	0.00	0.00	0.01
0.4	0.00	0.00	0.01	0.00	0.00	0.02
0.6	0.00	0.00	0.03	0.00	0.00	0.04
0.8	0.00	0.00	0.05	0.00	0.00	0.06
1.0	0.01	0.00	0.07	0.00	0.00	0.09
2.0	0.02	0.00	0.23	0.01	0.02	0.27
3.0	0.04	0.00	0.40	0.03	0.03	0.46
4.0	0.07	0.01	0.53	0.05	0.06	0.62
5.0	0.11	0.03	0.64	0.08	0.09	0.74
6.0	0.15	0.05	0.72	0.11	0.13	0.82
7.0	0.19	0.07	0.78	0.15	0.18	0.88
8.0	0.24	0.10	0.82	0.19	0.23	0.92
9.0	0.28	0.13	0.85	0.25	0.28	0.95
10.0	0.31	0.17	0.88	0.30	0.34	0.97

Note: from Scott et al. (1978)

particle size, tidal volume and breathing rate respectively. Results exhibited considerable scatter, but, as noted previously, can be represented by:

$$M = 20 \ \log_{10} D^2_{ad} F - 40.7$$

where $D^2_{ad} F$, in units of $\mu m^2 \ l \ min^{-1}$, has a value of more than 108.4.
    The data presented by Heyder and Rudolf (1975) and Hounam et al. (1971) have been analysed theoretically by Scott et al. (1978) using a five component model of the nasal passages. These regions are summarised below:

Region I   -   the section of the nasal passages where the nasal hairs are present.

Region II   -   the converging section of the passageway which forms the nasal valve.

Region III   -   the expansion area after the nasal valve.

Region IV   -   the turbinate region.

Region V   -   the curved back portion of the nasal passage.

Filtration efficiencies for these various regions, as calculated by Scott et al. (1978) are listed in Table 6.7 and fractional depositions in Table 6.8.
    Yu et al. (1981) discussed intra- and inter-subject variability and their effects on deposition in the nose and mouth. Mean efficiencies and depositions were represented as functions of $pD^2_{ad} F$.

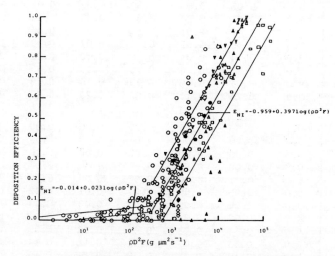

FIGURE 6.26. DEPOSITON OF PARTICLES IN THE HEAD FOR NASAL INSPIRATION AS A FUNCTION OF pD^2F. THE EQUATIONS OF E_{NI} AND THEIR σ_{NI} ARE GIVEN BY SOLID LINES. From Yu et al. (1981).

TABLE 6.8

REGIONAL DEPOSITION IN THE NOSE FOR
DIFFERENT PARTICLE SIZES

Particle diameter (m)	D_I	D_{II}	D_{III}	D_{IV}	D_V
A. Flow 10 L/min					
0.2	0.00	0.00	0.00	0.00	0.00
0.4	0.00	0.00	0.01	0.00	0.00
0.6	0.00	0.00	0.01	0.00	0.00
0.8	0.00	0.00	0.02	0.00	0.00
1.0	0.00	0.00	0.03	0.00	0.00
2.0	0.01	0.00	0.09	0.00	0.00
3.0	0.02	0.00	0.18	0.01	0.01
4.0	0.03	0.00	0.27	0.01	0.01
5.0	0.04	0.00	0.36	0.02	0.02
6.0	0.06	0.00	0.43	0.02	0.02
7.0	0.07	0.01	0.49	0.02	0.02
8.0	0.10	0.02	0.53	0.02	0.03
9.0	0.12	0.03	0.56	0.02	0.03
10.0	0.14	0.04	0.58	0.03	0.03
B. Flow - 20 L/min					
0.2	0.00	0.00	0.00	0.00	0.00
0.4	0.00	0.00	0.01	0.00	0.00
0.6	0.00	0.00	0.02	0.00	0.00
0.8	0.00	0.00	0.03	0.00	0.00
1.0	0.00	0.00	0.05	0.00	0.00
2.0	0.01	0.00	0.16	0.01	0.01
3.0	0.03	0.00	0.29	0.01	0.02
4.0	0.05	0.00	0.41	0.02	0.02
5.0	0.07	0.01	0.50	0.02	0.02
6.0	0.10	0.02	0.55	0.02	0.03
7.0	0.14	0.03	0.58	0.03	0.03
8.0	0.17	0.05	0.58	0.03	0.03
9.0	0.21	0.06	0.58	0.02	0.02
10.0	0.24	0.08	0.56	0.02	0.02
C. Flow = 30 L/min					
0.2	0.00	0.00	0.00	0.00	0.00
0.4	0.00	0.00	0.01	0.00	0.00
0.6	0.00	0.00	0.03	0.00	0.00
0.8	0.00	0.00	0.05	0.00	0.00
1.0	0.01	0.00	0.07	0.00	0.00
2.0	0.02	0.00	0.22	0.01	0.01
3.0	0.04	0.00	0.38	0.02	0.02
4.C	0.07	0.01	0.49	0.02	0.02
5.0	0.11	0.02	0.56	0.02	0.03
6.0	0.15	0.04	0.58	0.03	0.03
7.0	0.19	0.06	0.58	0.03	0.03
8.0	0.24	0.08	0.56	0.02	0.02
9.0	0.28	0.10	0.53	0.02	0.02
10.0	0.31	0.12	0.50	0.02	0.02

Note: from Scott et al. (1978)

Expressing this quantity as x, in units of g μm^2 s^{-1}, the following relationships were proposed:

Inspiratory nasal mean efficiency:

$$E_{NI} = -0.014 + 0.023 \log_{10}x \qquad x < 337$$

$$= -0.959 + 0.397 \log_{10}x \qquad x > 337$$

Expiratory nasal mean efficiency:

$$E_{NE} = 0.033 + 0.003 \log_{10}x \qquad x < 215$$

$$= -0.851 + 0.399 \log_{10}x \qquad x > 215$$

Inspiratory mouth efficiency:

$$E_{MI} = 0 \qquad x < 3000$$

$$= -1.117 + 0.324 \log_{10}x \qquad x > 3000$$

The variability of the data about these relationships is shown in Fig. 6.26 to 6.28.

Recent data, not included in the analyses of Yu et al. (1981) have been presented by Emmett et al., (1982) and Stahlhofen et al. (1983).

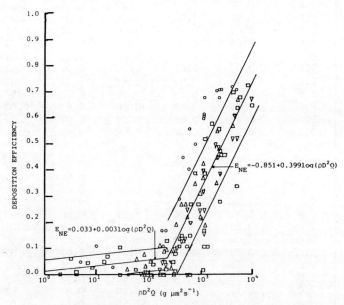

FIGURE 6.27. DEPOSITION OF PARTICLES IN THE HEAD FOR NASAL EXPIRATION AS A FUNCTION OF $\rho D^2 Q$. THE EQUATIONS OF E_{NE} AND THEIR σ_{NE} ARE GIVEN BY SOLID LINES.
From Yu et al. (1981).

Emmett et al. (1982) recorded limited data on oral deposition for mouth breathing of polystyrene particles of 3.5 to 10 μm diameter, but these add little to the extensive studies discussed above. Stahlhofen et al. (1983) presented curves of extrathoracic deposition against particle size for various breathing patterns, but did not include a discussion of the data on which these were based.

Finally, note should be taken of the recent theoretical analysis by Martonen (1983), in which the following functions were proposed for calculating deposition percentage as a function of $\rho D_{ad}^2 F$ (referred to as x and having units of g μm² s⁻¹).

Mouth breathing:

$$P_M = 0 \qquad\qquad\qquad\qquad\qquad\qquad x < 1670$$

$$= -0.496 + 0.154 \log_{10}x \qquad 1670 < x < 10000$$

$$= -2.988 + 0.777 \log_{10}x \qquad 10000 < x < 83000$$

Nose Breathing:

$$P_N = 0 \qquad\qquad\qquad\qquad\qquad\qquad x < 282$$

$$= -1.15 + 0.47 \log_{10}x \qquad\qquad 282 < x < 10000$$

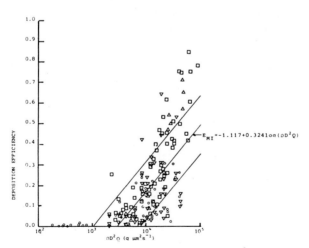

FIGURE 6.28. DEPOSITION OF PARTICLES IN THE HEAD FOR MOUTH INSPIRATION AS A FUNCTION OF $\rho D^2 Q$. THE EQUATION OF E_{MI} AND σ_{MI} IS GIVEN BY SOLID LINES.
From Yu et al. (1981).

6.3.6.   Tracheo-bronchial deposition

Because of the relatively simple dichotomous tubular branch-ing structure of the tracheo-bronchial region, there has been con-siderable interest in developing theoretical approaches to the study of particle deposition in this region. It is emphasised that while the theoretical problems involved in such studies are not insuperable, neither are exact calculations simple (e.g. Yu and Thiagarajan, 1978; Carpenter and Taulbee, 1980; Ingham, 1981; Chang and El Masry, 1982).

In particular, simultaneous consideration of the sedimenta-tion and diffusion of small particles is difficult. In practice, most theoretical calculations make the approximation that these two mecha-nisms are uncoupled. This approximation can lead to significant over-estimates of deposition (Goldberg, 1981).

Furthermore, numerous assumptions are included in the theo-retical models relating to the smoothness of the tubes, the physical structure of the branch regions and the pattern of branching. For these reasons, it is not advisable to rely too heavily upon purely theoretical calculations.

6.3.6.1   Theoretical and model studies

Theoretical studies of tracheo-bronchial deposition have become considerably refined in recent years and comparisons have been made with model systems. Thus, Johnston et al. (1977) studied the deposition of homogeneous monodisperse aerosols in simple bend systems of differing geometries and in five models of bifurcating airways. For an airway branching angle of 30°, the experimental results were in good agreement with the theoretical work of Landahl (1950), but at larger angles there was substantial disagreement. The authors commen-ted that it would be necessary to investigate the distribution of branching angles withing each generation of airways, the effects of pulsed and expiratory flow, the effects of one bifurcation on another, and the effects of asymmetry, before complete estimates of particle deposition in the lung could be made.

In a later study, Johnston and Schroter (1979) demonstrated that Landahl's generalised expression for impaction efficiency:

$$I = x/(i + x)$$

where $x = \rho d^2 \bar{v}.\sin\theta/9\eta\sigma$, could be modified to fit their experimental results in model bifurcations by redefining:

$$x = \rho(d/D)^2 \ Re.\sin\theta.$$

In these expressions:

$\bar{v}$ is the average velocity in the parent tube;

D   is the parent tube diameter;

d   is the particle diameter;

ρ   is the particle density;

σ   is the fluid density;

η   is the fluid viscosity;

Re   is Reynold's number $(\bar{v}\sigma D/\eta)$; and

θ   is the semi-inclusive branching angle.

Gerrity et al. (1979) used the Landahl deposition model, together with the Weibel 'A' lung model, to calculate the percentage of various size iron oxide aerosols (1 to 10 µm diameter) passing the glottis that deposit in the various airway generations. Results (Fig. 6.29) are as would be expected, with smaller particles penetrating deeper into the lung. The calculations were carried out for an inspiratory flow rate of 500 cm^3 s^{-1}, a tidal volume of 700 cm^3 and a breathing frequency of 15.8 min^{-1}. The flow pattern was assumed to follow a square wave with constant flow on inspiration and expiration equal to the average inspiratory flow. A breath pause of 0.5 s was included between inspiration and expiration. Other respiratory characteristics and breathing regimes would, of course, give somewhat different distribution patterns. Similar calculations were undertaken by Hofmann (1982a) for polydisperse aerosols.

Schum and Yeh (1980) summarised relevant deposition equations and calculated deposition probabilities in rat lung for comparison with experiment. Adequate agreement was achieved for gross deposition in the pulmonary, tracheo-bronchial and nasopharyngeal regions over a range of aerodynamic diameters from 0.2 to 3.0 µm. In a later paper, Cheng and Yeh (1981) proposed an aerosol model for the human tracheo-bronchial tree based on impaction and sedimentation. In this model, total tracheo-bronchial deposition, TB, is given by:

$$TB = TB_I + TB_G$$

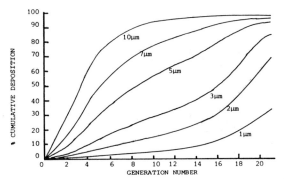

Note: Percentages are expressed for aerosol passing the glottis.

FIGURE 6.29. CUMULATIVE DEPOSITION OF IRON OXIDE PARTICLES OF 1, 2, 3, 5, 7, AND 10µm. From Gerrity et al. (1981).

where

   TB_I is deposition due to impaction; and

   TB_G is deposition due to sedimentation.

In turn:

   $$TB_I = D_{ad}^2 \, IQ$$

   $$TB_G = D_{ad}^2 \, G/Q$$

where

   D_{ad} is the aerodynamic diameter, and

   Q is the mean flow rate.

Values of I and G were found to be subject dependent. For three normal subjects, values of I were 1.27×10^{-5}, 1.18×10^{-5} and 5.74×10^{-6} s cm^{-5}. Corresponding values of G were 0.584, 0.753 and 1.30 cm s^{-1}.

   Cheng and Yeh (1981) pointed out that I is related to the effective radius of the airways comprising the tracheo-bronchial tree. Specifically:

   $$I = 0.478 \times 10^{-8} \rho_0 / 18 \mu \pi R^3$$

where

   ρ_0 is unit density;

   μ is the viscosity of air; and

   R is the average deposition size due to impaction.

The value of R is a weighted average over all generations of conducting airways, i.e.

   $$R = \left[\sum_{i=2}^{16} (1/N_i R_i^3) \right]^{-0.333}$$

where

   N_i is the number of airways in generation i; and

   R_i is the radius of the airways in generation i.

   Values of R for the three subjects studied by Cheng and Yeh (1981) were 0.330, 0.339 and 0.431 cm respectively. Calculated values of R are 0.263 cm for the Weibel 'A' model and 0.376 cm for the model of Yeh and Schum (1980).

   Chan et al. (1980) reported that, experimentally, there is a 'hot spot', for particles with mass median aerodynamic diameters of more than 2 μm, within the trachea at 2 cm below the larynx. This enhancement of deposition within the trachea was studied in a hollow cast and an idealised model. The larynx was found to have a significant effect on the flow field in the trachea and this effect was found to extend beyond the tracheal bifurcation. In theoretical studies, Hamill (1979) emphasised that turbulent flow is to be expected in the trachea even in the absence of laryngeal effects.

Empirically, Chan et al. (1980) reported that the deposition efficiency in the trachea for particles larger than 2 μm was well correlated with Stokes number ($St = \rho D^2 v/18\mu R$) according to:

$$E_{TRACHEA} = 2.536 \, St^{1.231} \text{ for } St > 3\times10^{-3}$$

In the larynx, deposition efficiencies were well fitted by:

$$E_{LARYNX} = 4.702 \, St + 0.0277 \text{ for } St > 7\times10^{-3}$$

It is noted that these expressions require information on air velocities in the trachea and larynx. Such velocities depend both on anatomical dimensions and breathing patterns. As such, they are not readily available for in vivo exposures.

In a later paper, Chan and Lippmann (1980) reported further on their hollow cast studies and presented deposition efficiencies against Stokes number for all bronchi down to generation 6 (see also Schlesinger et al., 1977). These results (Fig. 6.30) exhibit con-

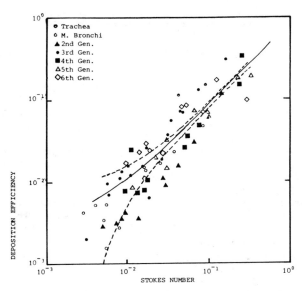

Note: The solid line represents the best fit linear correlation: η=0.803St+0.0023. The dotted lines represent the 95% confidence band for the regression line. St=Stoke's number.

FIGURE 6.30. LOG-LOG PLOT OF MEAN PARTICLE DEPOSITION EFFICIENCY IN THE AIRWAYS OF THE HUMAN TRACHEOBRONCHIAL CAST BY AIRWAY GENERATION VS. STOKES NUMBER IN EACH GENERATION. From Chan and Lippmann (1980).

siderable scatter, but are well fitted by:

$$E = 0.803St + 0.0023$$

The observed linear dependence on Stokes number is consistent with the aerodynamic theory of impaction in laminar flow which is discussed elsewhere (Section 6.3.3.1).

Yu and Diu (1983) used a continuous deposition model to calculate tracheo-bronchial deposition fractions for different flow rates and particle sizes (Fig. 6.31). The results show a very limited dependence on flow rate. Results also show a very limited dependence on mean residence time of air in the lungs.

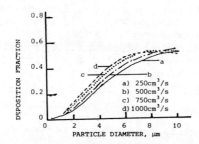

Note: Particle density=0.91 g cm^3

FIGURE 6.31. CALCULATED REGIONAL DEPOSITION AS A FUNCTION OF PARTICLE DIAMETER IN MOUTH BREATHING FOR VARIOUS FLOW RATES. From Yu and Diu (1983).

Yu and Diu (1982) also considered the inter-subject variability in tracheo-bronchial deposition which occurs even under well-controlled breathing conditions. To explain this variability they proposed a probabilistic lung model in which two random scaling factors were introduced to account for inter-subject differences in tracheo-bronchial and alveolar air space dimensions. Results of the model, and a comparison with the data of Chan and Lippmann (1980) for spontaneous breathing, at a tidal volume of 1000 cm^3 and a breathing rate of 14 min^{-1}, are shown in Fig. 6.32.

In respect of theoretical analyses of tracheo-bronchial deposition, three other studies require mention. Ingham (1981) developed methods for calculating deposition of charged particles in the tracheo-bronchial tree, Martonen and Wilson (1983) considered the effects of hygroscopic growth during passage through the tree, and Goldberg and Smith (1981) considered the theory of settling and diffusion of particles in the respiratory system during breath holding. This last topic is of particular interest in some planned respiratory manoeuvres and is discussed in more detail below.

The above discussion has emphasised the various theoretical approaches to studying tracheo-bronchial deposition, often by individual airway generation. However, this resolution is somewhat finer

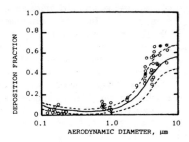

FIGURE 6.32. COMPARISON OF CALCULATED TRACHEOBRONCHIAL
DEPOSITION IN MOUTH BREATHING WITH EXPERIMENTAL
DATA. From Yu and Diu (1982).

than is required in a model concerned with occupational or environmental exposure to ambient aerosols. It is, therefore, also relevant
to reconsider the experimental data upon which such models are based
as input into a simpler representation of tracheo-bronchial deposition. This review is, therefore, concentrated upon results from
normal breathing studies, but, for completeness, a brief account is
given also of some results from a variety of special respiratory
manoeuvres.

6.3.6.2   Tracheo-bronchial deposition in planned respiratory manoevres

In the context of tracheobronchial deposition, the planned
respiratory manoeuvres normally relate to breath holding. Thus,
Palmes et al. (1973) determined the effect of depth of aerosol
inhalation on persistence in the respiratory tract by a respiratory
manoevre in which an aerosol bolus was inhaled followed by 200 to
800 cm^3 of clean air to a lung volume slightly below the total lung
capacity. The breath was then held for 0.5 to 20s after which a
forced exhalation was made and aerosol recovery measured. As was
shown by Landahl (1950), settling of an aerosol in a randomly oriented
infinitely long tube as a function of time is given by:

$$-\log_e(1-S) = 3.6 \times 10^5 \rho d^2 (1 + 1.8 \times 10^{-5}/d)\ (t/D)$$

where

S	is the fraction removed by settling;
ρ(g cm^{-3})	is the particle density;
d(cm)	is the particle diameter;
t(s)	is the containment time; and
D(cm)	is the diameter of the tube.

On this basis, the fractional recovery should decrease exponentially with time and the rate of decrease can be used to compute the effective diameter of the tube. While this equation is not exact, and is dependent upon the initial concentration profile, it is sufficiently accurate for estimation of tube diameters (see Goldberg and Smith, 1981). This was done by Palmes et al. (1973), who reported diameters which were typically rather larger than would have been expected on the basis of calculations for the Weibel 'A' lung model (Fig. 6.33). More recent data using this technique have been obtained by Heyder (1983) who gave the following data for average airway radius at various depths (see also Palmes, 1973).

| Subject | Average airway radius (µm) at lung depth (cm³) of | | | | Functional residual capacity (cm³) |
	120	200	400	600	
6	630	380	225	205	2200
2	1400	780	350	270	3000
3	790	390	240	190	2800
4	630	460	320	280	4200
5	640	340	185	175	2090
6	980	505	210	165	3400

These results indicate considerable inter-subject variability in gross averaged morphometric properties of the human tracheo-bronchial tree.

Alternatively, breath holding may be used not to estimate morphometric characteristics of the respiratory tract, but rather to deliver aerosols to a predefined depth (Thomson and Pavia, 1974; Pavia et al., 1977; Dolovich et al., 1981; Newman et al., 1981; 1982). Such studies give little information on deposition probabilities during normal breathing, but are of interest in evaluating clearance from particular levels of the lung. They are, therefore, considered in that context elsewhere in this review.

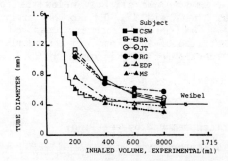

FIGURE 6.33. EQUIVALENT TUBE DIAMETER AS A FUNCTION OF INHALED VOLUME FOR BOLUS EXPERIMENT COMPARED TO DIAMETERS OF THE AIRWAY MODEL "A" OF WEIBEL. From Palmes et al.(1973).

6.3.6.3   Tracheo-bronchial deposition during normal breathing

        Extensive studies on this subject have been reported by
Lippmann and his co-workers.   The data of Lippmann and Albert (1969)
discussed above (Section 6.3.4) indicated that tracheo-bronchial deposition was related to $\rho d^2 Q$ (see also Foord et al., 1977) but the scatter on the data was large.   Later studies (Albert et al., 1973) showed

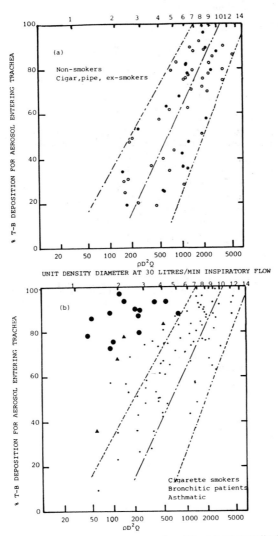

Note: Limit lines for non-cigarette smokers from (a) are reproduced in (b).

FIGURE 6.34.   TRACHEOBRONCHIAL DEPOSITION FOR SMOKERS AND NON-SMOKERS,
        From Albert et al. (1973).

little difference in deposition between smokers and non-smokers, but did indicate that deposition is enhanced in bronchitic and asthmatic patients (Fig. 6.34). Bohning et al. (1975), considering deposition of monodisperse aerosols in monozygotic twins, developed the concept of a deposition parameter y. This parameter was determined from the relationship:

$$D_A = [1/(1 + yd^2)]^{16}$$

where

D_A is the fractional alveolar deposition; and

d   is the particle diameter.

This expression implicitly assumes 16 generations of conducting airways.

Values of y were found to be similar in twins, indicating a genetic component in deposition and, therefore, presumably in lung structure and/or respiratory characteristics.

The deposition parameter y was also used by Palmes and Lippmann (1977) in a study of aerosol deposition in non-smokers and cigarette smokers. On the basis of the data presented, no difference can be recognised between the two groups for aerodynamic particle diameters over the entire range studied (2-12 μm).

More recently, Chan and Lippmann (1980) have pointed out that the parameter y does not include allowance for respiratory flow rate. For this reason, a new parameter, the bronchial deposition size (BDS), was defined. This quantity was given by:

$$D_{TB} = 8.14 \times 10^4 [d^2 Q/(BDS)^3] + 0.037$$

where

D_{TB} is the fractional tracheo-bronchial deposition;

d(cm)   is the aerodynamic diameter of the particle; and

$Q(l \min^{-1})$ is the average inspiratory flow rate.

Values of BDS for various populations were given by Chan and Lippmann (1980) and are summarised below:

Group	No. of subjects	No. of tests	Particle size range (μm)	BDS (cm)	Coeff. of variation
Non-smokers	26	34	1.0-7.5	1.20	0.23
Cigarette smokers	46	122	3.5-13.0	1.02	0.22
Mild bronchitics	19	74	2.0-5.0	0.90	0.20
Severe bronchitics	6	15	1.0-4.0	0.60	0.31

The trend to bronchial constriction in bronchitis is clear, whereas it is not possible to determine whether asymptomatic smokers exhibit any broncho-constriction relative to non-smokers.

Other groups have also studied tracheobronchial deposition. The results of Stahlhofen et al. (1983) are discussed in Section 6.3.4, as are those of Kimura (1971) and Emmett et al. (1982), while the work of Gerrity et al. (1979) is discussed in Section 6.3.6.1.

Braun et al. (1979) studied the ratio of tracheo-bronchial to pulmonary deposition in normal individuals and a variety of patients including those with normal ventilatory function, restrictive disease and obstructive disease. In patients with normal ventilatory function tracheo-bronchial deposition was increased relative to pulmonary deposition, but in restrictive and obstructive disease results were much more variable.

Finally, with respect to submicronic particles, James (1977) has shown, for pig lungs in vitro, that deposition of condensation nuclei (diameter $\sim$0.1 μm), in the first six bronchial generations, is strongly affected by the detailed shape of the vocal cords.

6.3.7   Deposition in the respiratory region

6.3.7.1   Theoretical considerations

Morrow (1974) discussed various data relevant to aerosol deposition in the respiratory region of the lung. He pointed out that technically the measurement of alveolar, or parenchymal, deposition is difficult and usually indirect. However, on the basis of studies by Landahl (1950; 1963) he concluded that particles smaller than 1 μm which enter the trachea deposit almost exclusively in the parenchymal region and that the major deposition sites are the alveolar ducts rather than the terminal air sacs.

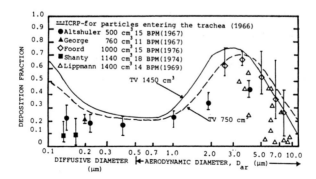

FIGURE 6.35. SELECTED DATA REPORTED FOR PULMONARY DEPOSITION OF MONODISPERSE AEROSOLS INHALED THROUGH THE MOUTH BY PEOPLE COMPARED WITH PREDICTED VALUES CALCULATED BY THE ICPP TASK GROUP ON LUNG DYNAMICS(1966). From Raabe(1982).

Raabe (1982) summarised data on alveolar deposition and compared them with the ICRP (1966) lung model (Fig. 6.35). The model gave an adequate representation of deposition for aerosols with aerodynamic diameters of more than 0.5 μm, but gave substantial overestimates of deposition for particles with diffusive diameters of less than 0.2 μm.

As Morrow (1974) pointed out, in the sub-micronic regime there is little deposition in the oropharyngeal and tracheo-bronchial regions of the lungs. Thus, alveolar and total deposition may be taken to be essentially identical for such particles (see also Heyder, 1982). Heyder et al. (1983) used monodisperse aerososls of di(2-ethyl-hexyl) sebacate with particle diameters of 0.08 and 0.10 μm and studied total deposition in the respiratory tracts of three subjects who inspired aerosols at a flow rate of 250 cm^3 s^{-1} over periods of 2, 4, 6 and 8 seconds. Total deposition was almost exactly proportional to the diffusion length and could be approximated by:

$$DE = 0.0064(\psi t)^{0.5}$$

where

DE   is the fractional deposition; and

ψt   has units of μm^2 (ψ being the diffusion constant).

Heyder et al. (1983) showed that this expression was equivalent to what would be expected for diffusional loss from long cylindrical tubes with a radius of 180 μm.

In the above expression, D can be calculated from the formula given by Morrow (1974), i.e.

$$D = kTC/6\pi\eta r$$

where

k   is Boltzmann's constant;

T   is the absolute temperature;

C   is the slip correction factor;

η   is the viscosity of air; and

r   is the particle radius.

Substituting appropriate values in this expression, gives;

$$D = 12.28 \, C/r \; \mu m^2 \; s^{-1}$$

where

r   is specified in units of μm.

On this basis:

$$DE = 0.02243 \, (Ct/r)^{0.5}$$

where

t   is in seconds;   and

r   is µm.

The date for submicron aerosols shown in Fig. 6.35 are typically for 3 to 6 second breathing cycles and for 0.15 to 0.25 µm diameter particles. Taking t = 4 and r = 0.1, DE is calculated to be 0.25, a value slightly higher than the mean of the available data, but not inconsistent with, those data.

It is also relevant to note that Yu and Diu (1982; 1983) have undertaken calculations of alveolar deposition based on more sophisticated models. However, these add little to the results discussed above.

6.3.7.2   Experimental studies

Studies on alveolar deposition divide into those undertaken as planned respiratory manoeuvres and those undertaken in normal breathing regimes. Studies using special breathing manoeuvres are discussed elsewhere (Section 6.3.6.2). Such studies have been used to measure airspace dimensions in chronic obstructive lung disease (Palmes, 1973). For the work, Gebhart et al. (1981) concluded that optimal conditions were obtained with boluses of monodisperse aerosols with particles between 1 and about 1.5 µm diameter, though larger particles have been used (Camner and Philipson, 1978). Much of the work on normal breathing regimes is discussed in the context of total and regional deposition (Section 6.3.4) or tracheo-bronchial deposition (Section 6.3.6). For particles of 2 µm aerodynamic diameter or

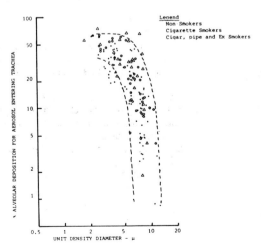

Notes: Eye-fit upper and lower limit lines are drawn through the nonsmoker data. In this region of the respiratory tract, the intersubject variability is much greater than the intrasubject.

FIGURE 6.36.   ALVEOLAR DEPOSITION. From Albert and Lippmann (1972).

larger, the review of Albert and Lippmann (1972) provides a useful summary of alveolar deposition results (Fig. 6.36). It is noted that Bohning et al. (1976) reported that aerosol deposition patterns may be correlated with pre-test temperature and humidity, but this is likely to be a small effect in most occupational and environmental situations.

Wolff et al. (1981) emphasised the lack of experimental data on ultrafine aerosols (Section 6.3.7.1) and noted that chain aggregated aerosols are often found in the environment. Their studies on beagle dogs indicate that the alveolar deposition of ultrafine aggregated aerosols can be predicted from spherical diameters calculated on an equivalent volume basis.

6.4   Clearance

The clearance of deposited materials from the lungs is most conveniently considered in terms of the same regions as used for deposition. To a large extent, such clearance is mediated by mucociliary transport, which was mentioned in Section 6.4.1 and is discussed in detail below. Other mechanisms of clearance, e.g. transport to lymph nodes and solubilisation, are discussed in the reviews of clearance of particular regions of the lung.

6.4.1   The mucociliary transport mechanism

As noted in Section 6.2.2, parts of the nasopharyngeal region and virtually all the lumenal surfaces of the tracheo-bronchial region are lined with ciliated cells which are covered by a layer of mucus. In general terms, the beating of the cilia propels the mucus, associated particulate material and associated cells, such as alveolar macrophages, toward the oropharynx where the material can be swallowed or expectorated. This transport mechanism is often termed the ciliary escalator.

Last (1982) has given a detailed review of the composition and structure of mucus, the nature of the secretory mechanism, and the operation of the ciliary escalator. Much of the following summary is based on that review, though earlier reviews (Hilding, 1963; Gilboa and Silberberg, 1976; Clarke and Pavia, 1980) have also been consulted.

Little or nothing is known about the composition of tracheo-bronchial mucus from direct analyses of this material and inferences have to be drawn from studies of mucus from ovarian cysts, salivary glands and the gastrointestinal tract, as well as from sputum. There is a striking contrast between the complex chemical composition of sputum, or tracheo-bronchial lavage fluids, and the simpler fluids produced by various glands and epithelial cells.

The conventional model of mucus structure suggests that tracheo-bronchial mucus exists as two layers, a lower sol and an upper gel. The gel, which may not constitute a continuous layer, contains primarily mucus glycoproteins and their counter-ions. The lower serous layer, through which the cilia beat, is assumed to be an aqueous isotonic salt solution.

Mucus is found to be extremely viscous at low levels of dissolved solute, as well as exhibiting elastic properties.   While changes in the viscoelastic properties of mucus appear to be inducable by various toxic materials, the effects of such changes in properties upon mucociliary transport are not clear.

Mucus is secreted in the tracheo-bronchial tree both by surface epithelial cells and by submucosal glands of the trachea and large bronchi.   The submucosal glands are under parasympathetic cholinergic nervous control.   Thus, either parasympathetic nerve stimulation or parasympathomimetic drugs can increase the volume and glycoprotein content of mucus secreted.   Increases in mucus transport rates are elicited by catecholamines, acetylcholine, and nicotine; decreases are elicited by cholinergic antagonists, α- and β-receptor blockers and some tranquillisers.   It is not clear whether these changes are due to effects on mucus secretion, on ciliary beat frequency, or on both processes (Last, 1982).

In man, there are approximately 250 cilia per ciliated cell. Each cilium, is ∿6 μm long and ∿0.3 μm wide (Gil, 1982).   The biochemical basis of their beating action is strikingly similar to that of muscle and ciliary disfunction in humans has, so far, been linked to absence of specific structural components in the structure of the cilium (e.g. Kartagener's sydrome).   In normal subjects, beat frequencies are typically 700 to 1000 min^{-1} (Clarke and Pavia, 1980).

Rates and directions of mucus flow in various regions of the respiratory tract are discussed in subsequent sections of this review.

6.4.2   Mucus and particle transport in the nasal passages

For particles that do not quickly dissolve or react with body fluids, clearance from the nasal passages is mechanical.   The anterior third of the nose in non-ciliated and does not clear except by blowing, wiping, sneezing, or other extrinsic means.   In contrast, in the posterior parts of the nose, including the nasal turbinates,

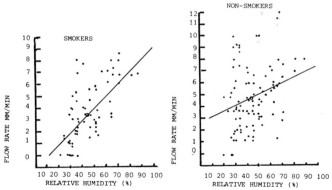

FIGURE 6.37. MUCUS FLOW RATES IN THE HUMAN NOSE.
From Ewert (1965).

particles are moved by mucociliary clearance to the throat where they are swallowed or expectorated (Tremble, 1948; Raabe, 1982).

Early quantitative studies on mucociliary clearance from the nasal passages were reported by Van Ree and Van Dishoeck (1962). In these studies, the mucous film near the entrance of the nose was labelled by blowing coloured powder just behind the head of the concha inferior and onto the opposite side of the nasal septum. The time for transport to the pharynx was measured and found to be 6 to 16 minutes in 100 normal individuals. The mean transport time was 10 minutes, corresponding to a transport velocity of 5 mm min^{-1}. The authors reported that the transport time was not influenced by the inclination of the head, nor by breathing pattern. However, supplementary experiments indicated that the inhalation of cold air (-6 to -8°C) could increase transit times to up to 30 minutes. Transit times were also longer in individuals sensitised to pollen and measured out of season, as well as in individuals exhibiting bacterial allergies. From the data presented, it is not possible to determine whether the allergy is a cause, or an effect, of the increased transit time.

A very extensive study on mucus flow rates in the human nose was reported by Ewert (1965). By direct observation of particles deposited on the nasal mucosa she was able to measure flow rates for smokers and non-smokers. Although the results (Fig. 6.37) showed considerable inter-subject variation, there was a distinct effect of relative humidity in both smokers and non-smokers.

Using I-131 labelled macroaggregated albumin, Proctor and Wagner (1965) reported that the linear velocity of particles through the human nasal passage was, typically, ∿6 mm min^{-1}, but rates varied from 3 to 9 mm min^{-1}. Proctor and Wagner (1965) noted that the rates recorded were not constant for an individual.

Bang et al. (1967) also used I-131 labelled materials and visual observation to calculate conveyance times for materials from the anterior ciliated nasal septum to the pharyngeal border. Average transit times were 4.4 to 4.8 minutes, corresponding to average transport rates of 10.4 to 11.3 mm min^{-1}. However, it is noted that these times and velocities relate to the initial observation of material at

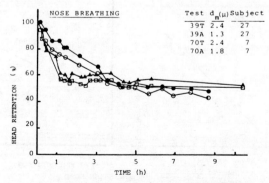

FIGURE 6.38. NASAL PARTICLE RETENTION FOR FOUR TESTS ON TWO SUBJECTS. From Lippmann (1970).

the pharyngeal boundary and that the range of velocities recorded in this study was 4.0 to 100 mm min^{-1}.

Bang et al. (1967) also reported some functional aberrancies in the anatomy of three of the subjects. Thus, in one subject about half the tracer moved anteriorly and was deposited at the mucocutaneous junction; even collecting in the external nostril. An initial placing of the tracer 1 mm further posterior eliminated this phenomenon.

Lippmann (1970) reported on the clearance of an inhaled monodisperse ferric oxide aerosol from the nasal passages. Deposition was partitioned between the unciliated anterior nares (UAN), the ciliated nasal passages (CNP) and the oral pharynx and larynx (OPL). These deposition fractions are summarised below for the four studies for which head retention data were presented for two nose breathing subjects.

Study	Particle diameter (μm)	Deposition (% total deposit) UAN	CNP	OPL
39T	2.38	24.9	69.9	0
39A	1.34	23.0	61.9	5.8
70T	2.42	31.6	19.6	5.8
70A	1.79	25.0	13.7	2.1

Retention measurements from these studies (Fig. 6.38) demonstrated long-term retention of a fraction of the deposited aerosol. It is of

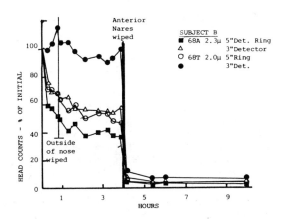

Note: Activity was mechanically removed from the outside of the nose and from the anterior unciliated nares at the times indicated.

FIGURE 6.39. DECAY-CORRECTED MEASUREMENTS OF RETAINED ACTIVITY VS. TIME AFTER INHALATION OF TAGGED TEST AEROSOL. From Lippmann (1970).

interest to note that this fraction is larger than the fractional
deposition on the unciliated anterior nares. This suggests that the
posterior to anterior migration observed by Bang et al. (1967) may
represent normal anatomical function.

It is emphasised that clearance of the anterior nares is
strongly affected by nose blowing and wiping. This is illustrated in
Fig. 6.39 (from Lippmann, 1970) which shows an order of magnitude
reduction in head retention with wiping of the anterior nares at 4 h
after inhalation. It will be noted that this figure emphasises that
the long-term retention observed in these studies is almost entirely
associated with the unciliated anterior nares.

The effects of nose blowing and swabbing were also investigated by Hounam (1975). Efficiencies were independent of particle
size, or flow rate at deposition, but did differ substantially between
subjects. Blowing the nose 10 min after inhalation removed 16.5 ±
9.4% ($\bar{x}$ ± s.d.) of the deposited material, whereas swabbing alone
removed 18.2 ± 6.5%. Swabbing immediately after the initial nose blow
gave a total recovery of 27.5%, whereas nose blowing after initial
swabbing gave a total recovery of 31.2%. Repeated swabbing only
removed a further 6% of the deposited activity. Efficiencies of nose
blowing decreased only slowly from 10 min to 15.5h after inhalation,
indicating the long period of potential retention in the unciliated
anterior nares. Hounam et al. (1983) reported further analyses of the
efficiency of nose blowing, but this paper added little to the discussion given by Hounam (1975).

Andersen and his co-workers (Andersen et al., 1971; 1974;
1974a; 1974b; Proctor et al., 1973) used Tc-99m tagged particles of
ion exchange resin to study nasal mucociliary clearance. Andersen
et al. (1971) placed the particles just beyond the initial prominence
of the inferior turbinate at 4.1 to 6.6 cm posterior to the nasal tip.
In studies on 58 subjects, three groups could be identified;

- 32 exhibited rapid uninterrupted particle movement;

- 14 exhibited a stop, or slow down, in particle movement after an
  initial normal flow; and

- 10 who exhibited constantly slow particle movement, or stasis,
  throughout the experiment.

In the first group, transport rates ranged from 2.3 to 23.6 mm min^{-1},
with an average of 8.4 mm min^{-1}. Andersen et al. (1971) noted that
there was an association of slow transport with recent upper respiratory tract infection, but this topic was not investigated further
(see also Proctor et al., 1973). Andersen et al. (1971) also commented that there is undoubtedly an area in the anterior nares from which
mucociliary clearance moves particles forward and emphasised that this
area occurs in that part of the nasal passage which exhibits a restricted cross section. Because of the high local linear velocity of
air, deposition is enhanced in this region.

Andersen et al. (1974) studied the effects of relative
humidity on nasal mucociliary clearance and found no significant
changes in nasal mucus flow rates during 78 h at 9% RH. In contrast,
Andersen et al. (1974a) found a significant decrease in nasal mucus
flow rates during 6 h exposures to 5 and 25 ppm of SO_2. No decrease

was observable as a result of exposure to SO_2 at a concentration of 1 ppm in air.

Andersen et al. (1974b) compared nasal clearance in mono-zygotic twins using both resin particles and saccharine particles. Results were compared with measurements of tracheo-bronchial clearance using a 6 μm Teflon aerosol. On the basis of these studies it was concluded that it does not seem possible to gain information relevant to tracheo-bronchial transport by studies of mucociliary clearance in the nose.

Black et al. (1974) also used single resin beads labelled with Tc-99m. In this case, the beads were deposited at the anterior end of the middle turbinate. These studies were conducted on nine woodworkers from the furniture industry and 12 controls, none of whom had been occupationally exposed to wood dust. Clearance rates in controls ranged from 1.9 to 18.5 mm min^{-1}, with a mean value of 6.8 mm min^{-1}. In contrast, only one of the woodworkers had a rate which fell within the normal range, in four, rates were less than 1 mm min^{-1} and in three there was almost complete stasis.

Fry and Black (1973) investigated the clearance of inhaled 2-10 μm diameter, Tc-99m labelled, monodisperse aerosols of poly-styrene from the human nose. At least 45% of the retained material was deposited in the anterior region of the nasal passages and the site of maximum deposition was 2-3 cm behind the tip of the nose. Fry and Black (1973) classified clearance patterns from the anterior nares as either one or two component exponential functions. Results of these studies are summarised below:

Two-phase-clearance:

		Component 1		Component 2	
Particle diameter (μm)	Method of deposition	Percent of deposit	Half-life (min)	Percent of deposit	Half-life (h)
7	Forced aspiration	64	4	36	3
7	"	21	19	79	8
7	"		17		
7	"		18		
7	"		18		
5	Normal breathing	36	8	64	>12
5	"	54	7	46	>12
5	"	20	6	80	>12
2.5	"	59	4	41	>12
7	"	17	15	83	>12
10	"	20	16	80	>12

Single Phase Clearance:

Particle diameter(µm)	Method of deposition	Half-life (h)
7	Forced aspiration	7
7	"	6
7	"	5
7	"	5
5	Normal breathing	3
5	"	12
5	"	8
5	"	>12
5	"	11
5	"	12
2.5	"	>12
2.5	"	>12
7	"	5
10	"	>12

The authors noted that considerable inter-and intra-subject variability occurred in respect of the magnitude and half-lives of the components of retention, but provided only limited, illustrative, data on this topic.

There has been very little work on absorption of material deposited in the nasal region. However, Cuddihy and Ozog (1973) administered CsCl, SrCl$_2$, BaCl$_2$, and CeCl$_3$ to the anterior nasal membranes of Syrian hamsters via a flexible tube. Fractional nasal absorptions ($\bar{x}$ + s.d.) were 54 ± 8%, 63 ± 9%, 51 ± 14% and 1.8 ± 0.9% for caesium, strontium, barium and cerium respectively.

6.4.3   Transport in the tracheo-bronchial region

6.4.3.1   Mucus flow

There have been numerous studies of mucus flow in the tracheo-bronchial region. However, many of these have employed aerosol techniques and are, therefore, considered in the context of particle transport (Section 6.4.3.2). This section concentrates on direct observations of mucus flow and on mucus flow rates measured by non-aerosol techniques.

The conventional picture of mucus flow is of a two layer system with a gel layer overlying a sol layer in which the cilia beat. However, Van As and his co-workers (Iravani, 1971; Iravani and Van As, 1972; Van As and Webster, 1972; 1974; Van As, 1977) have produced substantial evidence to suggest that the gel phase of the system is discontinuous. This evidence is based on observations of an in vitro test system which was prepared as summarised below (Iravani and Van As, 1971).

Wistar rats were killed by injection of 250 mg per kg of pentobarbital. Before respiration ceased, the trachea was cannulated and the abdomen opened. The lungs were inflated to the position of deep inspiration. The thorax and diaphragm were rapidly isolated and immersed in ice-cold saline, and the dissection continued under these conditions. The rib cage was removed leaving the trachea, lungs and intrathoracic cardiovascular system intact. The pulmonary vein drain-ing the left lobe was catheterised, the inferior vena cava and aorta occluded, and the pulmonary artery, supplying the cardiac lobe, open-ed. This lobe was gently perfused with ice-cold Kreb's solution to render it almost bloodless. Once the preparation had been dissected off the vertebral column, all the other lung lobes were ligated and removed, as were the cardio-vascular system, oesophagus and residual connective tissues. The specimen was bathed in circulating Kreb's solution at 2°C and oriented to give a view through the membranous wall of the trachea. Adherent peribronchial tissues were dissected off the trachea and lobar bronchus. The course of the lobar bronchus was followed by teasing the alveolar tissues apart. If care was taken not to rupture bronchioles of any significant size, the entire lobar bronchus with at least 12 side branches could be exposed. Once dis-section was complete the temperature of the bath was raised slowly to 37-38°C and a period of 1h allowed to elapse before mucus transport was studied with a stereoscopic microscope. Specimens were seen to remain viable for at least 5h after rewarming.

Such preparations are clearly highly artificial, but on rewarming new mucus production and transport was observed. For this reason, while it would not be appropriate to develop quantitative

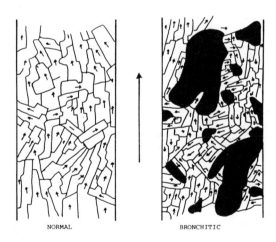

NORMAL   BRONCHITIC

Notes: The metachronal fields are outlined and the direction of ciliary beat
in them is indicated by the small arrows. The over-all direction of
ciliary beat is shown by the large arrow between the models. In normal
rats the over-all direction of ciliary beat is cranially, whereas in
bronchitic animals reversal of the direction of ciliary beat is seen in
abnormal areas. The shaded areas represent zones of ciliary inactivity.

FIGURE 6.40. METACHRONAL FIELDS DIAGRAMMATICALLY DEPICTED IN
THE PULMONARY MUCOUS MEMBRANE OF NORMAL AND BRONCHITIC
RATS. From Van As and Webster (1972).

models on the basis of such studies, they are likely to be relevant to the mechanisms of transport. The two main observations in these studies were that mucus is transported as droplets or flakes and that ciliary activity is organised in numerous metachronal fields (Van As and Webster, 1972). Within each field, ciliary beating is character-ised by synchronisation at right angles to the effective stroke of the ciliary beat. Diagrammatic illustrations of metachronal fields in normal and bronchitic rats are given in Fig. 6.40. This indicates that, while the general direction of transport is cranial, this is achieved by transport along tortuous paths and that, in bronchitic animals, trapping in zones of stasis may occur.

More recently, Van As (1977) has noted that in the main bronchi and trachea the flakes of mucus aggregate to form streams of up to 100 µm wide which coursed up the trachea, but did not become confluent to form a single layer.

It is noted that the concepts advanced by Van As and co-workers have not gone unchallenged. Luchtel (1978), on the basis of scanning electron microscopic studies of the major airways of rats has claimed that the mucus layer is continuous varying in thickness, in the airways studied, from 15 to a few tenths of a micron. However, Luchtel (1978) noted that a hypophase layer was not always distin-guishable, though an epiphase, in which the cilia were enmeshed, was always present. It is possible, therefore, that these observations are consistent with those of Van As and co-workers, which must neces-sarily refer to the hypophase, or gel, layer.

Several studies on tracheal mucus velocity have been con-ducted by Wanner and co-workers using cinebronchofibroscopy of Teflon discs (Sackner et al., 1973; Wanner et al., 1973; Santa-Cruz et al., 1974; Wood et al., 1975; Serafini et al., 1976; Goodman et al., 1978; Mezey et al., 1978). In dogs, Sackner et al. (1973) reported that 59 out of 78 exhibited tracheal mucus motion and that malnourished ani-mals often had slow, or no, mucus motion. The mean velocity of all particles, including those with zero motion, was 5.7 mm min^{-1} and, over a 6h period, tracheal mucus velocities remained fairly constant. In a subsequent study, Wanner et al. (1973) reported that tracheal mucus velocities were significantly reduced in smoking dogs relative to control dogs. Respiratory and various physiological indices were not significantly different between the two groups of animals and the authors concluded that the suppression of mucociliary activity assoc-iated with cigarette smoking may precede abnormalities of pulmonary function as determined by conventional methods. In man, Santa-Cruz et al. (1974) reported average tracheal mucus velocities ($\bar{x} \pm$ s.d.) of 21.5 ± 5.5 mm min^{-1} in normal volunteers and 1.7 ± 0.8 mm min^{-1} in pa-tients with chronic obstructive lung disease. In these patients, many regions of the tracheal mucosa failed to exhibit clearance. Santa-Cruz et al. (1974) also reported that the β-adrenergic agent terbutaline increased tracheal mucus velocities in the patients with chronic obstructive lung disease, but not in normal volunteers.

Similarly, Wood et al. (1975) reported reduced tracheal mucus velocities in patients with cystic fibrosis ($\bar{x}$ = 2.6 mm min^{-1}) and noted an increase in velocity in patients treated with terbutaline ($\bar{x}$ = 5.5 mm min^{-1}). However, it should be noted that Yeates et al. (1976) have found that patients with cystic fibrosis, as studied using inhaled albumin aerosols, fall into three groups:

-    those in whom no abnormal mucus transport is detected in the
     trachea;

-    those in whom normal transport rates occur, but who also exhibit
     abnormalities such as cessation or reversal of bolus movement;

-    those in whom normal transport rates are not observed.

In asymptomatic patients with allergic asthma, Mezey et al. (1978)
determined that baseline tracheo-bronchial mucus velocities are reduced and that inhalation of specific antigen causes a marked decrease
in tracheal mucus velocity independent of the degree of bronchospasm.
        Goodman et al. (1978) showed that tracheal mucus velocities
are higher in young non-smokers than they are in old non-smokers.
Tracheal mucus velocities were often, but not invariably, depressed in
young smokers relative to age-matched non-smoking controls. In selected smokers, tracheal mucus velocities were measured just before,
and ten minutes after, smoking one cigarette; no consistent changes
were observed in these studies on anaesthetised subjects. The authors
concluded that reduction of tracheal mucus velocity and small airway
disease appear to be the earliest signs of functional impairment in
cigarette smokers and may present together or separately. Reduced
tracheal transport velocities in smokers relative to non-smokers were
also recorded by Chopra et al. (1979) in studies in which albumin
microspheres were deposited at the carina via a catheter under topical
anaesthesia of the airways.
        Serafini et al. (1976) extended their tracheal studies to
the first 3 generations of major bronchi in eleven anaethetized mon-
grel dogs and after treatment with aminophyllin. Aminophyllin was
found to have no significant effect upon velocities. Results for
control dogs are summarised below (generation 0 = trachea).

Mucus velocity

Airway generation	Mean	Standard error(n=11)	Minimum	Maximum
0	4.90	0.92	2.06	8.46
1	3.02	0.37	1.60	5.11
2	2.19	0.35	1.45	4.53
3	1.65	0.40	0.72	3.12

Decreasing velocities with increasing generation number are indicated
clearly by these data, as they were by the earlier, in vitro, studies
of dog airways by Asmundsson and Kilburn (1970).
        It is important to note that studies of tracheobronchial
clearance undertaken on anaethetised subjects have to be viewed with
some caution. Thus, Patrick and Stirling (1977) studied the clearance
of $BaSO_4$ particles injected as a suspension into the tracahea of rats.
They reported that, compared with clearance up the trachea in con-
scious rats, the effect of halothane, thiopental and pentobarbital was
to inhibit clearance. With halothane, clearance was prevented entirely under anaethesia, but resumed normal values within a few minutes of
recovery. In contrast, thiopental and pentobarbital gave rise to
significant effects long after the recovery of consciousness. Similar

results for depression of tracheal mucus velocities under halothane anaesthesia were reported for dogs by Forbes (1976).

6.4.3.2   Tracheo-bronchial clearance

Because of the branching structure of the tracheo-bronchial tree, particles deposited distally have longer distances to travel up the mucociliary escalator than do particles deposited proximally. As Raabe (1982) has noted, this implies that clearance of material from the tracheo-bronchial tree cannot be described by a single rate. He interprets data from experimental studies as indicating that larger airways are cleared with a half-time of about 0.5 h, intermediate airways with a half-time of 2.5 h, and finer airways with a half-time of 5 h. Similarly, Morrow (1974) suggested transit times ranging from 4 h to 2 mins for the peripheral and hilar regions respectively.

Though movement up the mucociliary escalator is the major mechanism of clearance, coughing can also be effective in the larger airways, particularly in patients with lung disease. In the context of the depth to which coughing may be effective, it is noted that below the fifth bronchial generation there are no cough receptors present (Matthys and Köhler, 1981; Camner, 1981a).

Also, it is noted that not all material deposited on the mucociliary escalator is necessarily transported up it. Thus, Gore and Patrick (1982) reported that in a study in which rats either inhaled UO_2, or received $BaSO_4$ by intratracheal instillation, by 24h after administration UO_2 particles were present $\sim$10 μm below the bronchial surface and $BaSO_4$ particles were present 10 to 15 μm below the surface of the trachea. Gore and Patrick (1982) attributed this migration into the bronchial wall to particulate material engulfed in macrophages (see also Stirling and Patrick, 1980). This localisation of particles in the bronchial wall is thought to account for the long-term component of retention observed in rats after intratracheal injection (Patraick and Stirling, 1977a; Patrick, 1979). This retention is particularly notable at the first bifurcation (Gore and Patrick, 1978). A component of long-term retention (half-life 39h) is also observed at the first bifurcation in rabbits (Svartengren et al., (1981) and results on the uptake of Fe_2O_3 into the airway walls are consistent with the observations for UO_2 (Watson and Brain, 1979).

Although a review of tracheo-bronchial clearance can depend largely on human studies, it is relevant to note some of the animal studies that have been undertaken. These include the studies of Lippmann and co-workers on retention in donkeys. Thus, Spiegelman et al. (1968) observed no impairment of bronchial clearance in donkeys exposed for 30 minutes to up to 300 ppm of SO_2, whereas higher concentrations produced severe cough and either slowing or transient arrest of bronchial clearance. These results are consistent with those of Friberg and Holma (1967) who showed no effects of 10 ppm of SO_2 on early respiratory clearance in rabbits.

Albert et al. (1969; 1974) investigated the effects of cigarette smoke in donkeys and reported (Albert, 1974) that low levels of cigarette smoke accelerated clearance from the distal bronchi. Intermediate levels of exposure to whole and filtered smoke caused generalised, but transient, impairment of tracheobronchial clearance. At higher levels, whole cigarette smoke had twice the effectiveness of filtered smoke for causing sustained impairment of clearance (see also Lippmann et al., 1977). Similarly, Rylander (1971), in studies on guinea pigs, reported that smoking levels of 4 cigarettes per day caused a decrease in the clearance of killed, S-35 labelled E.coli bacteria and Holma (1969) reported that, in rabbits, the smoking of 6 cigarettes decreased early clearance of an aerosol composed of 7 μm polystyrene particles.

Sulphuric acid mists were also found to effect bronchial clearance in donkeys, causing slowing or erratic patterns of clearance

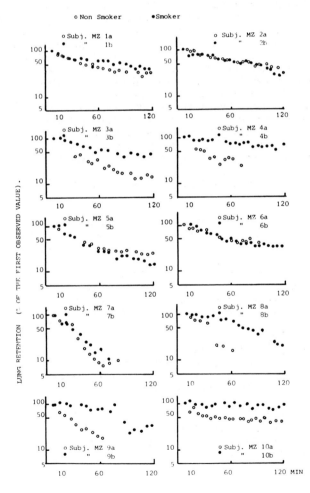

FIGURE 6.41. CLEARANCE PATTERNS IN 10 PAIRS OF MONOZYGOTIC TWINS, EACH PAIR BEING DISCORDANT WITH REGARD TO CIGARETTE SMOKING. From Camner (1971).

at exposure levels of above 100 µg m^{-3} (Schlesinger et al., 1978; 1979). In rabbits, 1 h exposures to H_2SO_4 aerosols at concentrations of 260 to 2155 µg m^{-3} produced a concentration-related effect on the clearance of tagged particles from the bronchial tree, with clearance acceleration at the lower exposures and retardation at the higher exposures (Chen and Schlesinger, 1983). Chen and Schlesinger (1983) also reported that high levels of sodium sulphite accelerated clearance and that exposure to a transition metal-sulphite complex had no effect on clearance.

Phalen and his co-workers (Frager et al., 1979; Phalen et al., 1980; Kenoyer et al., 1981) have studied the effects of sulphate aerosols and ozone on tracheo-bronchial clearance in rats. Frager et al. (1979) reported that a brief challenge to 1.2 ppm ozone following particle deposition caused a substantial delay in mucociliary clearance in rats. However, this delay was eliminated by a brief pre-exposure to 0.8 ppm of ozone three days prior to deposition of the particles. Pre-exposure at 13 days before particle exposure did not eliminate the ozone-induced delay. Phalen et al. (1980) reported that ozone slowed clearance over the period 0 - 50 h post-exposure, but stimulated clearance over the period 2 to 17 d (see also Kenoyer et al. 1981). High humidity amplified these effects, but the simultaneous presence of sulphate aerosols caused little change.

Undoubtedly, the most extensive studies of tracheo-bronchial clearance in the period immediately after inhalation of an aerosol (0-120 minutes post-exposure) are those of Camner and his co-workers. These studies have, almost exclusively, employed 6 µm Teflon particles tagged with Tc-99m. Early work by this group was summarised by Camner (1971) and some illustrative clearance curves from that paper are shown in Fig. 6.41.

Camner (1971) made several points which were important for his later work. These were as follows.

-    Clearance patterns varied considerably among the persons studied, but were quite reproducable within individuals. Thus, for investigations aimed at elucidation of the short term effect of an agent on mucociliary transport, the method of choice is to study a person first when he is not exposed to an agent and secondly when he is exposed to the agent. Observed differences in clearance patterns should then be due to differences in mucociliary transport, provided that the person is exposed to the agent after the inhalation of the test aerosol.

-    Clearance patterns within pairs of monozygotic twins were strikingly similar, but not those within dizygotic pairs. This indicates that clearance patterns are determined constitutionally to a high degree (see also Camner et al., 1972).

-    In ten pairs of smoking-discordant monozygotic twins, five pairs had quite similar clearance patterns and in the other five pairs the smokers had far slower clearance than the non-smokers (Fig. 6.41 and Camner and Philipson, 1972).

An indication of early clearance half-times over the first 30 to 120 minutes post-exposure was given by Camner et al. (1971).

All the data were interpretable in terms of a single exponential and the biological half-times were as listed below:

| | Half-time (min) | |
Subject	Exposure 1	Exposure 2
1	11.1	12.0
2	21.5	16.7
3	30.1	60.2
4	12.5	15.8
5	33.4	60.2
6	5.7	3.0
7	7.3	5.9
8	37.6	33.4

The importance of inter-subject variation, relative to intra-subject variation, is illustrated by these figures.

Camner et al. (1971a) compared tracheo-bronchial clearance in smokers who refrained from smoking, or who chain smoked throughout the period of the clearance study. The mean half-life of clearance in the absence of smoking was 43.9 min, but during chain smoking the mean value was 22.8 min. On average, tracheo-bronchial clearance diminished further in smokers who abstained from smoking for a week, (half-life 61.6 min), but this decrease was not statistically significant (confidence level not specified). Further studies (Camner et al., 1973a) demonstrated that clearance was faster in smokers three months after they had stopped smoking than it was in the first week after stopping smoking. With respect to other agents, Camner et al. (1973) reported that simultaneous exposure to carbon dust was found to enhance clearance in some subjects, but the effects were not marked.

Camner et al. (1973a) also demonstrated that, relative to healthy individuals, early tracheo-bronchial clearance was slowed in individuals with influenza studied one week after onset of symptoms. In individuals studied one and three months after onset of the symptoms, clearance was not significantly slower than in controls. However, these studies were limited to 6 individuals and revealed considerable inter-subject variability. In comparison, infection with Mycoplasma pneumoniae led to impairment of clearance at 10-15 d after onset of the disease and some residual impairment appeared still to be present up to 15 months after onset (Jarstrand et al., 1974; Camner et al., 1978). Other studies on patients with immunoglobulin deficiency indicated that chronic infection of the airways, if severe enough, will damage the mucociliary transport system, but that this damage is not necessarily irreversible (Mossberg et al., 1982).

Camner et al. (1973b) studied early tracheo-bronchial clearance in chronic obstructive lung disease (bronchitis) and reported that, whereas clearance was reduced in patients who could refrain from coughing over the test period, it was normal in patients who could not refrain. Clearance was also normal in two patients with emphysema, but without symptoms of chronic bronchitis. In these studies, it was not possible to factor out the effects of differences in deposition in chronic obstructive lung disease. However, the data clearly indicate that cough can largely compensate for decreased mucociliary transport, at least for particles deposited high up the tracheo-bronchial tree. In a later study, Camner et al. (1979) reported that in six healthy subjects coughing produced no substantial elimination of particles. Six out of eight patients with lung disease produced expectorate and also eliminated particles from the lungs by coughing. The other two patients had no phlegm, did not produce any expectorate and did not eliminate any particles by coughing. In patients, the effects of coughing were stated to be fairly reproducible.

In respect of control of the rate of mucociliary transport, Camner et al. (1974) reported that bethanechol chloride, a cholinergic compound with predominantly post-ganglionic action, produced an increase in mucociliary transport. The authors argued that this implied that vagal stimulation would also be expected to increase transport and that this could explain previously reported results with cigarette smoke and carbon dust. Camner et al. (1974) also noted that methyl-scopolamine produced marked anti-cholinergic effects on salivary excretion and heart rate, but produced, on average, no significant reduction in mucociliary transport. This was interpreted as indicating that the basal rate of mucociliary transport is not under the influence of vagal activity to any great extent.

Several studies investigated the effects of the β-adrenoceptor stimulating drug terbutaline (see Camner et al., 1976), Mossberg et al. (1976) reported that terbutaline caused less acceleration of clearance in asthmatics than in normal subjects. They suggested that this might be because of effects of asthma on the transport system, or that earlier drug treatments had produced tolerance. In patients suffering from chronic bronchitis, terbutaline enhanced clearance in some, but not all (Mossberg et al., 1976a). Other studies (Sadoul et al. 1981) have failed to demonstrate an effect of oral terbutaline

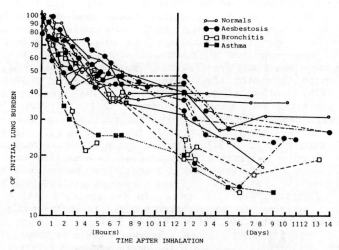

FIGURE 6.42. AEROSOL CLEARANCE FROM THE LUNG IN HEALTH AND IN OBSTRUCTIVE AIRWAY DISEASE AND ASBESTOSIS. From Thomson and Short (1969).

on clearance in bronchitics.   Because three of the four patients who showed a marked increase in clearance had less ventilatory impairment than the other seven patients, Mossberg et al. (1976a) suggested that this may indicate that the mucociliary transport mechanism is less severely damaged in the early stages of the disease than it is in the later stages.

Other studies by Mossberg and co-workers have investigated patients suffering from cystic fibrosis, or the immolite cilia syndrome.   Impaired clearance was demonstrated in both groups, but coughing was found to be an effective clearance mechanism in cystic fibrosis (Mossberg et al., 1978; Kollberg., et al 1978).

Pavia, Thomson and co-workers have conducted an extensive series of studies using inhaled 5 µm polystyrene spheres labelled with Tc-99m.   In early studies (Thomson and Short, 1969), both Tc-99m and Cr-51 were used as labels, permitting clearance to be studied to 14 days after inhalation (Fig. 6.42).   No distinctions in clearance efficiency were found between normal subjects and patients suffering from obstructive lung disease or asthma. However, more recent studies have indicated more rapid clearance in obstructive lung disease, probably due to more central deposition (Thomson and Pavia, 1974, Pavia et al., 1977a) and clearance has been observed to be impaired in mild asthma, but not in remission (Bateman et al., 1979).   Also, Short et al. (1979) have demonstrated distinctions in early retention between the central and peripheral regions of the lung in smokers, non-smokers and patients with chronic obstructive lung disease.   These data indicate limited clearance in the patients in association with more central deposition.   Limited clearance of centrally deposited aerosols in some, but not all, chronic bronchitics is also indicated by the data of Bertrand and Puchelle (1977) from studies employing aerosols of 8.1 µm monodisperse particles of resin labelled with Tc-99m.

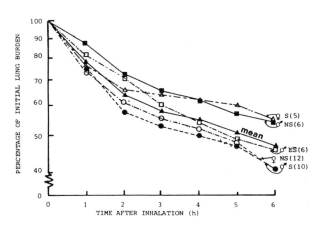

FIGURE 6.43. MEAN AEROSOL CLEARANCE FROM THE LUNG OF MALE SMOKERS
EX SMOKERS AND NON-SMOKERS , FEMALE SMOKERS AND
NON-SMOKERS AND THE GRAND MEAN FOR ALL SUBJECTS.
From Pavia et al.(1970).

More recent studies by Pavia and co-workers have typically been of a few hours duration and have usually involved distinct control and experimental groups. Thus Pavia et al. (1970) reported no significant differences in tracheo-bronchial clearance in male and female smokers and non-smokers studied to 6 h after inhalation of the tagged aerosol. Biphasic clearance was observed (Fig. 6.43). Examination of these data indicates a first phase of clearance with a half-life of less than 1 h, accounting for ∿30% of the initial lung burden. The remainder of the lung burden appears to have been cleared with a half-life of 10h or more. Although no long-term impairment of clearance was demonstrable in smokers, Pavia et al. (1971) were able to demonstrate transient decreases in rates of clearance, to 6 h post-exposure, during smoking. These results contrast with the transient increases found by Camner and his co-workers for the first 2 h post-exposure and suggest that responses to smoking may be different at different levels of the tracheo-bronchial tree. In this respect, it is noted that Albert et al. (1975) reported that upper bronchial clearance of Fe_2O_3 aerosols was not modified in short-term smoking studies, but that lower bronchial clearance was enhanced.

Pavia and Thomson (1971) reported that hyoscine inhibited mucociliary clearance to 5 h after inhalation, but the experiment did not permit them to distinguish whether this was due to direct inhibition of ciliary motion, or inspissation of mucus, or both. In contrast, Guaiphenesin, a widely used expectorant, was found to enhance tracheo-bronchial clearance in both aged 'healthy' volunteers and chronic bronchitics (Thomson et al., 1973). Again in elderly

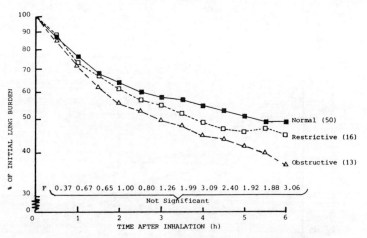

Notes: F= Snedecor's F: the value required for significance here at the 5% level is 3.11.

FIGURE 6.44. MEAN CLEARANCE CURVES FOR NORMAL SUBJECTS, SUBJECTS WITH AIRWAY OBSTRUCTION AND RESTRICTIVE IMPAIRMENT OF THE LUNGS. From Thomson and Pavia (1973).

subjects, Thomson and Pavia (1973) demonstrated marginally more rapid clearance in restrictive and obstructive lung disease than in healthy individuals (Fig. 6.44). However, the results were not significant at the 5% confidence level and Thomson and Pavia (1973) were unable to demonstrate any significant differences in clearance between smokers, non-smokers and ex-smokers in either the healthy or restricted venti- lation groups. Data on two patients with cystic fibrosis indicated that clearance is not substantially modified as a result of this disorder (Thomson et al., 1973a) and this is in agreement with the work of Sanchis et al. (1973) which also indicated more rapid clear- ance in children with cystic fibrosis than in adults.

Bateman et al. (1979a) demonstrated that circadian rhythm, physical activity and posture have no effect, whereas sleep reduces tracheobronchial clearance in the normal subject.

Other studies from Pavia, Thomson and co-workers relate to therapy-induced modifications of early tracheo-bronchial clearance. Thus, Thomson et al. (1974) found that bromhexine had a very limited effect, Francis et al. (1977) recorded no effect of the anticholiner- gic drug ipratropium bromide, Clarke et al. (1979) reported no signi- ficant effect with the mucolytic agent 2-mercapto-ethane sulphonate and Pavia et al. (1980) reported no significant effects of terbutaline and ipratropium bromide in patients with chronic obstructive bronchi- tis. In contrast, Pavia et al. (1978) reported that inhalation of an aerosol of hypertonic saline enhanced both sputum production and early tracheobronchial clearance, but did not affect the rate of coughing.

Albert and co-workers have conducted a number of studies using aerosols of Fe_2O_3, labelled with Cr-51, Au-198 and Tc-99m. Early studies (Albert and Arnett, 1955; Albert et al., 1967) revealed monophasic or biphasic bronchial clearance curves with both 3 and 5 μm particles. For 3 μm particles, 23 to 63% of the deposit was associa- ted with a clearance rate which averaged $0.19\ h^{-1}$ and 37 to 77% of the deposit was associated with a rate of $\sim0.08\ h^{-1}$. With 5 μm particles, 53 to 100% of the deposit was associated with a clearance rate of $0.18\ h^{-1}$ and 0 to 47% with a clearance rate of $0.033\ h^{-1}$.

Albert et al. (1969) studied the clearance of 0.8 to 7.9 μm monodisperse aerosols in 117 experiments on 37 subjects and identified two phases of bronchial clearance, with the first usually completed within one to two hours and the second within four to ten hours after inhalation. The fraction cleared in each phase was strongly dependent on the size of the particles. While quantitative data were not given, figures in the paper suggest that $\sim20\%$ of 1 μm particles and $\sim80\%$ of 4 μm particles were rapidly cleared. However, considerable inter- subject variation was present (see Albert et al., 1973).

Bohning et al. (1975) reported that mucociliary clearance characteristics were qualitatively and quantitatively similar for non-smoking- and smoking-concordant monozygotic twins. In twin pairs discordant with respect to smoking, upper bronchial clearance rates were greater in the non-smoking twin. These results were reported as being substantially in agreement with those of Camner and his co- workers (discussed above). However, Lourenco et al. (1971), using 2 μm iron oxide aerosols, demonstrated some delay in clearance in smokers relative to non-smokers, though total clearance to 5 h was very similar in both groups.

Lippman et al. (1981) studied the effects of exposure to sub-micron aerosols of H_2SO_4 and reported that such aerosols can slow mucociliary transport in small airways while at the same time accelerating mucus transport in the larger airways. Concentrations of H_2SO_4 in these studies were 100 to 1280 $\mu g\ m^{-3}$. It is noted that the effects reported were of very limited magnitude (see also Leikauf et al., 1981).

In other studies with iron oxide aerosols, Venizelos et al. (1981) reported that acute alcohol ingestion, at levels similar to those achieved during social drinking, alters mucociliary clearance, but direction and magnitude of the changes vary between individuals and no consistent trend was observed at any time in the first 4.5 h after inhalation. Also, Foster et al. (1980; 1981) used iron oxide aerosols to demonstrate that the ratio of tracheal to large bronchial mucociliary clearance rates is 2.7:1; that tracheal velocities are close to the maximum that can be stimulated by β-adrenergic aerosols, but that velocities in the main bronchi are only 40% of maximum and that β-adrenergic aerosols stimulate peripheral clearance.

Dolovich and co-workers conducted a series of studies using I-131 or Tc-99m labelled albumin aerosols. Using this technique, Sanchis et al. (1971) reported that in smokers there is considerable slowing of the first, fast, phase of bronchial clearance and speeding of the second phase of clearance. It is noted that these results were obtained in smokers that exhibited substantial depositional evidence of small airway obstruction. This renders interpretation of the results difficult (see also Sanchis et al., 1974).

Wolff et al. (1977) studied the effects of SO_2 and exercise on tracheo-bronchial clearance in the first 2.5 h after inhalation. They concluded:

-    clearance was highly reproducible in individuals in repeat control studies;

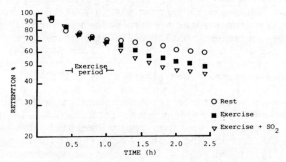

Note. Conditions identical in the half hour prior to exercise.

FIGURE 6.45. MEAN RETENTION RESULTS FOR TEN SUBJECTS AS AFFECTED BY EXERCISE AND SO_2 EXPOSURE. From Wolff et al.(1977).

- acute exposure to 5 ppm SO_2 resulted in a small transient speeding of mucociliary clearance at rest;

- exercise alone speeded clearance significantly ($p<0.05$);

- exercising in 5 ppm SO_2 showed a significant speeding in clearance beyond that found in air breathing exercising controls
  ($p<0.05$).

Results from this study, which extended one reported previously (Wolff
et al., 1975), are summarised in Fig. 6.45. Similar results for SO_2
and H_2SO_4 exposure have been reported by the same group of workers
(Newhouse et al., 1978).

Oldenburg et al. (1979) investigated the effects of postural
drainage, exercise and cough on mucus clearance in patients with
chronic bronchitis. Coughing greatly accelerated total and peripheral
clearance. Exercise had much smaller effects and postural drainage in
the absence of coughing did not alter clearance.

With respect to the effects of drugs, Lippmann et al. (1977)
reported that isoproterenol, a β-adrenergic stimulant, accelerated
clearance, as did epinephrine (adrenaline), an adrenergic stimulant
that affects both α- and β-receptors. Also, the parasympathetic
blocking drug atropine was found to slow clearance and atropine plus
isoproterenol was found to enhance clearance relative to atropine
alone. These experiments were all conducted on healthy non-smoking
volunteers. Yeates et al. (1975), using inhaled, Tc-99m labelled,
albumin microspheres demonstrated that mucociliary tracheal transport
rates in man are decreased by atropine and also by the sypathomimetic
drug Th1165a. Chronic and acute smoking had no appreciable effect on
mucociliary tracheal transport rates.

Yeates et al. (1973) used a mist of NaCl labelled with
Tc-99m as sodium pertechnetate to study clearance. The mass median
diameter of the droplets was 5 μm and clearance was studied using
gamma camera techniques. In the supine position, clearance half-times
were uniform over the entire lung and ranged from 7 to 13 minutes in
different subjects. For erect subjects clearance half-times in the
lower lung were comparable with those observed in supine subjects, but
clearance half-times were increased near the apex. These results give
an indication of half-times for absorption of ionic substances from
the lung to the pulmonary circulation.

Other studies on tracheal clearance have involved the use of
Tc-99m labelled sulphur colloid (Ross et al., 1979); insufflated
tantalum powder (Gamsu et al., 1973), Cr-51 tagged polystyrene particles (Luchsinger et al., 1968) and I-131 labelled carbon particles
(Toigo et al., 1963). These studies add little to the information
reviewed above.

Finally, some theoretical studies of tracheo-bronchial
clearance require consideration. Yeates et al. (1978) used the Horsfield morphonetric model (Section 6.2.1), a tracheal mucus velocity of
5 mm min^{-1} and a bronchial transport rate which varied inversely with
the total surface area of each order of bronchi. This model gave
clearance of the bronchi and large airways in ∿2 to 3 h and complete
clearance of the tracheo-bronchial tree in ∿7 h. This work was extended to predicting the clearance of particles from realistic deposition
patterns by Lee et al. (1979). The model was fitted to data for

7.9 μm aerosols and found to give a good representation of those data with a tracheal mucus velocity of 5.5 mm min^{-1}. Similar modelling studies have also been reported by Yu (1981).

6.4.4   Transport in the respiratory region

Several mechanisms are thought to be responsible for clearance of particles deposited distal to the end of the mucociliary escalator. Thus, the ICRP (1966) associated four compartments with this region of the lung. These compartments represented:

- rapid movement of particles to the mucociliary escalator;

- slow, and probably macrophage mediated, migration of particles to the mucociliary escalator;

- migration to respiratory lymph nodes; and

- translocation to blood as a result of solubilisation processes.

In this context, it can immediately be noted that subsequent work by Stahlhofen et al. (1980) has demonstrated a lack of rapid alveolar clearance in man. Thus, this pathway can reasonably be discounted, recognizing, however, that some macrophage involvement and the initiation of a limited amount of macrophage transport may occur within a few minutes of the inhalation of inert particles (Ferin, 1972; 1976). Also, studies on ultrafine material have indicated that dissolution is not a necessary prerequisite for transfer to the systemic circulation (Brightwell and Carter, 1977; Smith et al., 1977). The maximum size of particles participating in rapid lung to blood transfers is probably somewhere between 1 and 10 nm diameter (see also Kanapilly and Diel, 1980). Such particles are only of interest in a very limited number of specific situations.

Extensive reviews of alveolar clearance have been provided by Casarett (1972) and by Lauweryns and Baert (1977). Brief summaries are given by Morrow (1973; 1974), Lippmann et al. (1980) and Raabe (1982) and an interesting review of historical studies is given by Brundelet (1965).

Lauweryns and Baert (1977) enumerated and illustrated potential pathways of clearance from, or movement in, the alveolar region of the lungs. These comprised the following:

- particle clearance from the alveolar lumen via the tracheo-bronchial tree;

- particle absorption in the alveolar lumen by alveolar macrophages which could leave the alveoli either via the tracheo-bronchial tree or via the interstitium to the pulmonary lymphatics;

- interiorization of particles by large alveolar epithelial cells;

- absorption of particles by small epithelial cells, leading either to accumulation or transport to the interstitium;

- removal of particles from the interstitium via pulmonary blood capillaries or via the pulmonary lymphatics;

-     absorption of particles in the interstitium by interstitial
      connective tissue cells.

            On the basis of electron microscopic studies of carbon and
ferritin, together with a critical review of the literature, Lauweryns
and Baert (1977) listed various pathways and mechanisms by which, in
their view, particles can be cleared from the lung alveoli.   These
pathways and mechanisms comprised:

-     movement up the tracheo-bronchial tree with the mucociliary esca-
      lator;

-     endocytosis and digestion by non-ciliated bronchiolar epithelium;

-     endocytosis and digestion by the alveolar macrophages, which
      leave the alveolar lumen via the airways;

-     endocytosis and digestion by the neutrophilic granulocytes, which
      leave the alveolar lumen via the airways;

-     phagocytosis by the large alveolar (type II) epithelial cells;

-     endocytosis and either digestion or transcellular transport to
      the interstitium by small alveolar epithelial cells;

-     transport into pulmonary blood capilaries by mechanisms involving
      micropinocytosis;

-     transport into pulmonary lymphatics either via the main pathway
      of open endothelial junctions, or via endocytosis;

-     retention in pulmonary capillary or lymphatic endothelium.

            On the basis of the various reviews discussed above, it
seems that clearance of the non-ciliated, respiratory, region of the
lung can be best considered in terms of the following:

-     macrophage involvement, including phagocytosis and subsequent
      migration;

-     particle solubilisation;

-     dynamics of retention in the lung and transfers to other tissues.

6.4.4.1   Macrophage involvement

            Many of the data relevant to macrophages in the lung have
been discussed by Lauweryns and Baert (1977) and by Bowden (1981).
Under normal conditions, numbers are extremely low, but increases
occur after challenge with foreign substances (see also Bingham
et al., 1977), though phagocytic ability per cell may be reduced
(Brain and Corkery, 1977) and limited amounts of inert dusts may cause
little increase in macrophage populations (Strecker, 1967).   The
alveolar macrophage is thought to be of haemopoietic origin, but
proliferation is thought to occur in the alveolar interstitium and
mature cells cross the alveolar epithelium to enter the lumen of the
alveoli.   It is noted that the concept of substantial interstitial
division of macrophages is not supported by the data of Matutionis

(1979; 1979a) on mice challenged with cigarette smoke. However, interstitial division, in an unspecified animal species, was reported by Adamson and Bowden (1979).

The alveolar macrophages possess pronounced endocytic activity and a highly developed lysosomal system. They act mainly at the alveolar surface, rather than in connective tissue, and can absorb a wide range of materials, including micro-organisms, cell debris, inert and toxic particles (Lauwenryns and Baert, 1977).

Phagocytosis of inhaled particles by macrophages is rapid, typically occurring in a few hours (Sanders, 1969; Sanders and Adee, 1968; 1970) and rapid increases in macrophage numbers as well as some evidence of early clearance may be observed (see LaBelle and Brieger, 1960; Ferin, 1972; 1976). Tobacco smoke has measurable effects on alveolar macrophages in vitro (Drath et al., 1981) and these may include effects on phagocytosis (Haroz and Mattenberger-Kreber, 1977). Alveolar macrophage populations and cell characteristics have been observed to differ substantially between smokers and non-smokers (Harris et al., 1970). In emphysema, increases in the number of alveolar macrophages can result in enhanced loss of particles from the lungs in the first few days after exposure, but the presence of focal accumulations of dust-laden macrophages may be associated with a slowing of long-term clearance (Hahn and Hobbs, 1979).

Removal of alveolar macrophages from the lungs has been described by Lauweryns and Baert (1977). Movement to the ciliated airways undoubtedly occurs, but movement of macrophages up the mucociliary escalator may be very much slower than for free particles deposited on the airways (Gore and Thorne, 1977; Gore, 1983). Studies on rats by Ferin (1982) have indicated that alveolar clearance to the mucociliary escalator may occur on a time-scale of ∿7 d and theoretical analyses by Gross and Miller (1979) indicate that such motion must be directed rather than being the result of random non-directional migration.

With respect to clearance to the lymphatics, Lauweryns and Baert (1977) noted that while transfer of particle-loaded alveolar macrophages to the lymphatics is disputed, there is substantial evidence that such transfers do occur. While transfers beyond the pulmonary lymphatics probably occur, experimental evidence on this topic appears to be non-existent.

6.4.4.2   Particle solubilisation

Mercer (1967) emphasised the importance of particle solubilisation as a lung clearance mechanism and developed equations representing the time-dependence of mass loss for a log-normal distribution of particle sizes. More recently, Moss and Kanapilly (1980) have given a more extensive account of particle solubilisation, based on similar principles to the work of Mercer (1967).

The basis of the dissolution model is illustrated by considering dissolution of a single particle. In this case, for conditions in which solubility is not limiting:

$$\frac{dr}{dt} = -\frac{K}{\rho}$$

where

r (cm) is the particle radius;

t (s) is time;

K ($g\ cm^{-2}\ s^{-1}$) is the dissolution rate; and

ρ ($g\ cm^{-3}$) is the particle density.

Integrating this expression yields:

$$r = r_0 - Kt/\rho \quad \text{for } t \leq r_0\rho/K$$

$$= 0 \qquad\qquad \text{for } t > r_0\rho/K$$

Mercer (1967) considered the case of polydisperse, log-normal, distributions and showed that dissolution in such cases could be represented adequately by:

$$M/M_0 = f_1 \exp(-\lambda_1\beta) + f_2 \exp(-\lambda_2\beta)$$

where

M is the mass of material undissolved at time t;

M_0 is the original mass of material; and

f_1, f_2, λ_1 and λ_2 are constants which depend only on the geometric standard deviation, σ_g, of the distribution.

Values of β are given by:

$$\beta = \alpha_s Kt/\sigma_v \rho D_m$$

where

α_s is the surface shape factor;

α_v is the volume shape factor;

D_m is the mass median diameter of the original distribution; and

other quantities are as defined previously.

Particle shape factors are defined by:

$$\alpha_s = S/D^2 \quad \alpha_v = m/\rho D^3$$

where

S is the surface area of the particle;

m is its mass; and

D is its diameter.

Thus, for an aerosol composed of spherical particles $\alpha_s/\alpha_v=6$ and $\beta=6Kt/\rho D_m$.

Values of f_1, f_2, λ_1 and λ_2 were given by Mercer (1967) for various values of $\log_e \sigma g$ and are listed below.

$\log_e \sigma_g$	f_1	f_2	λ_1	λ_2
0.5	1.0	0	1.18	-
0.7	0.62	0.38	1.76	0.65
0.85	0.75	0.25	1.533	0.425
1.0	0.77	0.23	1.536	0.33

Thus, for aerosols with σ_g values of less than 1.65, clearance from the respiratory region by solubilisation should be representable by a single exponential clearance term. Studies on the dissolution of materials in simulated lung fluids (e.g. Thein et al., 1982) should allow determination of this half-time of clearance. Alternatively, Thomas (1971) has used Mercer's dissolution theory, together with observed clearance curves, to estimate the size distribution characteristics of aluminosilicate particles deposited in the lungs of dogs and rats.

6.4.4.3   Retention in, and clearance from, the respiratory region

In interpreting data for retention in, and clearance from, the respiratory region, it is convenient to have a model framework.

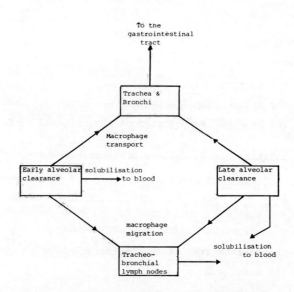

FIGURE 6.46. CONCEPTUAL MODEL OF THE CLEARANCE OF PARTICULATE
MATERIAL INITIALLY DEPOSITED IN THE RESPIRATORY
REGION OF THE LUNG.

The data reviewed above suggest that the minimum complexity that is likely to given an adequate representation of the processes involved is as shown in Fig. 6.46. In this model, early alveolar clearance is distinguished from late clearance to include provision for dealing with the components of retention with half-lives ~7 d. It is envisaged that these components relate to material engulfed by macrophages near the bottom of the mucociliary escalator. The main distinction between this model and that of the ICRP (1966) is that clearance processes are taken to be competitive in each compartment, rather than separate compartments being specified for each clearance process. No clearance from the tracheo-bronchial lymph nodes has been specified, other than by solubilisation, since there does not appear to be any experimental evidence for such a pathway.

       In order to utilise this model, it is necessary to derive rate coefficients for the various pathways. The degree of solubilisation will clearly depend both on the aerosol characteristics and on the chemical form of the inhaled material. However, macrophage transport via the mucociliary escalator and macrophage migration to the regional lymph nodes may also depend on particle size and chemical characteristics (see Morrow, 1972), since these could determine phagocytic and proliferative responses. Also, the presence of toxic materials in macrophages may enhance, or retard, their movement, and/or may induce cell lysis. If macrophage cell death is a significant phenomenon, secondary phagocytosis may also be important.

       In the remainder of this section, brief consideration is

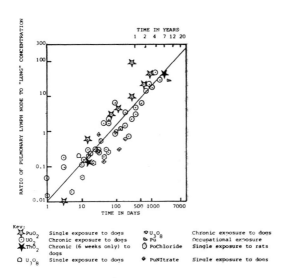

FIGURE 6.47. LYMPH NODE TO LUNG RATIOS FOR VARIOUS INHALATION EXPOSURE CONDITIONS. From Thomas (1968).

given to the retention of highly insoluble materials in the respiratory system, as an indication of the rate coefficients which might be
associated with macrophage-mediated transport.

In respect of transport of dust to tracheo-bronchial lymph
nodes, Thomas (1968) analysed ratios of lymph node to lung concentrations for a large number of human and animal studies. Results
(Fig. 6.47) indicate a relatively well-defined relationship between
this ratio and time from commencement of exposure. These data were
analysed in terms of two components of retention in the lung (90% of
deposited material being retained with a half-life of 350 d and 10%
with a half-life of 10,000 d). Material entering the lymph nodes was
assumed to be retained there indefinitely. Taking the tracheo-bronchial lymph nodes to comprise ∿1.5% of the mass of the lung (ICRP,
1974), the analysis presented by Thomas (1968) indicates that ∿20% of
material initially deposited in the respiratory region is translocated
to the tracheo-bronchial lymph nodes.

Pfleger et al. (1969) gave data on tracheo-bronchial lymph
node burdens in dogs exposed to Zr-95/Nb-95 labelled ZrO_2 aerosols.
In non-lavaged control dogs killed 30 d after exposure, 0.12 to 0.22%
of the initial lung burden was present in the lymph nodes. In dogs,
subject to single or repeated lavage treatments, 0.17 to 0.90% of the
initial lung burden was translocated to the tracheo-bronchial lymph
nodes.

Leach et al. (1970; 1973) studied the retention of UO_2 in
the respiratory systems of monkeys, dogs and rats. Data from these
studies were summarised by Leach et al. (1973) and are listed in
Table 6.9. Taking the mass of the tracheo-bronchial lymph nodes to be
1.5% of the mass of the lungs, the data on dogs exposed for one year,
indicate that up to 50% of material lost from the lungs may be transferred to the tracheo-bronchial lymph nodes. In monkeys, the comparable figure is ∿20% and in rats 6 to 15%. Data on dogs exposed to
PuO_2 (Sanders and Park, 1971) also indicate that ∿50% of the inital

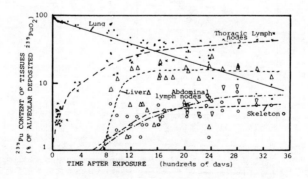

FIGURE 6.48. RETENTION AND TRANSLOCATION OF INHALED, ALVEOLARLY
DEPOSITED $^{239}PuO_2$ IN THE DOG. From Sanders and Park (1971).

TABLE 6.9

URANIUM CONCENTRATIONS IN LUNG AND LYMPH NODES FOR
CHRONICALLY EXPOSED DOGS, MONKEYS AND RATS

No. of animals	Exposure time(y)	Post-exposure time(mo)	µg U per g (f.w.) TBLN	Lung	TBLB:lung ratio
DOGS					
6	5	0	50000	1770	28
3	5	12	42000	773	54
1	5	18	43000	1150	37
1	5	22	10500	194	54
2	5	28	5400	550	9.8
1	5	54	14200	209	68
3	5	67	12500	206	61
2	5	75	3400	56	61
3	2	0	29000	2170	13
1	2	55	2300	135	17
2	2	75	5900	41	143
6	1	0	6730	1090	6.2
1	1	3	35000	1040	34
2	1	6	14800	412	36
2	1	18	16400	560	29
2	1	37	32900	450	73
4	1	60	16800	139	121
6	1	70	9800	130	75
MONKEYS					
1	4.7	0	57000	3870	15
2	5	12	21600	1650	13
1	5	73	20000	80	250
3	5	78	36400	228	160
1	1	0	14400	2750	5.2
2	1	71	45500	213	214
RATS					
5	1	0	1580	882	1.8
5	1	1	3900	754	5.2
5	1	3	3800	586	6.5
2	1	6	8700	865	10.0
10	1	0	190	708	0.27
5	1	6	505	404	1.3
5	1	9	260	329	0.79
6	1	12	2800	348	8.0

Note: from Leach et al. (1973); TBLN = tracheobronchial lymph
nodes.

lung burden may be transferred to the tracheo-bronchial lymph nodes
and show no evidence of clearance from those nodes (Fig. 6.48). A
phase of rapid uptake to the lymph nodes, paralleling early loss from
the lung, is also evidenced in these data, as it is in studies with
Y-90 incorporated into fused clay particles (Barnes et al., 1972).
    Weller and Ulmer (1972) studied the dust content of lungs
and pulmonary lymph nodes of rats exposed to coal dust. Their results
indicated that ∿14% of the lung deposit of dust was transferred to the
pulmonary lymph nodes during a period of chronic exposure lasting
22 months. In rats exposed to a heat-treated cerium hydroxide aerosol
labelled with Ce-144, maximum concentrations of Ce-144 in the tracheo-
bronchial lymph nodes were typically similar to, or a few times larger
than, those found in the lungs (Thomas et al., 1972). However, in
these studies transfers to liver, skeleton and kidneys were rapid and
substantial, indicating that solubilisation of the material played a
major role.
    In studies on dogs exposed to insufflated tantalum, Morrow
et al. (1976) reported the following data for initial lung burden
(ILB) and final lymph node burden (LNB).

Duration of study (d)	ILB (mg)	LNB (mg)	LNB:ILB
143	2890	39.4	0.014
149	3256	34.5	0.011
156	1478	5.86	0.004
240	7230	46	0.006
247	3410	22	0.006
253	347	3.5	0.010
317	2021	8.7	0.004
336	500	5.34	0.011
387	1649	0.09	-
468	4160	3.9	0.001
547	29	0.4	0.014
816	49	1.81	0.037

    Other data, for different size aerosols, gave similarly
limited lymph node uptakes, but these data have to be interpreted with
caution because of the mode of application of the aerosol.
    Also in dogs, Boecker et al. (1977) reported data indicating
that no more than 1 to 3% of the inital lung burden of Cs-137, inhaled
in fused aluminosilicate clay particles, is transferred to the
tracheo-bronchial lymph nodes in ∿300 d.
    Mewhinney et al. (1982) reported data for Am-241 uptake by
tracheo-bronchial lymph nodes following inhalation of a polydisperse
aerosol of AmO_2. The data presented indicate that ∿1% of the initial
lung content was transferred to the tracheo-bronchial lymph nodes in
the first 64 d after administration. Data at later times are difficult to interpret because of the rapid translocation of Am-241 to the
systemic circulation. On the basis of these data, Mewhinney and
Griffith (1982) gave a rate constant, for transfer from lung to lymph
nodes, of $0.0001 \, d^{-1}$.
    Snipes (1980) reported the following data for rates of
transfer of fused aluminosilicate particles to the tracheo-bronchial
lymph nodes of dogs and rats after inhalation exposure.

Particle size (aerodynamic diameter; μm)	Fraction per day	
	Dog	Rat
0.7	0.00006	0.00001
1.5	0.0001	0.00001
2.8	0.00012	0.00001
Polydisperse	0.00008	0.000005

In a later note, Snipes (1983) estimated a mechanical clearance rate from lung to lymph nodes in dogs of 0.0002 d^{-1} for fused aluminosilicate particles (see also Snipes et al., 1983).

Nolibé et al. (1977) plotted lung to lymph node burdens as a function of survival time in baboons exposed to high levels of [Pu-239]O_2. These data indicated that up to ∿30% of the initial lung burden could be transferred to the tracheo-bronchial lymph nodes in the first 10^3 d after exposure.

Clearance of insoluble dusts from the respiratory region of the lung has been the subject of a large number of studies and only relevant human data are considered in this review. In considering these studies, attention has to be given to possible solubility effects and the possibility of leaching of radioactive labels from inhaled aerosols. It is noted that the potential effects of leaching have to be considered carefully in respect of such studies. Thus, Stahlhofen et al. (1981) reported half-lives of iron oxide and Teflon particles in human lung of 60 d and 105 to 128 d respectively. Differences between half-lives of 105 d for In-111 labelled Teflon particles and 128 d for Au-198 labelled Teflon particles indicate that leaching effects cannot be ignored for this material. It is noted that these studies did not extend to more than 20 d after inhalation, so the presence of longer-term components of retention cannot be excluded on the basis of this study.

Watts (1975) reviewed published data on "in vivo" and bioassay measurements made after [Pu-239]O_2 inhalation by men and large animals. She concluded that three components of retention are present with biological half-lives of ∿1, 30 and 500 d. Examination of the faecal excretion data reviewed by Watts (1975) indicate that the 30 d component only represents a small fraction of total retention. More recently, Ramsden et al. (1978) and Ramsden, (1979) have suggested that high-fired PuO$_2$ exhibits two components of lung retention with half-lives of 30 and 300 d.

On the basis of a variety of data, Thomas (1968) postulated that 90% of material deposited in the respiratory region is cleared with a half-life of 350 d and 10% with a half-life of 10000 d. He commented that such a long-term component had not been observed experimentally.

West and Scott (1969) analysed data on the long-term retention of uranium in the chests of four accidently exposed individuals and reported half-lives of between 550 and 1500 d. Lack of knowledge of the materials involved, and the possibility of uptake in the ribs, limits interpretation of these data.

Hesp and Coote (1970) reported that the half-life of retention of Ru-106 in subjects who had accidently inhaled ruthenium oxide was 206±30 d. The urinary excretion data given indicate that this loss was largely due to solubilisation and systemic uptake.

Waligora (1971) reported on pulmonary retention of Nb-95 following on accidental exposure to labelled zirconium oxide. The long-term pulmonary half-life ($\bar{x} \pm 1$ s.d.) was estimated as 224 (122 to 1390) d. The error range is assymetric in this case because of the need to correct for radioactive decay of Nb-95.

In long-term studies with sub-micron aerosols of iron oxide labelled with Cr-51 and Pu-237 (Waite and Ramsden, 1971; 1971a) there was little evidence of any lung clearance over the period 20 to 60 d after inhalation. In comparison, data presented by Le Bouffant et al. (1972) indicated a half-life in the lung ~270 d for Fe-59 labelled iron oxide. Later results by this group (Le Bouffant and Henin, 1974) demonstrated considerable inter-subject variation in Fe-59 retention, with half-lives varying from 197 to 582 d in three subjects. It is not clear to what extent these values were determined by solubility considerations.

In a case of tantalum oxide accidently inhaled by a radiation worker, studies over 424 d indicated a half-life in the thoracic region of 1400 d (Newton, 1977).

Bohning et al. (1982) used Sr-85 tagged polystyrene microspheres in inhalation studies on man and reported the following long-term half-lives of retention in the lung.

Groups	Half-life (d)
Non-smokers	292 ± 48
Ex-smokers	296 ± 98
Smokers	270 - 1169
Subjects with obstructive lung disease	300 - 1404

Other data indicating that smoking impairs long-term clearance from the lung were given by Cohen et al. (1979) for individuals exposed to Fe_3O_4 and studied by a technique of remnant magnetisation measurements. A similar technique was used by Kalliomäki et al. (1978) who estimated clearance rates of 10 to 20% per year for inhaled welding fume.

Other studies on lung retention in man have been conducted by Bailey and co-workers using radioactively labelled fused aluminosilicate clay particles (Bailey et al., 1981; 1982; Fry et al., 1983). Bailey et al. (1982) analysed their data in terms of a two-component retention function and concluded that the half-times of the two components were ~20 and 400 d respectively. Approximately 8% of 1.2 μm particles and 40% of 3.9 μm particles were removed in the rapid clearance phase, indicating that proximity to the mucociliary escalator is likely to be a significant consideration in determining the partitioning of long-term retention in the respiratory region.

On the basis of the data discussed above, it seems appropriate to assume that 10% of particles deposited in the respiratory region are cleared with a half-life of 25 d and that 90% are cleared with a half-life of 400 d. It is also reasonable to take 10% of both the rapidly cleared and slowly cleared material as going to regional lymph nodes. Rates of loss of pulmonary derived material from the tracheo-bronchial region are not known for man, but data on rats (Gore and Thorne, 1977) indicate that a half-life of 15 d is not unreasonable.   It is emphasised that some materials may be retained with a half-life of up to, or in excess of, 1000 d in the respiratory region of some individuals.

The proposed model structure and associated rate constants are shown in Fig. 6.49.   The only element dependent value is λ_s, the rate of solubilisation.   Values of λ_s, derived from Jackson and Thorne (1983) are listed below.

Element	Form	λ_s (d^{-1})
As	All	0.07
Be	Oxides, halides, nitrates and ores	0.0005
	Sulphate	0.005
	Citrate	1.4
Cd	Oxide	0.009
Pb	All except motor exhaust	1.4
Ni	Oxides, hydroxides, carbides, Ni_3S_2 and NiS	0.01
	Other common compounds, excluding nickel carbonyl	1.4
Cr	Oxides and hydroxides	0.0001
	Halides and nitrates	0.01
	All other compounds	1.4

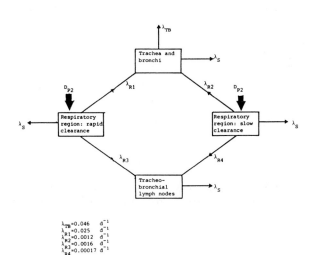

$\lambda_{TB} = 0.046$ d^{-1}
$\lambda_{R1} = 0.025$ d^{-1}
$\lambda_{R2} = 0.0012$ d^{-1}
$\lambda_{R3} = 0.0016$ d^{-1}
$\lambda_{R4} = 0.00017$ d^{-1}

λ_s is element dependent; D_{P1} is 10% of the total deposit in the respiratory region and D_{P2} is 90% of the total deposit.

FIGURE 6.49.   MODEL FOR CLEARANCE FROM THE RESPIRATORY REGION.

6.5   Model structure

6.5.1   Deposition

Total deposition in mouth breathing is estimated from the studies of Heyder (Section 6.3.4), except for sub-micron particles where the model is thought to underestimate. In this region, the data of Giacomelli-Maltoni (1972) are preferred. For a respiration rate of 12 min^{-1} and a minute volume of 20 litres, the following total deposition fractions are calculated.

Aerodynamic diameter (µm)	Fractional deposition
0.1	0.2
0.3	0.2
0.7	0.2
1.0	0.2
2.0	0.4
5.0	0.9
10.0	0.95

Mouth deposition in each case is best calculated using the formulation developed by Foord et al. (1978) on the basis of their own data, i.e.

$$D_M = 20 \log_{10} D^2 F - 40.7$$

where

D   (µm) is the aerodynamic diameter; and

F   (1 min^{-1}) is the average inspiratory flow rate.

Values of D_M and total deposition less mouth deposit, D_{T-M}, are listed below.

Aerodynamic diameter (µm)	D_M	D_{T-M}
0.1	0.00	0.20
0.3	0.00	0.20
0.7	0.00	0.20
1.0	0.00	0.20
2.0	0.03	0.37
5.0	0.19	0.71
10.0	0.31	0.64

Tracheo-bronchial deposition probabilities for material entering the trachea are given by the model of Chan and Lippmann (1980).

$$P_{TB} = 8.14 \times 10^{-4} [D^2F/(BDS)^3] + 0.037$$

where

    BDS   is taken as 1.1 cm in normal individuals;

    D   (μm) is the aerodynamic diameter; and

    F   (1 min^{-1}) is the mean inspiratory flow rate.

       Alveolar (pulmonary) depositions are obtained by difference. Thus, for a breathing rate of 12 min^{-1} and a minute volume of 20 litres, the following deposition fractions are obtained.

Aerodynamic diameter (μm)	Mouth	Fractional deposition Trachea and Bronchi	Alveolar	Total
0.1	0.00	0.04	0.16	0.20
0.3	0.00	0.04	0.16	0.20
0.7	0.00	0.05	0.15	0.20
1.0	0.00	0.06	0.14	0.20
2.0	0.03	0.13	0.24	0.40
5.0	0.19	0.53	0.18	0.90
10.0	0.31	0.64	0.00	0.95

       In the case of nose breathing, percentage deposition in the nose is calculated using:

$$D_N = -1.658 + 0.66 \log_{10} D^2 F^{1.5}$$

where

    D   (μm) is the aerodynamic diameter; and

    F   (1 min^{-1}) is the average inspiratory flow rate.

Correcting other depositions for nasal relative to mouth penetration gives the following deposition fractions.

Aerodynamic diameter (μm)	Nasal passages	Fractional deposition Trachea and Bronchi	Alveolar	Total
0.1	0.00	0.04	0.16	0.20
0.3	0.00	0.04	0.16	0.20
0.7	0.00	0.05	0.15	0.20
1.0	0.00	0.06	0.14	0.20
2.0	0.33	0.09	0.17	0.59
5.0	0.85	0.10	0.03	0.98
10.0	1.00	0.00	0.00	1.00

       In respect of clearance, the overall model is shown in Fig. 6.50. Mouth deposits are assumed to enter the gastrointestinal tract without delay and are not included.

       Deposition in the nasal passages occurs in compartments 1 and 2. Deposition in compartment 1 is taken to be 45% of total nasal deposition, to include a contribution from material carried forward into the anterior unciliated region. On the basis of data from Fry and Black (1973), λ_{N1} is taken to be 1.5 d^{-1}, though it is clearly

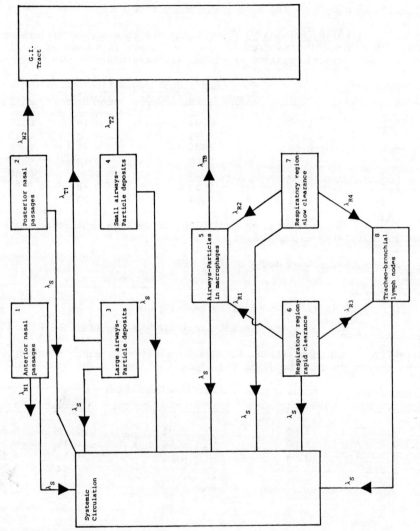

FIGURE 6.50. LUNG CLEARANCE MODEL.

strongly dependent upon personal habits. On the basis of data on nasal mucus flow rates, λ_{N2} is taken as 100 d^{-1}, corresponding to a mean residence time of 14 minutes for material deposited in this compartment.

Direct tracheo-bronchial deposition occurs to compartments 3 and 4. Partitioning between these compartments will depend upon particle size and respiratory characteristics. Assigning 40% of deposited material to compartment 3 is not likely to be substantially in error in most cases. On the basis of a wide variety of studies (Section 6.4.3.2), λ_{T1} taken as 25 d^{-1} and λ_{T2} is taken as 3 d^{-1}.

Values of λ_{TB}, λ_{R1}, λ_{R2}, λ_{R3} and λ_{R4} are discussed in Section 6.4.4.3 and are listed below.

$$\lambda_{TB} = 0.046 \ d^{-1}$$
$$\lambda_{R1} = 0.025 \ d^{-1}$$
$$\lambda_{R2} = 0.0012 \ d^{-1}$$
$$\lambda_{R3} = 0.0016 \ d^{-1}$$
$$\lambda_{R4} = 0.00017 \ d^{-1}$$

Values of λ_s are element and compound dependent. Appropriate values are given in Section 6.4.4.3 and are repeated below.

Element	Form	$\lambda_s \ (d^{-1})$
As	All	0.07
Be	Oxides, halides, nitrates and ores	0.0005
	Sulphate	0.005
	Citrate	1.4
Cd	Oxide	0.009
Pb	All except motor exhaust	1.4
Ni	Oxides, hydroxides, carbides Ni_3S_2 and NiS	0.01
	Other common compounds, excluding nickel carbonyl	1.4
Cr	Oxides and hydroxides	0.0001
	Halides and nitrates	0.01
	All other compounds	1.4

6.6 References

Adamson, I.Y.R. and Bowden, D.H., 1979. Alveolar macrophages, interstitial cells and monocytes: kinetic studies after carbon loading. Am. Rev. Resp. Dis., 119, p.198.

Albert, R.E. and Arnett, L.C. Clearance of radioactive dust from the human lung. AMA Arch. Industr. Health, 12, 99-106, 1955.

Albert, R.E., Berger, J., Sanborn, K. and Lippmann, M., 1974. Effects of cigarette smoke components on bronchial clearance in the donkey. Arch. Environ. Health, 29, 96-101.

Albert, R.E. and Lippmann, M., 1972. Factors influencing dust retention in the pulmonary parenchyma. Ann. N.Y. Acad. Sci., 200, 37-45.

Albert, R.E., Lippmann, M. and Briscoe, W., 1969. The characteristics of bronchial clearance in humans and the effects of cigarette smoking. Arch. Environ. Health, 18, 738-755.

Albert, R.E., Lippmann, M., Peterson, H.T., Berger, J., Sanborn, K. and Bohning, D., 1973. Bronchial deposition and clearance of aerosols. Arch. Intern. Med., 131, 115-127.

Albert, R.E., Lippmann, M., Spiegelman, J., Strehlow, G., Brisco, W., Wolfson, P. and Nelson, N., 1967. The clearance of radioactive particles from the human lung. In: Davies, C.N. (Ed.) Inhaled Particles and Vapours II, 361-378, Pergamon Press, Oxford.

Albert, R.E., Peterson, H.T., Bohning, D.E. and Lippmann, M., 1975. Short-term effects of cigarette smoking on bronchial clearance in humans. Arch. Environ. Health, 30, 361-367.

Albert, R.E., Spiegelman, J.R., Shatsky, S. and Lippmann, M., 1969. The effect of acute exposure to cigarette smoke on bronchial clearance in the miniature donkey. Arch. Environ. Health, 18, 30-41.

Altshuler, B., Yarmus, L., Palmes, E.D. and Nelson, N., 1957. Aerosol deposition in the human respiratory tract 1. Experimental procedures and total deposition. AMA Arch. Industr. Health, 15, 293-303.

Andersen, I., Camner, P., Jensen, P.L., Philipson, K. and Procter, D.F., 1974b. A comparison of nasal and tracheobronchial clearance. Arch. Environ. Health, 29, 290-293.

Andersen, I., Lundqvist, G.R., Jensen, P.L. and Proctor, D.F., 1974. Human response to a 78-hour exposure to dry air. Arch. Environ. Health, 29, 319-324.

Andersen, I., Lundqvist, G.R., Jensen, P.L. and Proctor, D.F., 1974a. Human response to controlled levels of sulfur dioxide. Arch. Environ. Health, 28, 31-39.

Andersen, I., Lundquist, G.R. and Proctor, D.F., 1971. Human nasal mucosal function in a controlled climate. Arch. Environ. Health, 23, 408-420.

Armbruster, L. and Breuer, H., 1982. Investigations into defining respirable dust. In: Walton, W.H. (Ed.) Inhaled particles V. Ann. occup. Hyg., 26, 21-32.

Asmundsson, T. and Kilburn, K.H., 1970. Mucociliary clearance rates at various levels in dog lungs. Am. Rev. Resp. Dis., 102, 388-397.

Asset, G., 1957. Effect of particle and wind speed on nasal penetration of wind-borne particles. AMA Arch. Industr. Health, 15, 119-123.

Bailey, M.R., Fry, F.A. and James, A.C., 1981. Pulmonary retention of inhaled particles in man. NRPB Radiol. Prot. Bull., 43, 13-20.

Bailey, M.R., Fry, F.A. and James, A.C., 1982. The long-term clearance kinetics of insoluble particles from the human lung. In: Walton, W.H. (Ed.) Inhaled Particles V. Ann. occup. Hyg., 26, 273-290.

Ballantyne, B. and Schwabe, P.H., 1981. Respiratory protection: an overview. In: Ballantyne, B. and Schwabe, P.H. (Eds.) Respiratory Protection: Principles and Applications, 3-38, Chapman and Hall, London.

Bang, B.G., Mukherjee, A.L. and Bang, F.B., 1967. Human nasal mucus flow rates. Johns Hopkins Medical Journal, 121, 38-48.

Barnes, J.E., McClellan, R.O., Hobbs, C.H. and Kanapilly, G.M., 1972. Toxicity in the dog of inhaled ^{90}Y in fused clay particles. Distribution, retention kinetics, and dosimetry. Radiat. Res., 49, 416-429.

Bateman, J.R.M., Pavia, D., Sheahan, N.F., Agnew, J.E. and Clarke, S.W., 1979. Tracheobronchial clearance in asthma. Thorax, 34, p.418.

Bateman, J.R.M., Sheahan, N.F., Pavia, D. and Clarke, S.W., 1979a. The effect of sleep, circadian rhythm, physical activity and posture on the clearance of secretions from the human lung. Am. Rev. Resp. Dis., 119, p.200.

Bertrand, A. and Puchelle, E., 1977. Mesure de la clearance muco-ciliaire des bronches proximales chez le bronchitique chronique. Pathol. Biol., 9, 623-627.

Bingham, E., Barkley, W., Murthy, R. and Vassallo, C., 1977. Investigation of aveolar macrophages from rats exposed to coal dust. In: Walton, W.H. (Ed.) Inhaled particles IV, 543-550, Pergamon Press, Oxford.

Black, A., Evans, J.C., Hadfield, E.H., Macbeth, R.G., Morgan, A. and Walsh, M., 1974.   Impairment of nasal mucociliary clearance in woodworkers in the furniture industry.   Brit. J. Industr. Med., 31, 10-17.

Boecker, B.B., Thomas, R.G. and McClellan, R.O., 1977.   Accumulation and retention of ^{137}Cs-labelled fused aluminosilicate particles by beagle dogs after repeated inhalation exposures.   In: Walton, W.H. (Ed.) Inhaled particles IV, 221-236, Pergamon Press, Oxford.

Bohning, D.E., Albert, R.E., Lippmann, M. and Cohen, V.R., 1976.   Effect of pretest temperature on aerosol penetration and clearance in donkeys.   J. Appl. Physiol., 41, 920-924.

Bohning, D.E., Albert, R.E., Lippmann, M. and Foster, W.M., 1975.   Tracheobronchial particle deposition and clearance: a study of the effects of cigarette smoking in monozygotic twins.   Arch. Environ. Health, 30, 457-462.

Bohning, D.E., Atkins, H.L. and Cohn, S.H., 1982.   Long term particle clearance in man: normal and impaired.   In: Walton, W.H. (Ed.) Inhaled particles V, Ann. occup. Hyg., 26, 259-271.

Bowden, D.H., 1981.   Reaction of the lung to injury.   In: Scadding, J.G., Cumming, G. and Thurlbeck, W.M. (Eds.) Respiratory Medicine, 529-545, W. Heinemann Medical Books Ltd., London.

Boyland, E., Gaddum, J.H. and McDonald, F.F., 1947.   Nasal filtration of airborne droplets.   J. Hyg., 45, 290-296.

Brain, J.D. and Corkery, G.C., 1977.   The effect of increased particles on the endocytosis of radiocolloids by pulmonary macrophages in vivo: competitive and toxic effects.   In: Walton, W.H. (Ed.) Inhaled Particles IV, 551-564, Pergamon Press, Oxford.

Braun, J.M., Gongora, G., Gongora, R., Roy, M., Bedu, M. Castillon du Perron, M., Jammet, H. and Drutel, P., 1979.   Dépositions trachéobronchique et pulmonaire mesurées par traceurs radioactifs.   Etude dans un groupe de sujets sains et pathologiques. Poumon, 35, 355-360.

Brightwell, J. and Carter, R.F., 1977.   Comparative measurements of the short-term lung clearance and translocation of PuO_2 and mixed Na_2O+PuO_2 aerosols in mice.   In: Walton, W.H. (Ed.) Inhaled Particles IV, 285-302, Pergamon Press, Oxford.

Brundelet, P.J., 1965.   Experimental study of the dust clearance mechanisms of the lung.   I. Histological study in rats of the intra-pulmonary bronchial route of elimination.   Acta Pathol. Microbiol. Scand. (Suppl.) 175, 1-141.

Camner, P., 1971.   The production and use of test aerosols for stud-
    ies of human tracheobronchial clearance.   Environ. Physiol., 1,
    137-154.

Camner, P., 1981.   Influence of nose and mouth breathing on particle
    deposition in the lung.   Health Phys., 40, 99-100.

Camner, P.,   1981a.   Clinical   aspects   on   lung   clearance.   In:
    Hauck, H. (Ed.) Int. Symp. Deposition and Clearance of Aerosols
    in   the   Human   Respiratory   Tract,   89-105,   Bad   Gleichenberg,
    Austria.

Camner, P. and Bakke, B., 1980.   Nose or mouth breathing?   Environ.
    Res., 21, 394-398.

Camner, P., Jarstrand, C. and Philipson, K., 1973a.   Tracheobronchial
    clearance in patients with influenza.   Am. Rev. Resp. Dis., 108,
    131-135.

Camner, P., Jarstrand, C. and Philipson, K., 1978.   Tracheobronchial
    clearance after infection with Mycoplasma pneumoniae.   Scand. J.
    Infect. Dis., 10, 33-35.

Camner, P., Mossberg, B. and Philipson, K., 1973b.   Tracheobronchial
    clearance and chronic obstructive lung disease.   Scand. J. Resp.
    Dis., 54, 272-281.

Camner, P.,   Mossberg, B.,   Philipson, K.   and Strandberg, K.,   1979.
    Elimination   of   test   particles   from   the   human   tracheobronchial
    tract by voluntary coughing.   Scand. J. Resp. Dis., 60, 56-62.

Camner, P., Strandberg, K. and Philipson, K., 1974.   Increased muco-
    ciliary   transport   by   cholinergic   stimulation.   Arch.   Environ.
    Health, 29, 220-224.

Camner, P. and Philipson, K., 1972.   Tracheobronchial clearance in
    smoking discordant twins.   Arch. Environ. Health, 25, 60-63.

Camner, P. and Philipson, K., 1978.   Human alveolar deposition of
    4 μm teflon particles.   Arch. Environ. Health, 33, 181-185.

Camner, P., Philipson, K. and Arvidsson, T., 1971a.   Cigarette smok-
    ing in man: short-term effect on mucociliary transport.   Arch.
    Environ. Health, 23, 421-426.

Camner, P., Philipson, K. and Arvisdsson, T., 1973.   Withdrawal of
    cigarette   smoking.   A   study   on   tracheobronchial   clearance.
    Arch. Environ. Health., 26, 90-92.

Camner, P.,   Philipson, K.   and Friberg, L.,   1972.   Tracheobronchial
    clearance in twins.   Arch. Environ. Health, 24, 82-87.

Camner, P., Philipson, K., Friberg, L., Holma, B., Larsson, B. and
Svedberg, J., 1971.   Human tracheobronchial clearance studies
with fluorocarbon resin particles tagged with [18]F.   Arch.
Environ. Health, 22, 444-449.

Camner, P., Strandberg, K. and Philipson, K., 1976.   Increased mucociliary transport by adrenergic stimulation.   Arch. Environ.
Health, 31, 79-82.

Carpenter, P.S. and Taulbee, D.B., 1980.   Time dependent gravitational sedimentation of aerosol particles from steady laminar flows
in channels and ducts.   J. Aerosol Sci., 11, 161-178.

Casarett, L.J., 1972.   The vital sacs: alveolar clearance mechanisms
in inhalation toxicology.   In: Hayes, W.J. (Ed.) Essays in
Toxicology, Vol.3, 1-36, Academic Press, New York.

Chan, T.L. and Lippmann, M., 1980.   Experimental measurements and
empirical modelling of the regional deposition of inhaled particles in humans.   Am. Ind. Hyg. Assoc. J., 41, 399-409.

Chan, T.L., Screck, R.M. and Lippmann, M., 1980.   Effect of the
laryngeal jet on particle deposition in the human trachea and
upper bronchial airways.   J. Aerosol. Sci., 11, 447-459.

Chang, H.K. and El Masry, O.A., 1982.   A model study of flow dynamics
in human central airways.   Part I: axial velocity profiles.
Respiration Physiology, 49, 75-95.

Chen, L.C. and Schlesinger, R.B., 1983.   Response of the bronchial
mucociliary clearance system in rabbits to inhaled sulfite and
sulfuric acid aerosols.   Toxicol. Appl. Pharmacol., 71, 123-131.

Chopra, S.K., Taplin, G.V., Elam, D., Carson, S.A. and Golde, D.,
1979.   Measurement of tracheal mucociliary transport velocity in
humans - smokers versus non-smokers.   Am. Rev. Resp. Dis., 119,
p.205.

Corrin, B., 1981.   The cellular constituents of the lung.   In:
Scadding, J.G., Cumming, G. and Thurlbeck, W.M. (Eds.) Scientific
Foundations of Respiratory Medicine, 78-91, W. Heinemann Medical
Books Ltd., London.

Clarke, S.W., Lopez-Vidriero, M.T., Pavia, D. and Thompson, M.L. 1979.
The effect of sodium 2-mercapto-ethane sulphonate and hypertonic
saline aerosols on bronchial clearance in chronic bronchitis.
Br. J. clin. Pharmac., 7, 39-44.

Clarke, S.W. and Pavia, D., 1980.   Lung mucus production and mucociliary clearance: methods of assessment.   Br. J. clin.
Pharmac., 9, 537-546.

Cohen, D., Arai, S.F. and Brain, J.D., 1979. Smoking impairs long-term dust clearance from the lung. Science, 204, 514-517.

Cuddihy, R.G., and Ozog, J.A., 1973. Nasal absorption of CsCl, $SrCl_2$, $BaCl_2$ and $CeCl_3$ in Syrian Hamsters. Health Phys., 25, 219-224.

Cumming, G., 1974. The morphometry of the human airways. INSERM, 29, 3-8.

Dautrebande, L., Beckmann, H. and Walkenhorst, W., 1959. Studies on deposition of submicronic dust particles in the respiratory tract. AMA Arch. Ind. Health, 19, 383-391.

Davies, C.N., 1972. Breathing of half-micron aerosols. II. Interpretation of experimental results. J. Appl. Physiol., 32, 601-611.

Davies, C.N., 1972a. An algebraical model for the deposition of aerosols in the human respiratory tract during steady breathing. Aerosol Sci., 3, 297-306.

Davies, C.N., 1974. Deposition of inhaled particles in man. Chemistry and Industry, 11, pp441-444.

Davies, C.N., 1980. An algebraic model for the deposition of aerosols in the human respiratory tract during steady breathing - addendum. J. Aerosol Sci., 11, 213-224.

Davies, C.N., 1981. The deposition and distribution in the lungs of inhaled particles. In: Ballantyne, B. and Schwabe, P.H. (Eds.) Respiratory Protection: Principles and Applications, 65-92, Chapman and Hall, London.

Davies, C.N., Heyder, J. and Subba Ramu, M.C., 1972. Breathing of half-micron aerosols. I. Experimental. J. Appl. Physiol., 32, 591-600.

Davies, C.N., Lever, M.J. and Rothenberg, S.J., 1977. Experimental studies on the deposition of particles in the human lungs. In: Walton, W.H. (Ed.). Inhaled Particles IV, 151-162, Pergamon Press, Oxford.

Dolovich, M., Ruffin, R.E., Roberts, R. and Newhouse, M.T., 1981. Optimal delivery of aerosols from metered dose inhalers. Chest, 80, 911-915.

Drath, D.B., Shorey, J.M. and Huber, G.L., 1981. Functional and metabolic properties of alveolar macrophages in response to the gas phase of tobacco smoke. Infection and Immunity, 34, 11-15.

Dunnill, M.S., 1962. Postnatal growth of the lung. Thorax, 17, 329-333.

Emmett, P.C., Aitken, R.J. and Hannan, W.J., 1982. Measurements of the total and regional deposition of inhaled particles in the human respiratory tract. J. Aerosol Sci., 13, 549-560.

Emmett, P.C., Aitken, R.J. and Muir, D.C.F., 1979. A new apparatus for use in studies of the total and regional deposition of aerosol particles in the human respiratory tract during steady breathing. J. Aerosol Sci., 10, 123-131.

Ewert, G., 1965. On the mucus flow rate in the human nose. Acta Oto-laryngol., Suppl. 200.

Ferin, J., 1972. Observations concerning alveolar dust clearance. Ann. N.Y. Acad. Sci., 200, 66-72.

Ferin, J., 1976. Lung clearance of particles. In: Aharonson, E.F., Ben-David, A. and Klingberg, M.A. (Eds.), Air Pollution and the Lung, 64-78, John Wiley and Sons, New York.

Ferin, J., 1982. Alveolar macrophage mediated pulmonary clearance suppressed by drug-induced phospholipidosis. Exp. Lung Res., 4, 1-10.

Ferin, J., Mercer, T.T. and Leach, L.J., 1983. The effect of aerosol charge on the deposition and clearance of TiO_2 particles in rats. Environ. Res., 31, 148-151.

Foord, N., Black, A. and Walsh, M., 1977. Pulmonary deposition of inhaled particles with diameters in the range 2.5 to 7.5 μm. In: Walton, W.H. (Ed.) Inhaled Particles IV, 137-149, Pergamon Press, Oxford.

Foord, N., Black, A. and Walsh, M., 1978. Regional deposition of 2.5-7.5 μm diameter inhaled particles in healthy male non-smokers. J. Aerosol Sci., 9, 343-357.

Forbes, A.R., 1976. Halothene depresses mucociliary flow in the trachea. Anaesthesiology, 45, 59-63.

Foster, W.M., Langenback, E. and Bergofsky, E.H., 1980. Measurement of tracheal and bronchial mucus velocities in man: relation to lung clearance. J. Appl. Physiol. (Resp. Environ. Exercise Physiol.), 48, 965-971.

Foster, W.M., Langenback, E.G. and Bergofsky, E.H., 1981. Respiratory drugs influence lung mucociliary clearance in central and peripheral ciliated airways. Chest, 80, 877-880.

Frager, N.B., Phalen, R.F. and Kenoyer, J.L., 1979. Adaptations to ozone in reference to mucociliary clearance. Arch. Environ. Health, 34, 51-57.

Francis, R.A., Thomson, M.L., Pavia, D. and Douglas, R.B., 1977. Ipratropium bromide: mucociliary clearance rate and airway resistance in normal subjects. Br. J. Dis. Chest, 71, 173-178.

Friberg, L. and Holma, B., 1967. Études expérimentales de l'épuration pulmonaire d'aerosols radio-actifs a l'aide du balayage de profil et du comptage intéressant la totalité de l'organisme. Le Poumon et le Coeur, 23, 1279-1291.

Fry, F.A., 1970. Charge distribution on polystyrene aerosols and deposition in the human nose. Aerosol. Sci., 1, 135-146.

Fry, F.A., Bailey, M.R. and James, A.C., 1983. Long-term pulmonary retention of inhaled particles in man. J. Aerosol Sci., 14, 199-201.

Fry, F.A. and Black, A., 1973. Regional deposition and clearance of particles in the human nose. Aerosol Sci., 4, 113-124.

Fuchs, N.A., 1964. The Mechanics of Aerosols. Pergamon Press, Oxford.

Gamsu, G., Wientraub, R.M. and Nadel, J.A., 1973. Clearance of tantalum from airways of different caliber in man evaluated by a roentgenographic method. Am. Rev. Resp. Dis., 107, 214-224.

Garrard, C.S., Gerrity, T.R., Schreiner, J.F. and Yeates, D.B., 1981. Analysis of aerosol deposition in the healthy human lung. Arch. Environ. Health, 36, 184-193.

Gebhart, J., Heyder, J. and Stahlhofen, W., 1981. Use of aerosols to estimate pulmonary air-space dimensions. J. Appl. Physiol. (Resp. Environ. Exercise Physiol.), 51, 465-476.

Gerrity, T.R., Lee, P.S., Hass, F.J., Marinelli, A., Werner, P. and Lourenco, R.V., 1979. Calculated deposition of inhaled particles in the airway generations of normal subjects. J. Appl. Physiol. (Resp. Environ. Exercise Physiol.), 47, 867-873.

Giacomelli-Maltoni, G., Melandri, C., Prodi, V. and Tarroni, G., 1972. Deposition efficiency of monodisperse particles in the human respiratory tract. Am. Ind. Hyd. Assoc. J., 33, 603-610.

Gil, J., 1982. Comparative morphology and ultrastructure of the airways. In: Witschi, H. and Nettesheim, P. (Eds.) Mechanisms in Respiratory Toxicology, Vol.1, 3-25, CRC Press, Boca Raton, Florida.

Gilboa, A. and Silberberg, A., 1976. Characterization of epithelial mucus and its function in clearance by ciliary propulsion. In: Aharonson, E.F., Ben-David, A. and Klingberg, M.A. (Eds.), Air Pollution and the Lung, 49-63, John Wiley and Sons, New York.

Goldburg, I.S., 1981.   Settling and diffusion of particles in small airways.   34th ACEMB Houston, Texas, Vol.23, p.36.

Goldberg, I.S. and Smith, R.B., 1981.   Settling and diffusion of aerosol particles in small airways during breath holding.   Ann. Biomed. Eng., $\underline{9}$, 557-575.

Goodman, R.M., Yergin, B.M., Landa, J.F., Golinvaux, M.H. and Sackner, M.A., 1978.   Relationship of smoking history and pulmonary function tests to tracheal mucus velocity in non-smokers, young smokers, ex-smokers, and patients with chronic bronchitis.   Am. Rev. Resp. Dis., $\underline{117}$, 205-214.

Gore, D.J., 1983.   The spatial and temporal distribution of inhaled UO_2 particles in the respiratory tract of the rat II.   The relative concentration of UO_2 between the intrapulmonary airways and the pulmonary tissue.   Radiat. Res., $\underline{93}$, 276-287.

Gore, D.J. and Patrick, G., 1978.   The distribution and clearance of inhaled UO_2 particles on the first bifurcation and trachea of rats.   Phys. Med. Biol., $\underline{23}$, 730-737.

Gore, D.J. and Patrick, G., 1982.   A quantitative study of the penetration of insoluble particles into the tissue of conducting airways.   In: Walton, W.H. (Ed.) Inhaled Particles V.   Ann. occup. Hyg., $\underline{26}$, 149-161.

Gore, D.J. and Thorne, M.C., 1977.   The distribution and clearance of inhaled uranium dioxide particles in the respiratory tract of the rat.   In: Walton, W.H. (Ed.) Inhaled Particles IV, 275-284, Pergamon Press, Oxford.

Gross, N.J. and Miller, I.F., 1979.   Models of emigration of macrophages from alveolar spaces: random versus tactic mechanisms. Am. Rev. Resp. Dis., $\underline{119}$, p.219.

Hahn, F.F. and Hobbs, C.H., 1979.   The effect of enzyme-induced pulmonary emphysema in Syrian hamsters on the deposition and long-term retention of inhaled particles.   Arch. Environ. Health, $\underline{34}$, 203-211.

Hamill, P., 1979.   Particle deposition due to turbulent diffusion in the upper respiratory system.   Health Phys., $\underline{36}$, 355-369.

Hansen, J.E. and Ampaya, E.P., 1975.   Human air space shapes, sizes, areas and volumes.   J. Appl. Physiol., $\underline{38}$, 990.

Haroz, R.K. and Mattenberger-Kreber, L., 1977.   Effects of cigarette smoke on macrophage phagocytosis.   In: Sanders, C.L., Schneider, R.P., Dagle, G.E. and Ragan, H.A. (Eds.) Pulmonary Macrophage and Epithelial Cells. 36-57.   ERDA Technical Information Center.

Harris, J.O., Swenson, E.W. and Johnson, J.E. III, 1970.   Human alveolar macrophages: Comparison of phagocytic ability, glucose utilisation and ultrastructure in smokers and non-smokers.   J. Clin. Invest., 49, 2086-2096.

Hesp, R. and Coote, J., 1970.   Body radioactivity studies on a series of cases in which ruthenium-106 oxide was inhaled.   UKAEA Report PG 979(W).

Heyder, J., 1982.   Alveolar deposition of inhaled particles in humans.   Am. Ind. Hyd. Assoc. J., 43, 864-866.

Heyder, J., 1983.   Charting thoracic airways by aerosols.   Clin. Phys. Physical Meas., 4, 29-37.

Heyder, J. and Davies, C.N., 1971.   The breathing of half-micron aerosols III.   Dispersion of particles in the respiratory tract. Aerosol Sci., 2, 437-452.

Heyder, J., Gebhart, J., Heigwer, G., Roth, C. and Stahlhofen, W., 1973.   Experimental studies of the total deposition of aerosol particles in the human respiratory tract.   Aerosol Sci., 4, 191-208.

Heyder, J., Gebhart, J., Rudolf, G. and Stahlhofen, W., 1980.   Physical factors determining particle deposition in the human respiratory tract.   J. Aerosol Sci., 11, 505-515.

Heyder, J., Gebhart, J., Roth, C., Scheuch, G. and Stahlhofen, W., 1983.   Diffusional transport of aerosol particles.   J. Aerosol Sci., 14, 279-283.

Heyder, J., and Rudolf, G. 1977.   Deposition of aerosol particles in the human nose.   In: Walton, W.H. (Ed.) Inhaled Particles IV. 107-126.   Pergamon Press, Oxford.

Hilding, A.C., 1963.   Phagocytosis, mucous flow, and ciliary action. Arch. Environ. Health, 6, 61-71.

Hiller, F.C., Mazumder, M.K., Wilson, J.D., McLeod, P.C. and Bone, R.C., 1982.   Human respiratory tract deposition using multimodal aerosols.   J. Aerosol. Sci., 13, 337-343.

Horsfield, K., 1981.   The structure of the tracheobronchial tree. In: Scadding, J.G., Cumming, G. and Thurlbeck, W.M. (Eds.) Scientific Foundations of Respiratory Medicine, 54-70, W. Heinemann Medical Books Ltd., London.

Hofmann, W., 1982.   Mathematical model for the postnatal growth of the human lung.   Respiratory Physiology, 49, 115-129.

Hofmann, W., 1982a.   The effect of polydispersiveness of natural radioactive aerosols on tracheobronchial deposition.   Radiat. Prot. Dos., 3, 97-101.

Holma, B., 1969.   The acute effect of cigarette smoke on the initial course of lung clearance in rabbits.   Arch. Environ. Health, 18, 171-173.

Horsfield, K. and Cumming, G., 1968.   Morphology of the bronchial tree in man.   J. Appl. Physiol., 24, 373-383.

Horsfield, K., Dart, G., Olson, D.E., Filley, G.F. and Cumming, G., 1971.   Models of the human bronchial tree.   J. Appl. Physiol., 31, 207-217.

Horsfield, K., Relea, F.G. and Cumming, G., 1976.   Diameter, length and branching ratios in the bronchial tree.   Respir. Physiol., 26, 351-356.

Hounam, R.F., 1975.   The removal of particles from the nasopharyngeal (NP) compartment of the respiratory tract by nose blowing and swabbing.   Health Phys., 28, 743-750.

Hounam, R.F., Black, A. and Morgan, A., 1983.   Removal of particles deposited in human nasal passages by nose blowing.   Health Phys., 44, 418-422.

Hounam, R.F., Black, A. and Walsh, M., 1969.   Deposition of aerosol particles in the nasopharyngeal region of the human respiratory tract.   Nature (Lond.), 221, 1254-1255.

Hounam, R.F., Black, A. and Walsh, M., 1971.   The deposition of aerosol particles in the nasopharyngeal region of the human respiratory tract.   Aerosol Sci., 2, 47-61.

Hughes, J.M.B., Hoppin, F.G. Jr. and Mead, J., 1972.   Effect of lung inflation on bronchial length and diameter in excised lungs.   J. Appl. Physiol., 32, 25-35.

ICRP Task Group on Lung Dynamics, 1966.   Deposition and retention models for internal dosimetry of the human respiratory tract. Health Phys., 12, 173-207.

ICRP Publication 23, 1974.   Report of the Task Group on Reference Man.   Pergamon Press, Oxford.

ICRP Publication 19, 1979.   The Metabolism of Compounds of Plutonium and other Actinides.   Pergamon Press, Oxford.

Ingham, D.B., 1981.   Precipitation of charged particles in human airways.   J. Aerosol Sci., 12, 131-135.

Iravani, J., 1971.   Clearance function of the respiratory ciliated epithelium in normal and bronchitic rats.   In: Walton, W.H. (Ed.) Inhaled Particles III, 143-148, Unwin Bros., London.

Iravani, J. and Van As, A., 1972.   Mucus transport in the tracheo-bronchial tree of normal and bronchitic rats.   J. Pathol., 106, 81-93.

James, A.C., 1977. Bronchial deposition of free ions and submicron particles studied in excised lung. In: Walton, W.H. (Ed.) Inhaled Particles IV, 203-219, Pergamon Press, Oxford.

Jarstrand, C., Camner, P. and Philipson, K., 1974. Mycoplasma pneumoniae and tracheobronchial clearance. Am. Rev. Resp. Dis., 110, 415-419.

Johnston, J.R., Isles, K.D. and Muir, D.C.F., 1977. Inertial deposition of particles in human branching airways. In: Walton, W.H. (Ed.) Inhaled Particles IV, 61-73, Pergamon Press, Oxford.

Johnston, J.R. and Schroter, R.C., 1979. Deposition of particles in model airways. J. Appl. Physiol., 47, 947-953.

Kalliomäki, P.L., Korhonen, O., Vaarenen, V., Kalliomäki, K. and Koponen, M., 1978. Lung retention and clearance of shipyard arc welders. Int. Arch. Occup. Environ. Health, 42, 83-90.

Kanapilly, G.M. and Diel, J.H., 1980. Ultrafine ^{239}PuO$_2$ aerosol generation, characterisation and short-term inhalation study in the rat. Health Phys., 39, 505-519.

Kenoyer, J.L., Phalen, R.F. and Davis, J.R., 1981. Particle clearance from the respiratory tract as a test of toxicity: effect of ozone on short and long term clearance. Exp. Lung Res., 2, 111-120.

Kimura, K., 1971. Experimental studies on the aerosol deposition in the human respiratory system. J. Science of Labour, 47, 668-675.

Kollberg, H., Mossberg, B., Afzelius, B.A., Philipson, K. and Camner, P., 1978. Cystic fibrosis compared with the immotile-cilia syndrome: a study of mucociliary clearance, ciliary ultrastructure, clinical picture and ventilatory function. Scand. J. Resp. Dis., 59, 297-306.

LaBelle, C.W. and Brieger, H., 1960. The fate of inhaled particles in the early post-exposure period II. The role of pulmonary phagocytosis. Arch. Environ. Health, 5, 423-427.

Landahl, H.D., 1950. On the removal of airborne droplets by the human respiratory tract: I. The lung. Bull. Math. Biophys., 12, 43-56.

Landahl, H.D. Particle removal by the respiratory system. Note on the removal of airborne particulates by the human respiratory tract with particular reference to the role of diffusion. Bull. Math. Biophys., 25, 29-39.

Landahl, H.D. and Black, S., 1947. Penetration of airborne particulates through the human nose. J. Indust. Hyg. Toxicol., 29, 269-277.

Landahl, H.D. and Tracewell, T., 1949.   Penetration of airborne particulates through the human nose II.   J. Indust. Hyg. Toxicol., <u>31</u>, 55-59.

Landahl, H.D., Tracewell, T.N. and Lassen, W.H., 1951.   On the retention of airborne particulates in the human lung II.   AMA Arch. Indust. Hyg., <u>3</u>, 359-366.

Last, J.A., 1982.   Mucus production and the ciliary escalator.   In: Witschi, H. and Nettesheim, P. (Eds.) Mechanisms of Respiratory Toxicology, Vol. 1, 247-268, CRC Press, Boca Raton, Florida.

Lauweryns, J.M. and Baert, J.H., 1977.   Alveolar clearance and the role of the pulmonary lymphatics.   Am. Rev. Resp. Dis., <u>115</u>, 625-683.

Leach, L.J., Maynard, E.A., Hodge, H.C., Scott, J.K., Yuile, C.L., Sylvester, G.E. and Wilson, H.B., 1970.   A five year inhalation study with natural uranium dioxide (UO_2) dust-I.   Retention and biological effect in the monkey, dog and rat.   Health Phys., <u>18</u>, 599-612.

Leach, L.J., Yuile, C.L., Hodge, H.C., Sylvester, G.E. and Wilson, H.B., 1973.   A five year inhalation study with natural uranium dioxide (UO_2) dust-II.   Postexposure retention and biologic effects in the monkey, dog and rat.   Health Phys., <u>25</u>, 239-258.

Le Bouffant, L. and Henin, J.P., 1974.   Mesure de l'epuration pulmonaire chez l'homme par des particules d'oxyde de fer marque. INSERM, <u>29</u>, 193-204.

Le Bouffant, L., Henin, J.-P., Martin, J.-C. and DaNiel, H., 1972. Etude expérimentale de l'epuration pulmonaire.   Action de l'empoussiérage sur la capacité d'épuration.   Application à l'homme. Lille Méd., <u>17</u>, 1091-1101.

Lee, P.S., Gerrity, T.R., Hass, F.J. and Lourenco, R.V., 1979.   A model for tracheobronchial clearance of inhaled particles in man and a comparison with data.   IEEE Trans. Biomed. Eng., <u>26</u>, 624-630.

Leikauf, G., Yeates, D.B., Wales, K.A., Spektor, D., Albert, R.E. and Lippmann, M., 1981.   Effects of sulfuric acid aerosol on respiratory mechanics and mucociliary particle clearance in healthy non-smoking adults.   Am. Ind. Hyg. Assoc. J., <u>42</u>, 273-282.

Lippmann, M., 1970.   Deposition and clearance of inhaled particles in the human nose.   Ann. Otol. Rhinol. Laryngol., <u>79</u>, 519-528.

Lippmann, M., 1972.   Aerosol sampling for inhalation hazard evaluations.   In: Mercer, T.T., Morrow, P.E. and Stöber, W. (Eds.) Assessment of Airborne Particles.   Fundamentals, Applications, and Implications to Inhalation Toxicity, 449-464, Chales C. Thomas, Springfield, Illinois.

Lippmann, M. and Albert, R.E., 1969. The effect of particle size on the regional deposition of inhaled aerosols in the human respiratory tract. Am. Ind. Hyg. Assoc. J., 30, 257-275.

Lippmann, M., Albert, R.E., Yeates, D.B., Berger, J.M., Foster, W.M. and Bohning, D.E., 1977. Factors affecting tracheobronchial mucociliary transport. In: Walton, W.H. (Ed.) Inhaled Particles IV, 305-319, Pergamon Press, Oxford.

Lippmann, M., Leikauf, G., Spektor, D., Schlesinger, R.B. and Albert, R.E., 1981. The effects of irritant aerosols on mucus clearance from large and small conductive airways. Chest, 80, 873-877.

Lippmann, M., Yeates, D.B. and Albert, R.E., 1980. Deposition, retention and clearance of inhaled particles. Brit. J. Indust. Med., 37, 337-362.

Lourenco, R.V., Klimek, M.F. and Borowski, C.J., 1971. Deposition and clearance of 2 μ particles in the tracheobronchial tree of normal subjects - smokers and non-smokers. J. Clin. Invest., 50, 1411-1420.

Love, R.G. and Muir, D.C.F., 1976. Aerosol deposition and airway obstruction. Am. Rev. Resp. Dis., 114, 891-897.

Luchsinger, P.C., Lagarde, B. and Kilfeather, J.E., 1968. Particle clearance from the human tracheobronchial tree. Am. Rev. Resp. Dis., 97, 1046-1050.

Luchtel, D.L., 1978. The mucous layer of the trachea and major bronchi in the rat. In: Scanning Electron Microscopy, Vol.II, 1089-1098, SEM Inc., O'Hare, Ill.

Martonen, T., 1983. Deposition of inhaled particulate matter in the upper respiratory tract, larynx, and bronchial airways: a mathematical description. J. Toxicol. Environ. Health, 12, 787-800.

Martonen, T.B. and Wilson, A.F., 1983. The influence of hygroscopic growth upon the deposition of bronchodilator aerosols in upper human airways. J. Aerosol. Sci., 14, 208-211.

Matthys, H. and Köhler, D., 1981. Diagnostic use of radioaerosols. In: Hauck, H. (Ed.) Int. Symp. Deposition and Clearance of Aerosols in the Human Respiratory Tract, 135-154, Bad Gleichenberg, Austria.

Matulionis, D.H., 1979. Reaction of macrophages to cigarette smoke. I. Recruitment of pulmonary macrophages. Arch. Environ. Health, 34, 293-298.

Matulionis, D.H., 1979a. Reaction of macrophages to cigarette smoke. II. Immigration of macrophages to the lungs. Arch. Environ. Health, 34, 298-301.

Melandri, C., Prodi, V., Tarroni, G., Formignani, M., De Zaiacomo, T., Bompane, G.F. and Maestri, G., 1977. On the deposition of unipolarly charged particles in the human respiratory tract. In: Walton, W.H. (Ed.) Inhaled Particles IV, 193-201, Pergamon Press, Oxford.

Melandri, C., Tarroni, G., Prodi, V., De Zaiacomo, T., Formignani, M. and Lombardi, C.C., 1983. Deposition of charged particles in the human airways. J. Aerosol Sci., 14, 184-186.

Melandri, C., Tarroni, G., Prodi, V., De Zaiacomo, T., Formignani, M. and Lombardi, C.C., 1983a. Deposition of charged particles in the human airways. J. Aerosol Sci., 14, 657-669.

Mercer, T.T., 1967. On the role of particle size in the dissolution of lung burdens. Health Phys., 13, 1211-1221.

Mewhinney, J.A. and Griffith, W.C., 1982. Models of Am metabolism in beagles and humans. Health Phys., 42, 629-644.

Mewhinney, J.A., Griffith, W.C. and Muggenburg, B.A., 1982. The influence of aerosol size on retention and translocation of ^{241}Am following inhalation of ^{241}AmO$_2$ by beagles. Health Phys., 42, 611-627.

Mercer, T.T., 1975. The deposition model of the Task Group on Lung Dynamics: a comparison with recent experimental data. Health Phys., 673-680.

Mezey, R.J., Cohn, M.A., Fernandez, R.J., Januszkiewicz, A.J. and Wanner, A., 1978. Mucociliary transport in allergic patients with antigen-induced bronchospasm. Am. Rev. Resp. Dis., 118, 677-684.

Michel, F.B., Marty, J.P., Quet, L. and Cour, P., 1977. Penetration of inhaled pollen into the respiratory tract. Am. Rev. Resp. Dis., 115, 609-616.

Mitchell, R.I., 1977. Lung deposition in freshly excised human lungs. In: Walton, W.H. (Ed.) Inhaled Particles IV, 163-173, Pergamon Press, Oxford.

Morrow, P.E., 1972. Lymphatic drainage of the lung in dust clearance. Ann. N.Y. Acad. Sci., 200, 46-65.

Morrow, P.E., 1973. Alveolar clearance of aerosols. Arch. Intern. Méd., 131, 101-108.

Morrow, P.E., 1974. Theoretical and experimental models for dust deposition and retention in man. Rev. Environ. Health, 1, 185-212.

Morrow, P.E., 1981. An evaluation of the physical properties of monodisperse and heterodisperse aerosols used in the assessment of bronchial function. Chest, 80, 809-813.

Morrow, P.E., 1981a.   Aerosol factors affecting respiratory deposition.   In: Hauck, H., (Ed.).   Int. Symp. Deposition and Clearance of Aerosols in the Human Respiratory Tract, 1-24, Bad
Gleichenberg (Austria).

Morrow, P.E., Kilpper, R.W., Bieter, E.H. and Gibb, F.R., 1976.
Pulmonary retention and translocation of insufflated tantalum.
Radiol., 121, 415-421.

Morrow, P.E., Mehrhof, E., Casarett, L.J. and Morken, D.A., 1958.   An
experimental study of aerosol deposition in human subjects.   AMA
Arch. Ind. Health, 18, 292-298.

Moss, O.R. and Kanapilly, G.M., 1980.   Dissolution of inhaled aerosols.   In: Willeke, K. (Ed.) Generation of Aerosols and Facilities for Exposure Experiments, 105-124, Ann Arbor Science Publishers Inc., Ann Arbor, Mich.

Mossberg, B., Björkander, J., Afzelius, B.A. and Camner, P., 1982.
Mucociliary clearance in patients with immunoglobulin deficiency.
Eur. J. Respir. Dis., 63, 570-578.

Mossberg, B., Strandberg, K., Philipson, K. and Camner, P., 1976.
Tracheobronchial clearance in bronchial asthma: response to
beta-adrenoceptor stimulation.   Scand. J. resp. Dis., 57,
119-128.

Mossberg, B., Strandberg, K., Philipson, K. and Camner, P. 1976a.
Tracheobronchial clearance and beta-adrenoceptor stimulation in
patients with chronic bronchitis.   Scand. J. resp. Dis., 57,
281-289.

Mossberg, B., Afzeluis, B.A., Eliasson, R. and Camner, P., 1978.   On
the pathogenesis of obstructive lung disease.   A study on the
immotile-cilia syndrome.   Scand. J. resp. Dis., 59, 55-65.

Newhouse, M.T., Dolovich, M., Obminski, G. and Wolff, R.K., 1978.
Effect of TLV levels of SO_2 and H_2SO_4 on bronchial clearance in
exercising man.   Arch. Environ. Health, 33, 24-32.

Newman, S.P., Pavia, D. and Clarke, S.W., 1981.   Improving the bronchial deposition of pressurized aerosols.   Chest, 80, 909-911.

Newman, S.P., Pavia, D., Garland, N. and Clarke, S.W., 1982.   Effects
of various inhalation modes on the deposition of radioactive
pressurised aerosols.   Eur. J. Respir. Dis. (Suppl. 119), 63,
57-65.

Newton, D., 1977.   Clearance of radioactive tantalum from the human
lung after accidental inhalation.   Am. J. Roentgenol., 129,
327-328.

Nolibé. D., Metivier, H., Masse, R. and Lafuma, J., 1977.   Thera-
    peutic effect of pulmonary lavage in vivo after inhalation of
    insoluble radioactive particles.   In: Walton, W.H. (Ed.)
    Inhaled Particles IV, 597-613, Pergamon Press, Oxford.

Ogden, T.L. amd Birkett, J.L., 1977.   The human head as a dust samp-
    ler.   In: Walton, W.H. (Ed.) Inhaled Particles IV, 93-105,
    Pergamon Press, Oxford.

Oldenburg, F.A., Dolovich, M.B., Montgomery, J.M. and Newhouse, M.T.,
    1979.   Effects of postural drainage, exercise, and cough on
    mucus clearance in chronic bronchitis.   Am. Rev. Resp. Dis.,
    120, 739-745.

Palmes, E.D., 1973.   Measurement of pulmonary air spaces using aero-
    sols.   Arch. Intern. Med., 131, 76-79.

Palmes, E.D., and Lippmann, M., 1977.   Influence of respiratory air
    space dimensions on aerosol deposition.   In: Walton, W.H. (Ed.)
    Inhaled Particles IV, 127-136, Pergamon Press, Oxford.

Palmes, E.D., Wang, C.-S., Goldring, R.M. and Altshuler, B., 1973.
    Effect of depth of inhalation on aerosol persistence during
    breath holding.   J. Appl. Physiol., 34, 356-360.

Patrick, G., 1979.   The retention of uranium dioxide particles in the
    trachea of the rat.   Int. J. Radiat. Biol., 35, 571-576.

Patrick, G. and Stirling, C., 1977.   Measurement of mucociliary
    clearance from the trachea of conscious and anaesthetized rats.
    J. Appl. Physiol., 42, 451-455.

Patrick, G. and Stirling, C., 1977a.   The retention of particles in
    large airways of the respiratory tract.   Proc. R. Soc. Lond. B,
    198, 455-462.

Pavia, D., Bateman, J.R.M., Sheahan, N.F. and Clarke, S.W., 1980.
    Clearance of lung secretions in patients with chronic bronchitis:
    effects of terbutaline and ipratropium bromide aerosols.   Eur.
    J. Respir. Dis., 61, 245-253.

Pavia, D., Short, M.D. and Thomson, M.L., 1970.   No demonstrable long
    term effects of cigarette smoking on the mucociliary mechanism of
    the human lung.   Nature (Lond.), 226, 1228-1231.

Pavia, D. and Thomson, M.L., 1971.   Inhibition of mucociliary clear-
    ance from the human lung by hyoscine.   Lancet, 449-450, Feb 27.

Pavia, D., Thomson, M.L. and Clarke, S.W.   Enhanced clearance of
    secretions from the human lung after adminstration of hypertonic
    saline aerosol.   Am. Rev. Resp. Dis., 117, 199-203, 1978.

Pavia, D., Thomson, M.L., Clarke, S.W., and Shannon, H.S., 1977. Effect of lung function and mode of inhalation on penetration of aerosol into the human lung. Thorax, 32, 194-197.

Pavia, D., Thomson, M.L., and Pocock, S.J., 1971. Evidence for temporary slowing mucociliary clearance in the lung caused by tobacco smoking. Nature (Lond.) 231, 325-326.

Pavia, D., Thomson, M. amd Shannon, H.S., 1977a. Aerosol inhalation and depth of deposition in the human lung: the effect of airway obstruction and tidal volume inhaled. Arch. Environ. Health, 32, 131-137.

Pfleger, R.C., Wilson, A.J., Cuddihy, R.G. and McClellan, R.O., 1969. Bronchopulmonary lavage for removal of inhaled insoluble materials from the lung. Dis. Chest, 56, 524-530.

Phalen, R.F., Kenoyer, J.L., Crocker, T.T. and McClure, T.R., 1980. Effects of sulfate aerosols in combination with ozone on elimination of tracer particles inhaled by rats. J. Toxicol. Environ. Health, 6, 797-810.

Phalen, R.F., Yeh, H.C., Schum, G.M. and Raabe, O.G., 1978. Application of an idealised model to morphometry of the mammalian tracheobronchial tree. Anat. Rec., 190, 167-176.

Pritchard, J.N., Black, A., Foord, N. and Walsh, M., 1980. A comparison of the regional deposition of monodisperse polystyrene aerosols in the respiratory tract of healthy male smokers and non-smokers. In: Aerosols in Science, Medicine and Technology; Physical and Chemical Properties of Aerosols, 245-250, Association for Aerosol Research.

Proctor, D.F., Andersen, I. and Lundqvist, G., 1973. Clearance of inhaled particles from the human nose. Arch. Intern. Med. 131, 132-139.

Proctor, D.F. and Wagner, H.N. Jr., 1976. Clearance of particles from the human nose. Arch. Environ. Health, 11, 366-371.

Raabe, O.G., 1982. Deposition and clearance of inhaled aerosols. In: Witschi, H. and Nettesheim, P. (Eds.) Mechanisms of Respiratory Toxicology, Vol.1, 27-76, CRC Press Inc., Bota Raton, Florida.

Ramsden, D., 1979. Direct comparisons of human and animal data for plutonium oxide inhalation. Health Phys., 36, 88-89.

Ramsden, D., Bains, M.E.D. and Fraser, D.C., 1978. A case study of multiple low level exposure to plutonium oxide. Health Phys., 34, 649-659.

Ross, I.T.H., Wallace, J.C. and Waite, D., 1979. A simplified method of monitoring muco-ciliary transport. Brit. J. Radiol., 52, 968-971.

Rudolf, G., Gebhart, J., Heyder, J., Scheuch, G. and Stahlhofen, W., 1983. Modelling the deposition of aerosol particles in the human respiratory tract. J. Aerosol. Sci., 14, 188-192.

Rylander, R., 1971. Lung clearance of particles and bacteria: effects of cigarette smoke exposure. Arch. Environ. Health, 23, 321-326.

Sackner, M.A., Rosen, M.J. and Wanner, A., 1973. Estimation of tracheal mucous velocity by bronchofiberscopy. J. Appl. Physiol., 34, 495-499.

Sadoul, P., Puchelle, E., Zahm, J-M., Jacquot, J., Aug, F. and Polu, J.-M., 1981. Effect of terbutaline on mucociliary transport and sputum properties in chronic bronchitis. Chest, 80, 885-889.

Sanchis, J., Dolovich, M., Chalmers, R. and Newhouse, M.T., 1971. Regional distribution and lung clearance mechanisms in smokers and non-smokers. In: Walton, W.H. (Ed.) Inhaled Particles III, 183-190, Unwin Bros., London.

Sanchis, J., Dolovich, M., Rossman, C. and Newhouse, M., 1974. Evaluation of bronchial clearance after inhalation of radioactive material. INSERM, 29, 79-88.

Sanchis, J., Dolovich, M., Rossman, C., Wilson, W. and Newhouse, M., 1973. Pulmonary mucociliary clearance in cystic fibrosis. New Engl. J. Med., 288, 651-654.

Santa-Cruz, R., Landa, J., Hirsch, J. and Sackner, M.A., 1974. Tracheal mucous velocity in normal man and patients with obstructive lung disease, effects of terbutaline. Am. Rev. Resp. Dis., 109, 458-463.

Sanders, C.L., 1969. The distribution of inhaled plutonium-239 dioxide particles within pulmonary macrophages. Arch. Environ. Health, 18, 904-912.

Sanders, C.L. and Adee, R.R., 1968. Phagocytosis of inhaled plutonium oxide - ^{239}Pu particles by pulmonary macrophages. Science, 162, 918-920.

Sanders, C.L. and Adee, R.R., 1970. Ultrastructural localisation of inhaled ^{239}PuO$_2$ particles in alveolar epithelium and macrophages. Health Phys., 18, 293-295.

Sanders, C.L. and Park, J.F., 1971. Pulmonary distribution of alpha dose from ^{239}PuO$_2$ and induction of neoplasia in rats and dogs. In: Walton, W.H. (Ed.) Inhaled Particles III, 489-498, Unwin Bros, London.

Schlesinger, R.B., Bohning, D.E., Chan, T.L. and Lippmann, M., 1977. Particle deposition in a hollow cast of the human tracheobronchial tree. J. Aerosol Sci., 8, 429-445.

Schlesinger, R.B., Halpern, M., Albert, R.E. and Lippmann, M., 1979. Effect of chronic inhaltion of sulfuric acid mist upon muco-ciliary clearance from the lungs of donkeys. J. Environ. Pathol. Toxicol., 2, 1351-1367.

Schlesinger, R.B., Lippmann, M. and Albert, R.E., 1978. Effects of short-term exposures to sulfuric acid and ammonium sulfate aero-sols upon bronchial airway function in the donkey. Am. Ind. Hyg. Assoc. J., 39, 275-286.

Schum, M. and Yeh, H.C., 1980. Theoretical evaluation of aerosol deposition in anatomical models of mammalian lung airways. Bull. Math. Biol., 42, 1-15.

Serafini, S.M., Wanner, A. and Michaelson, E.D., 1976. Mucociliary transport in central and intermediate size airways: effect of aminophyllin. Bull. europ. Physiopath. resp., 12, 415-422.

Short, M.D., Dowsett, D.J., Heaf, P.J.D., Pavia, D. and Thomson, M.L., 1979. A comparison between monodisperse Tc-99m labelled aerosol particles and Kr-81m for the assessment of lung function. J. Nucl. Med., 20, 194-200.

Smith, H., Stradling, G.N., Loveless, B.W. and Ham, G.J., 1977. The in vivo solubility of plutonium-239 dioxide in the rat lung. Health Phys., 33, 539-551.

Sneddon, S.L. and Brain, J.D., 1981. Persistent apex to base grad-ients of aerosol deposition in rats. Resp. Physiol., 46, 113-124.

Snipes, M.B., 1980. Long term retention of monodisperse and poly-disperse particles inhaled by beagle dogs, rats and mice II. In: Inhalation Toxicology Research Institute Annual Report, 1979-1980, 340-343, Lovelace Foundation, Albuquerque, NM.

Snipes, M.B., 1983. Retention of relatively insoluble particles inhaled by dogs, rats and mice. In: Fisher, D.R., (Ed.) Cur-rent Concepts in Lung Dosimetry, 73-79, USDOE Technical Inform-ation Center, CONF 820492, Pt.1.

Snipes, M.B., Muggenburg, B.A. and Bice, D.E., 1983. Translocation of particles from lung lobes or the peritoneal cavity to regional lymph nodes in beagle dogs. J. Toxicol. Environ. Health, 11, 703-712.

Spiegelman, J.R., Hanson, G.D., Lazarus, A., Bennett, R.J., Lippmann, M. and Albert, R.E., 1968. Effects of acute sulfur dioxide exposure on bronchial clearance in the donkey. Arch. Environ. Health, 17, 321-326.

Stahlhofen, W., Gebhart, J. and Heyder, J., 1980. Experimental determination of the regional deposition of aerosol particles in the human respiratory tract. Am. Ind. Hyg. Assoc J., 41, 305-398.

Stahlhofen, W., Gebhart, J. and Heyder, J., 1981.   Biological variability of regional deposition of aerosol particles in the human respiratory tract.   Am. Ind. Hyg. Assoc. J., 42, 348-352.

Stahlhofen, W., Gebhart, J., Heyder, J. and Scheuch, G., 1983.   New regional deposition data of the human respiratory tract.   J. Aerosol. Sci., 14, 186-188.

Stirling, C. and Patrick, G., 1980.   The localisation of particles retained in the trachea of the rat.   J. Pathol., 131, 309-320.

Stokinger, H.E., Steadman, L.T., Wilson, H.B., Sylvester, G.E., Dziuba, S. and LaBelle, C.W., 1951.   Lobar deposition and retention of inhaled insoluble particulates.   AMA Arch. Indust. Hyg. Occup. Med., 4, 346-353.

Strecker, F.I., 1967.   Tissue reactions in rat lungs after dust inhalation with special regard to bronchial dust elimination and to the penetration of dust into the lung interstices and lymphatic nodes.   In: Davies, C.N. (Ed.) Inhaled Particles II, 141-152, Pergamon Press, Oxford.

Stuart, B.O., 1973.   Deposition of inhaled aerosols.   Arch. Intern. Med., 131, 60-73.

Svartengren, M., Widtskiöld-Olsson, K., Philipson, K. and Camner, P., 1981.   Retention of particles on the first bifurcation and the trachea of rabbits.   Bull. europ. Physiopath. resp., 17, 87-91.

Swift, D.L., 1981.   Aerosol deposition and clearance in the human upper airways.   34th ACEMB Houston, Texas, Vol.23, p.38.

Swift, D.L., Cobb, J.A.C. and Smith, J.C., 1977.   Aerosol deposition in the dog respiratory tract.   In: Walton, W.H., (Ed.) Inhaled Particles IV, 237-245, Pergamon Press, Oxford.

Tarroni, G., Melandri, C., Prodi, V., De Zaiacomo, T., Formignani, M. and Bassi, P., 1980.   An indication on the biological variability of aerosol total deposition in humans.   Am. Ind. Hyg. Assoc. J., 41, 826-831.

Taulbee, D.B. and Yu, C.P., 1975.   A theory of aerosol deposition in the human respiratory tract.   J. Appl. Physiol., 38, 77-85.

Thein, M., Maitz, A.H., Austin, M.A., Rao, G.R. and Gur, D., 1982.   Dissolution rates of airborne uranium in simulated lung fluid.   Health Phys., 43, 587-590.

Thomas, R.G., 1968.   Transport of relatively insoluble materials from lung to lymph nodes.   Health Phys., 14, 111-117.

Thomas, R.G., 1971.   Estimation of particle size distribution parameters in animal lungs.   Aerosol Sci., 2, 393-400.

Thomas, R.L., Scott, J.K. and Chiffelle, T.L., 1972.   Metabolism and
toxicity of inhaled [144]Ce in rats.   Radiat. Res., 49, 589-610.

Thomson, M.L. and Pavia D., 1973.   Long-term tobacco smoking and
mucociliary clearance from the human lung in health and respiratory impairment.   Arch. Environ. Health, 26, 86-89.

Thomson, M.L. and Pavia D., 1974.   Particle penetration and clearance
in the human lung.   Results in healthy subjects and subjects
with chronic bronchitis.   Arch. Environ. Health, 29, 214-219.

Thomson, M.L., Pavia, D., Gregg, I. and Stark, J.E., 1974.   Bromhexine and mucociliary clearance in chronic bronchitis.   Brit.
J. Dis. Chest, 68, 21-27.

Thomson, M.L., Pavia, D. and McNicol, M.W., 1973.   A preliminary
study of the effect of quaiphenesin on mucociliary clearance from
the human lung.   Thorax, 28, 742-747.

Thomson, M.L., Pavia, D., Short, M.D. and Norman, A.P., 1973a.   Lung
clearance in two patients with cystic fibrosis.   New Eng. J.
Med., 289, 749-750.

Thomson, M.L. and Short, M.D., 1969.   Mucociliary function in health,
chronic obstructive airway disease, and asbestosis.   J.
Appl. Physiol., 26, 535-539.

Thorne, M.C. and Jackson, D., 1983.   Models for the Metabolism of
Chemical Carcinogens in Man.   ANS Report No. 347.

Toigo, A., Imarisio, J.J., Murmall, H. and Lepper, M.N., 1963.
Clearance of large carbon particles from the human tracheo-
bronchial tree.   Am. Rev. Resp. Dis., 87, 487-492.

Tremble, G.E., 1948.   Clinical observations on the movement of nasal
cilia.   An experimenal study.   Laryngoscope, 58, 206-224.

Van As, A., 1977.   Pulmonary airway clearance mechanisms: a reapp-
raisal.   Am. Rev. Resp. Dis., 115, 721-726.

Van As, A. and Webster, I., 1972.   The organisation of ciliary activity and mucus transport in pulmonary airways.   S.A. Medical
J., 46, 347-350.

Van As, A. and Webster, I., 1974.   The morphology of mucus in mammalian pulmonary airways.   Environ. Res., 7, 1-12.

Van Ree, J.H.L. and Van Dishoeck, H.A.E., 1962.   Some investigations
on nasal ciliary activity.   Pract. oto-rhino-laryng., 24,
383-390.

Venizelos, P.C., Gerrity, T.R. and Yeates, D.B., 1981.   Response of human mucociliary clearance to acute alcohol adminstration. Arch. Environ. Health, 36, 194-201.

Vincent, J.H. and Mark, D., 1982.   Applications of blunt sampler theory to the definition and measurement of inhalable dust.   In: Walton, W.H. (Ed.) Inhaled Particles V.   Ann. Occup. Hyg., 26, 3-19.

Waite, D.A. and Ramsden, D., 1971.   The inhalation of insoluble iron oxide particles in the sub-micron range.   Part I - chronium-51 labelled aerosols.   AEEW-R740.

Waite, D.A. and Ramsden, D., 1971a.   The inhalation of insoluble iron oxide particles in the sub-micron ranges Part II - plutonium-237 labelled aerosols.   AEEW-R741.

Waligora, S.J., 1971.   Pulmonary retention of zirconium oxide (^{95}Nb) in man and beagle dogs.   Health Phys., 20, 89-91.

Wanner, A., Hirsch, J.A., Greeneltch, D.E., Swenson, E.W. and Fore, T., 1973.   Tracheal mucous velocity in beagles after chronic exposure to cigarette smoke.   Arch. Environ. Health, 27, 370-371.

Watson, A.Y. and Brain, J.D., 1979.   Uptake of iron oxide aerosols by mouse airway epithelium.   Lab. Invest., 40, 450-459.

Watts, L., 1975.   Clearance rates of insoluble plutonium-239 compounds from the lung.   Health Phys., 29, 53-59.

Weibel, E.R., 1963.   Morphometry of the human lung.   Springer-Verlag, Berlin.

Weller, W. and Ulmer, T., 1972.   Inhalation studies of coal-quartz dust mixture.   Ann. N.Y. Acad. Sci., 200, 142-154.

West, C.M. and Scott, L.M., 1969.   Uranium cases showing long chest burden retention - an updating.   Health Phys., 17, 781-791.

Wolff, R.K., Dolovich, M., Obminski, G. and Newhouse, M.T., 1977. Effect of sulphur dioxide on tracheobronchial clearance at rest and during exercise.   In: Walton, W.H. (Ed.) Inhaled Particles IV, 321-332, Pergamon Press, Oxford.

Wolff, R.K., Dolovich, M., Rossman, C. and Newhouse, M.T., 1975. Sulphur dioxide and tracheobronchial clearance in man. Arch. Environ. Health, 30, 521-527.

Wolfsdorf, J., Swift, D.L. and Avery, M.E., 1969.   Mist therapy reconsidered; an evaluation of the respiratory deposition of labelled water aerosols produced by jet ultrasonic nebulizers. Pediatrics, 43, 799-808.

Wolff, R.K., Kanapilly, G.M., DeNee, P.B. and McClellan, R.O., 1981. Deposition of 0.1 μm chain aggregate aerosols in beagle dogs. J. Aerosol. Sci., 12, 119-129.

Wood., R.E. Wanner, A., Hirsch, J. and Farrell, P.M., 1975. Tracheal mucociliary transport in patients with cystic fibrosis and its stimulation by terbutaline. Am. Rev. Resp. Dis., 111, 733-738.

Yeates, D.B. and Aspin, N., 1978. A mathematical description of the airways of the human lungs. Respiration Physiology, 32, 91-104.

Yeates, D.B., Aspin, N., Bryan, A.C. and Levison, H., 1973. Regional clearance of ions from the airways of the lung. Am. Rev. Resp. Dis., 107, 602-608.

Yeates, D.B., Aspin, N., Levison, H., Jones, M.T. and Bryan, A.C., 1975. Mucociliary tracheal transport rates in man. J. Appl. Physiol., 39, 487-495.

Yeates, D.B., Sturgess, J.M., Kahn, S.R., Levison, H. and Aspin, N., 1976. Mucociliary transport in trachea of patients with cystic fibrosis. Arch. Dis. Childh., 51, 28-33.

Yeh, H.C., Phalen R.F. and Raabe, O.G., 1976. Factors influencing the deposition of inhaled particles. Environ. Health Perspect., 15, 147-156.

Yeh, H.C., and Schum, G.M., 1980. Models of human lung airways and their application to inhaled particle deposition. Bull. Math. Biol., 42, 461-480.

Yu, C.P., 1981. A model of particle clearance in human tracheo-bronchial tree. 34th ACEMB Houston, Texas, Vol.23, p.39.

Yu, C.P. and Diu, C.K., 1982. A probabilistic model for intersubject deposition variability of inhaled particles. Aerosol Sci. and Technol., 1, 355-362.

Yu, C.P. and Diu, C.K., 1983. Total and regional deposition of inhaled aerosols in humans. J. Aerosol Sci., 14, 599-609.

Yu, C.P., Diu, C.K. and Soong, T.T., 1981. Statistical analysis of aerosol deposition in nose and mouth. Am. Ind. Hyg. Assoc. J., 42, 726-733.

Yu, C.P. and Thiagarajan, V., 1978. Sedimentation of aerosols in closed finite tubes in random orientation. J. Aerosol Sci., 9, 315-320.

7
Method of calculation

7.1　General description of the model

The metabolism of twelve carcinogens is described in Section 4, where models are proposed for their retention in, and elimination from the body. The carcinogens studied can be divided into two groups. These groups are as follows:

- The metalloids and asbestos. These are inhaled as particulate matter and, thus, their absorption into the body from the lung depends on many parameters such as particle size, mucociliary and macrophage clearance, and dissolution. These processes are described in detail in Section 6.

- Organic compounds. These are assumed to enter the lung in the gaseous form, and so their uptake is determined by physico-chemical properties such as diffusion and solubility.

Data for retention of substances in the lungs and gastrointestinal (GI) tract and their uptake from these organs were reviewed by Committee 2 of the International Commission for Radiological Protection (ICRP). Models for these processes were proposed and used in conjunction with models of systemic metabolism in setting limits on intake for workers exposed to radionuclides (ICRP, 1979). As the models for lung and gastrointestinal tract were proposed nearly twenty years ago, it was thought appropriate that they should be re-evaluated to take into account later work. These reviews are included as Sections 5 and 6 of this report. The interactions of the model of systemic metabolism and those for respiratory and gastrointestinal retention are shown for a typical metalloid (lead) in Fig. 7.1. The ICRP lung and gut models are shown here but the same interrelationship between the three systems apply if the revised models are substituted. The transfer factors can be found in the appropriate sections (Thorne and Jackson, 1983 for lung and GI tract, Section 4 for systemic metabolism).

Similar models can be developed for the other metal-like carcinogens. However, for the organic carcinogens studied, it was not thought appropriate to use a basic lung and GI tract model in conjunction with that for systemic metabolism.   This is because the processes involved in the clearance of these substances from the lung are, for the most part, different from and occur much more quickly, than those involved in the clearance of particulates from the lung.   With respect to gastrointestinal absorption, these compounds are both lipid soluble and of low molecular weight and will therefore rapidly cross biologi- cal membranes.   For this reason, these compounds are assumed to be completely absorbed into the body, when ingested.

As can be seen from Fig. 7.1, the metabolism of carcinogens in the body can be interpreted in terms of a multi-compartment model. It is assumed that transfers between the various compartments obey first-order kinetics.   If this is the case, a single compartment model can be described mathematically by the following equation:

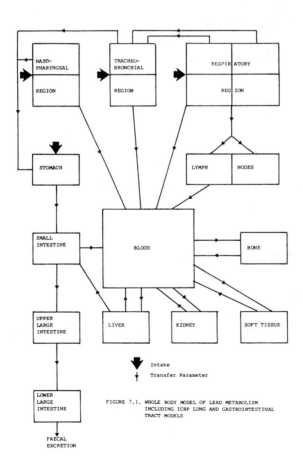

FIGURE 7.1. WHOLE BODY MODEL OF LEAD METABOLISM
INCLUDING ICRP LUNG AND GASTROINTESTINAL
TRACT MODELS

$$\frac{\delta}{\delta t} q(t) = I(t) - \lambda q(t) \tag{1}$$

where   q is the compartmental contents at time t, (mass);
           I is the rate of intake into the compartment at time t,
              (mass time^{-1});
           λ is the rate of loss from the compartment, (time^{-1}).

Most processes in the body are saturable, because of the limited number of sites available at which they can occur. The Michaelis-Menten rate equation can be used to describe any saturable process mathematically. Thus:

$$V_o = \frac{Vmax \ q}{Km + q} \tag{2}$$

when V_o is the initial rate of the process;

          Vmax is the maximum rate of the process, i.e. when it is

              saturated;

          q is the amount of substrate;

          Km is a constant which can be defined as being equal to the

              amount of substrate when $V_o = \frac{Vmax}{2}$

To illustrate the characteristics of a saturable process, consider two values of q.

a)   When q >> Km.

Eqn. 2 reduces to V_o = Vmax. Therefore, when the amount of substrate is very much greater than Km, the initial velocity equals V_{max} i.e. the process is saturated.

b)   When q<<Km.

Equation 2 now becomes:

$$V_o = \frac{Vmax \ q}{Km} \tag{3}$$

Vmax/Km is obviously constant and the initial velocity can be interpreted as the rate of change of substrate amount. So, Eqn. 3 can be rewritten as

$$\frac{\delta}{\delta t} q = K \ q .$$

Therefore, when the amount of substrate is very much less than Km, the process obeys first order kinetics.

So, as long as the transfer parameters on which the model is based are not approaching saturation, it is reasonable to assume that they can be described by first order kinetics.

The general form of equation 1 describing a multi-compartment system such as that shown in Fig. 7.1 is as follows.

$$\frac{\delta}{\delta t} q_i(t) = \sum_{i=1}^{n} \lambda_{ij} q_j(t) + I_i(t) \quad \text{for i=1 to n}$$

where q_i is the activity content of compartment i at time t;

λ_{ij}, with i=j, is the rate of transfer (time^{-1}) from compartment j to compartment i;

λ_{ij}, with i=j, is ≤ 0 and is the total rate of loss (time^{-1}) from compartment i;

I_i is the rate of intake of activity into compartment i from outside the system at time t; and

n is the number of compartments comprising the system.

Compartmental models can be solved by a variety of analytical and numerical techniques (Jacquez, 1972).

7.2   The computer code MOSAIC

The models for systemic metabolism of carcinogens described in Section 4 together with the relevant lung and GI tract models, where appropriate, have been implemented in a computer code that runs under the CP/M operating system on a Tandy TRS-80 MkII microcomputer. The code has been written in standard FORTRAN, with the exception of file handling routines. Referring to the relevant technical manual (Microsoft, Fortran80 Users Manual, 1979 in this case) should make the code wholly transportable to other installations.

Results are presented in a graphical form using a machine-dependent graphics plotter and software package. However, the post-processing section of the codes includes subroutines that plot histograms (for urinary and faecal contents) and graphs (for tissue concentrations) on a line printer.

The code is known by the mnemonic MOSAIC, standing for MOdel Simulation of Airborne Industrial Carcinogens. The operation of MOSAIC can be functionally divided into 3 sections; the pre-processor, the processor and the post-processor.

7.2.1   The pre-processor

This section of the code permits the user to specify parameters and define the type of simulation to be performed. The code runs interactively, prompting the user to enter the various parameters and specify options. It is divided into well defined sections, dealing with different areas of model operation such as output mode, exposure type and excretion patterns. There is also an editing option, allowing the user to alter model parameters.

FIGURE 7.2.   CODE GENERATED SCREEN DISPLAY AND ILLUSTRATIVE INPUT FOR THE
COMPUTER CODE MOSAIC

```
                                ARSENIC =  1
                             BERYLLIUM =  2
                               CADMIUM =  3
                                  LEAD =  4
                                NICKEL =  5
                              CHROMIUM =  6
                              ASBESTOS =  7
                               BENZENE =  8
                        VINYL CHLORIDE =  9
                             BENZIDINE = 10
              CARBON TETRACHLORIDE = 11
                         METHYL IODIDE = 12
                                   END = 13
```

```
WHICH CARCINOGEN?  :4

              THE MODEL CAN BE RUN IN THREE MODES

FULL DEBUGGING OUTPUT (PRINTS RESULTS AT EACH ITERATION)
STORE ORGAN CONCENTRATIONS ON FILE
STORE ALL COMPARTMENTAL CONTENTS ON FILE

              ALL THREE MODES CAN BE RUN SIMULTANEOUSLY
```

```
DO YOU REQUIRE FULL DEBUGGING MODE? (Y/N)  :N

DO YOU WISH TO SAVE ORGAN CONCENTRATIONS? (Y/N)   :Y
```

```
IN WHICH FILE ARE ORGAN CONCENTRATIONS TO BE STORED?  :LEAD1


ON WHICH DISK DRIVE IS THIS FILE LOCATED?
PRESENT DRIVE = 1  EXPANSION DRIVE = 2  :2

DO YOU WISH TO SAVE ALL COMPARTMENTAL CONTENTS? (Y/N)  :Y
```

```
IN WHICH FILE ARE COMPARTMENTAL CONTENTS TO BE STORED?  :LEAD2


ON WHICH DISK DRIVE IS THIS FILE LOCATED?
PRESENT DRIVE = 1  EXPANSION DRIVE = 2  :2
```

FIGURE 7.2. (cont.)

INHALATION PARAMETERS

ENTER MEAN PARTICLE DIAMETER (MICRONS)   :1.0

WHICH LUNG MODEL IS TO BE USED? ICRP = 0 NEW MODEL = 1   :1

INPUT INHALATION CLASS (D,W,Y) :W   WHICH BREATHING PATTERN? NOSE   0 MOUTH = 1   :1

DIETARY PARAMETERS

THE PRESENT VALUE OF F1 = 8.0000E-01
DO YOU WISH TO CHANGE THIS? (Y/N)   :N

THE PRESENT DIETARY INTAKE = 1.5000E-01 MG/DAY
DO YOU WISH TO CHANGE THIS? (Y/N)   :N

DO YOU WISH TO EDIT THE MODEL? (Y/N)   :Y

CHANGE EXISTING MODEL PARAMETERS = 1
ADD NEW MODEL PARAMETERS = 2
RETURN = 3

WHICH OPTION?   :1

EDIT INITIAL TIME STEP = 1
EDIT VALUE OF ERROR LIMIT = 2
EDIT VENTILATION RATE = 3
CONTINUE = 4

WHICH OPTION?   :3

THE PRESENT VENTILATION RATE = 2.0000E+01 M3/DAY

ENTER NEW VALUE FOR VENTILATION RATE (M3/DAY) :1.E+01

EDIT INITIAL TIME STEP = 1
EDIT VALUE OF ERROR LIMIT = 2
EDIT VENTILATION RATE = 3
CONTINUE = 4

WHICH OPTION?   :4

FIGURE 7.2.   (cont.)

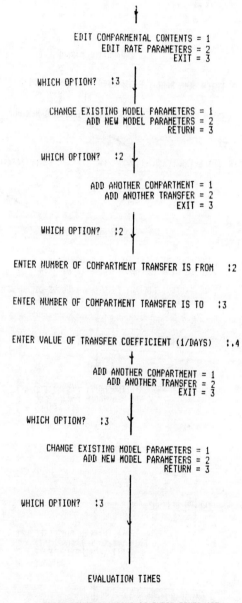

EDIT COMPARMENTAL CONTENTS = 1
EDIT RATE PARAMETERS = 2
EXIT = 3

WHICH OPTION?   :3

CHANGE EXISTING MODEL PARAMETERS = 1
ADD NEW MODEL PARAMETERS = 2
RETURN = 3

WHICH OPTION?   :2

ADD ANOTHER COMPARTMENT = 1
ADD ANOTHER TRANSFER = 2
EXIT = 3

WHICH OPTION?   :2

ENTER NUMBER OF COMPARTMENT TRANSFER IS FROM   :2

ENTER NUMBER OF COMPARTMENT TRANSFER IS TO   :3

ENTER VALUE OF TRANSFER COEFFICIENT (1/DAYS)   :.4

ADD ANOTHER COMPARTMENT = 1
ADD ANOTHER TRANSFER = 2
EXIT = 3

WHICH OPTION?   :3

CHANGE EXISTING MODEL PARAMETERS = 1
ADD NEW MODEL PARAMETERS = 2
RETURN = 3

WHICH OPTION?   :3

EVALUATION TIMES

ORGAN CONCENTRATIONS AT THESE TIMES ARE
TABULATED AT THE END OF THE SIMULTION

HOW MANY EVALUATION TIMES DO YOU REQUIRE?   :5

FIGURE 7.2.   (cont.)

ENTER EVALUATION TIME 1 (DAYS)   :1.

ENTER EVALUATION TIME 2 (DAYS)   :2.

ENTER EVALUATION TIME 3 (DAYS)   :3.

ENTER EVALUATION TIME 4 (DAYS)   :4.5

ENTER EVALUATION TIME 5 (DAYS)   :6.8

WHICH EXPOSURE REGIME? CHRONIC=0 ACUTE=1 :1

CHRONIC EXPOSURE

ENTER AIR CONCENTRATION (MG/M3) :50.25

ENTER ADDITIONAL INPUT TO TO GI TRACT(MG/DAY) :0.3

IS THE EXPOSURE TIME-DEPENDENT? (Y/N) :Y

THE INITIAL EXPOSURE IS TIME-DEPENDENT AND WILL
BE SCALED ACCORDING TO THE POLYNOMIAL :-
EXPOSURE(T)=EXPOSURE(0)*(K1+K2*T+K3*T**2...ETC)

ENTER ORDER OF POLYNOMIAL   :1

ENTER K1   :2

WHICH ACUTE EXPOSURE PATTERN? SHIFT=0 SPIKE=1 :0

SPIKE EXPOSURE

THIS OPTION SETS UP A DEFINED EXPOSURE REGIMEN

FOR A SPECIFIED NUMBER OF EXPOSURES

HOW MANY EXPOSURES ARE THERE? :2

ENTER TIME EXPOSURE 1 BEGINS (DAYS) :1.0
ENTER TIME EXPOSURE 1 ENDS (DAYS)   :2.0
ENTER AIR CONCENTRATION (MG/M3)   :5.25
ENTER EXTRA INPUT TO GI TRACT (MG/DAY) :2.30

SHIFT EXPOSURE

THIS OPTION SETS UP A DEFINED DIURNAL EXPOSURE REGIMEN
FOR A SPECIFIED NUMBER OF DAYS

THE CODE CANNOT CALCULATE OVERNIGHTSHIFT EXPOSURES
IF THIS FACILITY IS REQUIRED,ENTER THE EXPOSURE PATTERN AS

AN EXPOSURE UP TO 23.59 AND AN EXPOSURE FROM 00.00 THE NEXT DAY

HOW MANY DAYS DOES THIS EXPOSURE PATTERN LAST?   :5

HOW MANY EXPOSURES PER DAY ARE THERE?   :2

ENTER TIME EXPOSURE 1 BEGINS (24-HOUR CLOCK)   :8.30

ENTER TIME EXPOSURE 1 ENDS (24-HOUR CLOCK)   :12.30

ENTER AIR CONCENTRATION (MG/M3) :1.0

ENTER INPUT TO TO GI TRACT (MG) :0.0

ENTER INPUT TO SKIN (MG)   :0.0

ENTER TIME EXPOSURE 2 BEGINS (24-HOUR CLOCK)   :13.30

ENTER TIME EXPOSURE 2 ENDS (24-HOUR CLOCK)   :17.30

ENTER AIR CONCENTRATION (MG/M3) :1.0

ENTER INPUT TO TO GI TRACT (MG) :0.0

ENTER INPUT TO SKIN (MG)   :0.0

ANOTHER EXPOSURE PATTERN? (Y/N)   :N

FIGURE 7.2.   (cont.)

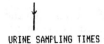

URINE SAMPLING TIMES

COLLECTION OF EXCRETION SAMPLES IS SIMULATED AT
THESE TIMES EACH DAY THROUGHOUT THE SIMULATION

HOW MANY URINE SAMPLES PER DAY?   :4

AT WHAT TIME IS SAMPLE 1 VOIDED? (24-HR CLOCK)   :8.00

AT WHAT TIME IS SAMPLE 2 VOIDED? (24-HR CLOCK)   :12.45

AT WHAT TIME IS SAMPLE 3 VOIDED? (24-HR CLOCK)   :17.30

AT WHAT TIME IS SAMPLE 4 VOIDED? (24-HR CLOCK)   :22.30

FAECAL SAMPLING TIMES

COLLECTION OF EXCRETION SAMPLES IS SIMULATED AT
THESE TIMES EACH DAY THROUGHOUT THE SIMULATION

HOW MANY FAECAL SAMPLES PER DAY   :1

AT WHAT TIME IS SAMPLE 1 VOIDED? (24-HR CLOCK)   :12.45

FIGURE 7.2.   (cont.)

The input specifications during the running of the code are described below. This should be read with reference to the relevant section of Fig. 7.2, which shows the code-generated displays together with user-supplied input.

The machine code version of MOSAIC is stored in the file MOSAIC.COM, and is loaded and executed under CP/M by typing MOSAIC<CR> (RETURN or ENTER is indicated by <CR>). After specifying an option or entering a parameter value, <CR> must always be entered, to return control to the central processing unit for execution to continue.

A brief description of the purpose of each section of the pre-processor, together with the form of the required input (except when this is obvious) is given below.

(a)   Select the carcinogen that is to be studied. Rate parameters for the code will be set up on the basis of the model described in Section 4. Enter the relevant number followed by <CR>.

(b)   Define the mode of output of the program. Three modes are available, all of which can be used simultaneously.
-   Full debugging output. With this option, the contents of each compartment are printed on the line printer, together with the time and total exposure, at each iteration of the program (see Section 7.2.2).
-   Save organ concentrations. This option permits organ concentrations at each iteration to be stored on file for post processing (see Section 7.3). If this option is specified, the user is prompted for the name of the file on which these results are to be stored. Files can have a maximum of eight characters in their name. The file extension (.DAT) is automatically supplied by the code. The disk drive on which this file is to be located must also be specified. If a file of this name does not exist on the specified drive, the CP/M operating system will automatically create one, if a file already exists, the contents of the file will be overwritten by the new results.
-   Save compartmental contents. This causes the contents of all compartments at each iteration to be stored on the specified file, for post-processing.

(c)   Define which lung model is to be used to calculate deposition and clearance of particulates. (This only applies to the metalloid carcinogens). Two options are provided, these being the ICRP lung model (ICRP, 1979) and the model proposed in Section 6. The mass median aerodynamic diameter (in microns) must be specified, and the type of cleearance, for each model. For the ICRP model, the inhalation class must be specified (D, W or Y). This refers to the time-scale of the slow phase clearance from the lungs (i.e. days, weeks or years). In the model proposed in Section 6, clearance is mainly determined by the solubility of the particle. Where different chemical forms of the metalloid carcinogens have different solubilities, the user is asked to specify the chemical species inhaled. Where only one value is quoted in the literature, this value is assumed to apply to all forms.

(d) Specify dietary parameters. Enter the fractional absorption of the compound and daily dietary intake (if values other than the default values are required).

(e) Editing option. A summary of existing model parameters that can be modified by the editor is output on the line printer upon request.   The required option should be specified.   There now follows a brief outline of the operation of each option.
  –   Change existing model parameters. This permits the user to change the values of parameters relevant to the operation of the code.   The initial time step, error limit (see section 7.2.2), ventilation rate and fractional uptake (for uptake of gaseous carcinogens only) can all be changed.   The code performs error and consistency checks on the edited data and requires the user to re-enter parameter values as appropriate.   Subsequent to editing parameter values, the user has the option of modifying initial compartmental contents, rates of intake or rate parameters already present in the model.
  –   Add new model parameters. This permits the user to add further compartments or transfer parameters to the model.

(f) Evaluation times.   Organ concentrations at these times are stored, and presented in tabulated form upon completion of the simulation.   The user enters the number of evaluation times, and then the value of each evaluation time.   These values must be entered as decimal fractions of days.   The code checks for self consistency, i.e. that each time is larger than the previous value.   The final time specified will signal the calculation module to terminate when this value has been reached (see Section 7.2.2).

(g) Exposure regime. Chronic or acute exposure must be specified.
  –   Chronic exposure. The code prompts the user for values of intestinal tract and skin exposure where applicable.   The code then derives intake rate to the relevant compartments on the basis of these values. As the heading implies, these intake rates are constant throughout the simulation.   However, a secondary option is available, which allows the user to specify time-dependent chronic exposure. If this is chosen, the initial intake rates calculated on the basis of the above values are scaled with time according to the polynomial.

$$\text{intake }(t) = \text{intake }(o) \ast \sum_{i=0}^{n} a_i \, t^i$$

The user is asked to specify the order of the polynomial and the relevant values of a_i.
  –   Acute exposure. Two sub-options are provided: Spike and shift exposure. Spike exposure, as its name implies, allows the user to define an exposure regime of one or more expo-

```
SUMMARY OF MODEL PARAMETERS FOR CADMIUM

FIRST STEP = 1.0000E-06 DAYS

ERROR LIMIT = 1.0000E-06

NUMBER OF COMPARTMENTS = 21

    INHALATION PARAMETERS

THE ICRP LUNG MODEL IS IMPLEMENTED FOR THIS SIMULATION

MEAN PARTICLE DIAMETER = 1.00E+00 MICRONS

INHALATION CLASS = W

VENTILATION RATE = 2.00E+01 M3/DAY

    DIETARY PARAMETERS

DAILY DIETARY INTAKE = 1.500E-01 MG

F1 = 5.00E-02

    INITIAL CONTENTS (MG) AND RATES OF INTAKE (MG/DAY)
```

COMPARTMENT	CONTENT	RATE OF ENTRY	COMPARTMENT	CONTENT	RATE OF ENTRY	COMPARTMENT	CONTENT	RATE OF ENTRY
1	0.0000E+00	0.0000E+00	2	0.0000E+00	0.0000E+00	3	0.0000E+00	0.0000E+00
4	0.0000E+00	0.0000E+00	5	0.0000E+00	0.0000E+00	6	0.0000E+00	0.0000E+00
7	0.0000E+00	0.0000E+00	8	0.0000E+00	0.0000E+00	9	0.0000E+00	0.0000E+00
10	0.0000E+00	0.0000E+00	11	1.1000E-03	0.0000E+00	12	0.0000E+00	0.0000E+00
13	0.0000E+00	0.0000E+00	14	0.0000E+00	0.0000E+00	15	0.0000E+00	0.0000E+00
16	0.0000E+00	0.0000E+00	17	2.5000E-03	0.0000E+00	18	2.6100E+01	0.0000E+00
19	4.1400E+00	0.0000E+00	20	7.1300E+00	0.0000E+00	21	0.0000E+00	0.0000E+00

FIGURE 7.3.   SUMMARY OF MODEL PARAMETERS OUTPUT TO THE LINE PRINTER AT THE END OF THE PRE-PROCESSER STAGE

```
11   1   6.9300E+01    11   11   6.9300E+01    12    1.3900E-02    12    2   1.7300E+00
12   4   3.4700E+00     4    4   3.4700E+00     9    1.3900E-02     9    8   1.3900E-02
15   8   0.0000E+00     8   13   1.3900E-02    14    2.4000E+01    14   13   6.0000E+00
15  14   1.8000E+00    11   12   3.1579E-01    11    3.1579E-01    11   18   6.0000E+00
11  19   1.0000E-05    16   13   1.0000E-05    17    1.0000E-05    17   20   1.0000E-05
17  17   2.0000E-01    19   19   2.0000E+00    20    3.2000E+00    20   17   8.0000E-01
21  17   2.0000E-01    16   11   2.0000E-01     1    1.0000E-05     1    5  -6.9300E+01
 2   2  -1.7300E+00    16   19  -6.9300E+01     5   -3.4700E+00     5    9  -1.3900E-02
 6   6  -6.9300E-01     3    4  -1.3900E-02     8   -1.3900E-02     9    9  -1.3900E-02
 6  10   0.0000E+00     7    8  -7.4000E+00     8   -2.4000E+01    13    9  -6.3158E+00
10  14  -1.8000E+00    11   12  -1.0000E+00    12   -2.0000E+01    17   13  -1.0000E+00
14  18  -1.0000E-05    15   16  -3.0000E-05    16   -2.0000E-05    21   21   0.0000E+00
```

TIMES OF EVALUATION (DAYS)

1.0000E+00 2.0000E+00 3.0000E+00 4.0000E+00 5.0000E+00 6.0000E+00 7.0000E+00 8.0000E+00 9.0000E+00 1.0000E+01

THIS IS A SIMULATION OF ACUTE EXPOSURE
THE EXPOSURE PATTERN IS AS FOLLOWS:-

T(START) (DAYS)	T(STOP) (DAYS)	AIR CONC (MG/M3)	EXP(GI TRACT) (MG/DAY)	SKIN EXPOSURE (MG/DAY)
3.7500E-01	5.2083E-01	1.0000E+00	0.0000E+00	0.0000E+00
5.6250E-01	7.0833E-01	1.0000E+00	0.0000E+00	0.0000E+00
1.3750E+00	1.5208E+00	1.0000E+00	0.0000E+00	0.0000E+00
1.5625E+00	1.7083E+00	1.0000E+00	0.0000E+00	0.0000E+00
2.3750E+00	2.5208E+00	1.0000E+00	0.0000E+00	0.0000E+00
2.5625E+00	2.7083E+00	1.0000E+00	0.0000E+00	0.0000E+00
3.3750E+00	3.5208E+00	1.0000E+00	0.0000E+00	0.0000E+00
3.5625E+00	3.7083E+00	1.0000E+00	0.0000E+00	0.0000E+00
4.3750E+00	4.5208E+00	1.0000E+00	0.0000E+00	0.0000E+00
4.5625E+00	4.7083E+00	1.0000E+00	0.0000E+00	0.0000E+00
5.5000E+00	5.5208E+00	0.0000E+00	0.0000E+00	0.0000E+00
6.5000E+00	6.5208E+00	0.0000E+00	0.0000E+00	0.0000E+00
7.3750E+00	7.5208E+00	1.0000E+00	0.0000E+00	0.0000E+00
7.5625E+00	7.7083E+00	1.0000E+00	0.0000E+00	0.0000E+00
8.3750E+00	8.5208E+00	1.0000E+00	0.0000E+00	0.0000E+00
8.5625E+00	8.7083E+00	1.0000E+00	0.0000E+00	0.0000E+00
9.3750E+00	9.5208E+00	1.0000E+00	0.0000E+00	0.0000E+00
9.5625E+00	9.7083E+00	1.0000E+00	0.0000E+00	0.0000E+00

ORGAN CONCENTRATIONS ARE STORED IN FILE CAD1 DAT
THIS FILE IS ON THIS DISK

FIGURE 7.3. (cont.)

sures, which are not diurnal. The user is asked to specify the "start" and "stop" times for each exposure. These must be entered as decimal fractions of days. The air concentration, additional non-dietary, gastrointestinal intake and skin intake must also be specified for each exposure.

Shift exposure permits an exposure pattern to be set up for a period of one or more days after specifying the exposure regime of the first day. The user is asked to specify the number of days this exposure pattern lasts, and the number of exposures per day. The code will then ask for the start and stop times of each exposure period. These must be input in the 24 hour clock notation in the form HH.MM. The code automatically converts these to their decimal equivalents.

Once again, air concentrations, extra GI intake and skin intake must be specified for each exposure period.

After the first day exposure regime has been input, the code automatically creates the same exposure regime for the following days specified. The code then gives the option of entering another exposure pattern to run after the one already defined. (Note that the code will only run up to the final evaluation time specified in (f)).

(h) Excretion sampling times. This section allows the code to simulate the collection of urine and faecal samples. A sampling regime is defined for the first day, and samples are then taken at the same times on the following days throughout the simulation. The code prompts for the number of samples per day, and then for each sampling time. These times must be input in the 24 hour clock format HH.MM. The code converts these to their decimal equivalent and calculates the sampling regime for the following days.

A summary of all parameters used by the code is then output to the line printer. An example of this is given in Fig. 7.3.

7.2.2   The processor

As discussed in Section 7.1, the metabolism of carcinogens in the body can be described by a set of first-order linear differential equations. The processor section of the code is used to calculate the time-dependent solution of this set of equations. The technique used is a hybrid of the Runge-Kutta and predictor-corrector methods. This hybrid method was developed specifically by ANS as a compact and rapid method of solution appropriate to micro-computer systems. The fourth-order Runge-Kutta routine used requires only the current value of the function, whereas the predictor-corrector method requires both the current and previous values. However, the predictor-corrector method gives an indication of the rapidity and adequacy of convergence, which is not readily available using the Runge-Kutta technique. Thus the predictor-corrector method is the standard method of solution and the Runge-Kutta is used when a change in step length is required.

The code uses a short Runge-Kutta step plus several predictor-corrector steps to change the overall step length, on convergence grounds, to reach a specified evaluation time, or to reach a time where the exposure pattern changes abruptly (acute exposure). Where no change in step-length is required, a single predictor-corrector step is used.

7.2.2.1   The Runge-Kutta method

This technique is used to perform one step in the solution of a set of first-order differential equations. The fourth order Runge-Kutta method used can be defined by the following five equations.

$$Y_{m+1} = Y_m + h(k_1 + 2k_2 + 2k_3 + k_4)/6$$

$$k_1 = f(x_m, Y_m)$$

$$k_2 = f(x_m + h/2, Y_m + hk_1/2)$$

$$k_3 = f(x_m + h/2, Y_m + hk_2/2)$$

$$k_4 = f(x_m + h, Y_m + hk_3)$$

where

Y_m is the vector of compartmental contents at time x_m;

Y_{m+1} is the vector of compartmental contents at time $x_m + h$;

$f(x_o, Y_o)$ is the first derivative of y with respect to x at time x_o for compartmental contents y_0, i.e.

$$f(x_o, Y_o) = \frac{d}{dx} Y(x) \Big|_{x=x_o}$$

7.2.2.2   The predictor-corrector technique

The method used is a second order technique, which performs one step in the solution of a set of first order differential equations. It can be defined by the following equations:

$$Y_{m+1}^{(o)} = Y_{m-1} + 2h\, f(x_m, Y_m)$$

$$Y_{m+1}^{(i)} = Y_m + 0.5h\, [f(x_m, Y_m) + f(x_{m+1}, Y_{m+1}^{(i-1)})]$$

where

$y_{m+1}^{(o)}$ is an initial estimate of the y vector at x_m + h,

y_m is the final estimate of the y vector at x_m,

y_{m-1} is the final estimate of the y vector at x_m-h,

$y_{m+1}^{(i)}$ is the i'th estimate of the y vector at x_m+h,

and f and h have values defined in Section 7.2.2.1.

Convergence of the y vector estimate is tested using

$$y_{m+1}^{(i+1)} - y_{m+1}^{(i)} \quad [max] \quad < \varepsilon$$

where [max] indicates the maximum component of the vector and the convergence criterion is given by:

$$\varepsilon = \phi \, [y_m]_{[max]} + 10^{-10}$$

where ϕ is the specified error limit (see Section 7.2.1).

The function f can be defined, for both techniques, as the first derivative of y with respect to t at time t. For a multicompartmental model, the vector dy/dt can be calculated using:

$$\frac{dy_i}{dt} = \Sigma \lambda_{ij} y_j + I_i$$

where:

y_i is the content of the i'th compartment at time t;

I_i is the rate of intake into compartment i at time t;

λ_{ij} for i≠j is the rate constant for transfer from compartment j to compartment i;

λ_{ii} is negative and is the overall rate of loss from compartment i.

If the convergence as defined above is very good, then the step length is increased; if it is poor, the step length is decreased.

7.2.2.3   Other methods of calculation used

For time dependent exposures, the intake rates into the various compartments are calculated at each iteration of the program. This is done by comparing the cumulative time (sum of step lengths) with the exposure regime defined in the pre-processor, for acute exposures, or by calculating the scaling factor or input rates on the basis of the polynomials (see Section 7.2.1), for time dependent chronic exposures.

Urinary and faecal excretion are calculated as follows. The value of the cumulative time at the end of a step length is compared with the excretion sampling regimen set up in the pre-processor. If a sampling time has been reached, the amount of substance excreted in the sample is calculated from the accumulation of the substance in the relevant excretion compartment since the last sample was voided. Since a sampling time will not usually be reached exactly, a scaling routine is used:

$$R = (T_S - T_{N-1})/(T_N - T_{N-1})$$

where

T_S is the sampling time;

T_N is the cumulative time after the nth (i.e. current) time step.

so $\quad Y_E = Y_{N-1} + R^*(Y_N - Y_{N-1})$

where

Y_E = total contents of excretion sample;

Y_N = contents of the excretion sample after the Nth (i.e. current) time step.

After a sampling time is reached, the excretion sample contents are reset to contain the difference $(Y_N - Y_E)$ from the above equation.

The excretion samples are normalised to concentrations by dividing by the total output of excreted material constituting that sample (see ICRP, 1975 and later in this section for values).

As was noted in Section 4.12, a special technique is required for calculating the rate constants for methyl iodide metabolism. Methyl iodide is rapidly broken down to iodide which is metabolized with the body iodine. The thyroid regulates its uptake of iodide by means of a negative feedback system with respect to total body iodine. Thus the parameter value for thyroid uptake has to be recalculated after each time step since the simulations performed with the code involve situations where the total amount of iodine in the body varies. Iodine in the blood is the major regulator of thyroid uptake of iodine, and as the half-life of iodine in blood is 6 hours, it seems reasonable to assume that thyroid uptake will be a function of the average intake into the body during the previous six hours.

On this basis, before each time step, an averaging routine is called to calculate the average iodine intake of the body during the previous six hours, and this value is used to calculate the thyroid uptake using the equation given in section 4.12.

7.2.3   The post-processor

This section is concerned with the presentation of results calculated by the processor. There are three sections.

a)   The values of organ concentrations at the specified evaluation
     time are output in tabulated form to the line printer. Organ
     concentrations are calculated by dividing the total amount of
     substance present in the organ by the mass of the organ. Organ
     weights are taken from "Reference Man" (ICRP, 1975) and are as
     follows:

Tissue	Weight (kg)
Whole body	70.0
Muscle	28.0
Adipose tissue	15.0
Bone	10.0
Blood	5.5
Liver	1.8
Kidney	0.31
Spleen	0.18
Thyroid	0.02

$$\text{Urinary output} = 1.4 \text{ litres day}^{-1}$$
$$\text{Faecal output} = 0.135 \text{ kg day}^{-1}$$

Concentrations are expressed as parts per million (ppm). Concentrations in "other tissues" are calculated by subtracting stated
organ masses from total body masses and dividing the compartmental contents by this value (see Fig. 7.4).

b)   Histograms of urinary and faecal excretion are output on the line
     printer. Excretion is presented as a concentration either mg/l
     (urine) on ppm (faeces) (wet weight). This assumes that urinary
     output is constant throughout the day (see Fig. 7.5).

c)   The code terminates after the histograms have been printed.
     However, a separate graph plotting routine is available which
     permits graphs of either compartmental contents or organ concen-
     trations to be plotted against time, with output to the line
     printer.

RESULTS AT SPECIFIED TIMES

COMPARTMENTAL CONCENTRATIONS IN PPM

TIME	BLOOD	LUNG	KIDNEY	LIVER	OTHERS	TOTAL (MG)
1.0000E+00	2.1432E-02	2.1466E+00	2.3082E+01	2.3629E+00	4.2810E-01	3.9954E+01
2.0000E+00	3.0221E-02	3.4022E+00	2.3326E+01	2.4395F+00	4.3169E-01	4.1692E+01
3.0000E+00	3.4074E-02	4.4079E+00	2.3648E+01	2.5194E+00	4.3544E-01	4.3193E+01
4.0000E+00	3.5821E-02	5.3177E+00	2.4003E+01	2.6007E+00	4.3926E-01	4.4603E+01
5.0000E+00	3.6696E-02	6.1804E+00	2.4375E+01	2.6829E+00	4.4311E-01	4.5970E+01
6.0000E+00	1.6359E-02	4.8689E+00	2.4677E+01	2.7038E+00	4.4409E-01	4.4738E+01
7.0000E+00	7.9372E-03	4.4294E+00	2.4822E+01	2.7117E+00	4.4446E-01	4.4334E+01
8.0000E+00	2.5227E-02	6.3716E+00	2.4970E+01	2.7789E+00	4.4761E-01	4.6732E+01
9.0000E+00	3.2521E-02	7.5071E+00	2.5248E+01	2.8586E+00	4.5135E-01	4.8367E+01
1.0000E+01	3.5741E-02	8.4288E+00	2.5591E+01	2.9412E+00	4.5522F-01	4.9799E+01

FIGURE 7.4.   TABULATED VALUES OF ORGAN CONCENTRATION AT SPECIFIED
              TIMES OUTPUT TO THE LINE PRINTER BY THE POST-PROCEESSO

HISTOGRAM OF URINARY EXCRETION

```
         TIME  +++++++++++++++++++++++++++++++++++++++++++++++++++++  OUTPUT(MG/L)
DAY 1   7:59  +X    ,     ,     ,     ,     ,     ,     ,     ,     +  3.365E-04
        12:45  +XX   ,     ,     ,     ,     ,     ,     ,     ,     +  1.072E-03
        17:30  +XXXX,XXXX,XXX ,     ,     ,     ,     ,     ,     ,  +  5.969E-03
        22:30  +XXXX,XXXX,XXXX,XXXX,XXXX,    ,     ,     ,     ,    +  1.117E-02
DAY 2   7:59  +XXXX,XXXX,XXXX,XXXX,XXXX,    ,     ,     ,     ,    +  1.135E-02
        12:44  +XXXX,XXXX,XXXX,XXXX,XX   ,     ,     ,     ,     ,  +  1.041E-02
        17:30  +XXXX,XXXX,XXXX,XXXX,XXXX,XXXX,    ,     ,     ,    +  1.412E-02
        22:30  +XXXX,XXXX,XXXX,XXXX,XXXX,XXXX,XXXX,XXXX,    ,     +  1.821E-02
DAY 3   7:59  +XXXX,XXXX,XXXX,XXXX,XXXX,XXXX,XXXX,XXXX,X    ,     +  1.694E-02
        12:44  +XXXX,XXXX,XXXX,XXXX,XXXX,XXXX,XX   ,     ,     ,  +  1.482E-02
        17:30  +XXXX,XXXX,XXXX,XXXX,XXXX,XXXX,XXXX,XXX  ,     ,   +  1.788E-02
        22:30  +XXXX,XXXX,XXXX,XXXX,XXXX,XXXX,XXXX,XXXX,XXXX,X     +  2.139E-02
DAY 4   7:59  +XXXX,XXXX,XXXX,XXXX,XXXX,XXXX,XXXX,XXXX,X    ,     +  1.943E-02
        12:44  +XXXX,XXXX,XXXX,XXXX,XXXX,XXXX,XXXX,XXXX,X    ,     +  1.677E-02
        17:30  +XXXX,XXXX,XXXX,XXXX,XXXX,XXXX,XXXX,XXXX,XX   ,     +  1.954E-02
        22:30  +XXXX,XXXX,XXXX,XXXX,XXXX,XXXX,XXXX,XXXX,XXXX,XXXX  +  2.281E-02
DAY 5   7:59  +XXXX,XXXX,XXXX,XXXX,XXXX,XXXX,XXXX,XXXX,XXXX,       +  2.055E-02
        12:44  +XXXX,XXXX,XXXX,XXXX,XXXX,XXXX,XXXX,XXXX,XXX  ,     +  1.766E-02
        17:30  +XXXX,XXXX,XXXX,XXXX,XXXX,XXXX,XXXX,XXXX,XXX  ,     +  2.031E-02
        22:30  +XXXX,XXXX,XXXX,XXXX,XXXX,XXXX,XXXX,XXXX,XXXX,XXXXX+  2.348E-02
DAY 6   7:59  +XXXX,XXXX,XXXX,XXXX,XXXX,XXXX,XXXX,XXXX,XXXX,      +  2.109E-02
        12:44  +XXXX,XXXX,XXXX,XXXX,XXXX,XXXX,XXXX,XX   ,     ,   +  1.732E-02
        17:30  +XXXX,XXXX,XXXX,XXXX,XXXX,XXXX,XX   ,     ,     ,  +  1.498E-02
        22:30  +XXXX,XXXX,XXXX,XXXX,XXXX,XXX  ,     ,     ,     ,  +  1.303E-02
DAY 7   7:59  +XXXX,XXXX,XXXX,XXXX,XX   ,     ,     ,     ,     ,  +  1.035E-02
        12:44  +XXXX,XXXX,XXXX,XXX  ,     ,     ,     ,     ,     +  8.329E-03
        17:30  +XXXX,XXXX,XXXX,    ,     ,     ,     ,     ,     ,  +  7.110E-03
        22:30  +XXXX,XXXX,XXX ,     ,     ,     ,     ,     ,     ,  +  6.192E-03
DAY 8   7:59  +XXXX,XXXX,X   ,     ,     ,     ,     ,     ,     ,  +  4.977E-03
        12:44  +XXXX,XXXX,    ,     ,     ,     ,     ,     ,     ,  +  4.839E-03
        17:30  +XXXX,XXXX,XXXX,XXXX,    ,     ,     ,     ,     ,  +  9.231E-03
        22:30  +XXXX,XXXX,XXXX,XXXX,XXXX,XXXX,    ,     ,     ,    +  1.402E-02
DAY 9   7:59  +XXXX,XXXX,XXXX,XXXX,XXXX,XXXX,    ,     ,     ,    +  1.368E-02
        12:44  +XXXX,XXXX,XXXX,XXXX,XXXX,X    ,     ,     ,     ,  +  1.236E-02
        17:30  +XXXX,XXXX,XXXX,XXXX,XXXX,XXXX,    ,     ,     ,    +  1.586E-02
        22:30  +XXXX,XXXX,XXXX,XXXX,XXXX,XXXX,XXXX,XXXX,XX   ,    +  1.977E-02
DAY10   7:59  +XXXX,XXXX,XXXX,XXXX,XXXX,XXXX,XXXX,XXXX,XXXX,      +  1.829E-02
        12:44  +XXXX,XXXX,XXXX,XXXX,XXXX,XXXX,XXXX,XXXX,    ,     +  1.600E-02
        17:30  +XXXX,XXXX,XXXX,XXXX,XXXX,XXXX,XXXX,XXXX,XXXX,     +  1.898E-02
        22:30  +XXXX,XXXX,XXXX,XXXX,XXXX,XXXX,XXXX,XXXX,XXXX,XXX  +  2.242E-02
              +++++++++++++++++++++++++++++++++++++++++++++++++++++
```

HISTOGRAM OF FAECAL EXCRETION

```
         TIME  +++++++++++++++++++++++++++++++++++++++++++++++++++++  OUTPUT( PPM)
DAY 1  12:45  +     ,     ,     ,     ,     ,     ,     ,     ,     +  5.771E-02
DAY 2  12:44  +XXXX,X    ,     ,     ,     ,     ,     ,     ,     +  2.161E+00
DAY 3  12:44  +XXXX,XXXX,XXXX,XXXX,XXX  ,     ,     ,     ,     ,  +  8.144E+00
DAY 4  12:44  +XXXX,XXXX,XXXX,XXXX,XXXX,XXXX,XXXX,XXX  ,     ,    +  1.314E+01
DAY 5  12:44  +XXXX,XXXX,XXXX,XXXX,XXXX,XXXX,XXXX,XXXX,XXXX,X     +  1.604E+01
DAY 6  12:44  +XXXX,XXXX,XXXX,XXXX,XXXX,XXXX,XXXX,XXXX,XXXX,XXXXX+  1.752E+01
DAY 7  12:44  +XXXX,XXXX,XXXX,XXXX,XXXX,XXXX,XXXX,XXXX,XXXX,XX   +  1.645E+01
DAY 8  12:44  +XXXX,XXXX,XXXX,XXXX,XXXX,XXXX,XX   ,     ,     ,  +  1.129E+01
DAY 9  12:44  +XXXX,XXXX,XXXX,XXXX,XXXX,    ,     ,     ,     ,  +  8.524E+00
DAY10  12:44  +XXXX,XXXX,XXXX,XXXX,XXXX,XXXX,XXX  ,     ,     ,  +  1.141E+01
              +++++++++++++++++++++++++++++++++++++++++++++++++++++
```

FIGURE 7.5.   HISTOGRAM OF FAECAL AND URINARY EXCRETION OUTPUT TO
              THE LINE PRINTER BY THE POST-PROCESSOR

GRAPH PLOTTER

FILE NAME ON WHICH RESULTS ARE STORED   :1OSPIKE

ON WHICH DISK DRIVE IS THIS FILE LOCATED?
PRESENT DRIVE = 1 EXPANSION DRIVE = 2   :1

THIS FILE CONTAINS THE CONTENTS OF THE FOLLOWING TISSUES :-


```
                        BLOOD      (1)
                        LIVER      (2)
                        METABOLITES (3)
                        GI CONTENTS (4)
                        TOTAL (MG) (5)
```

HOW MANY LINES DO YOU WANT TO PLOT? (MAX = 8)   :5

ENTER NUMBER OF REQUIRED PARAMETER FOR LINE 1

(COMPARTMENT NUMBER OR ORGAN LABEL)   :1

ENTER NUMBER OF REQUIRED PARAMETER FOR LINE 2

(COMPARTMENT NUMBER OR ORGAN LABEL)   :2

ENTER NUMBER OF REQUIRED PARAMETER FOR LINE 3

(COMPARTMENT NUMBER OR ORGAN LABEL)   :3

ENTER NUMBER OF REQUIRED PARAMETER FOR LINE 4

(COMPARTMENT NUMBER OR ORGAN LABEL)   :4

ENTER NUMBER OF REQUIRED PARAMETER FOR LINE 5

(COMPARTMENT NUMBER OR ORGAN LABEL)   :5

DO YOU WANT EXPOSURE PLOTTING? (Y/N)   :Y

DO YOU WISH TO CHANGE TIME RANGE? (Y/N) :N

ENTER TIME STEP FOR DATA PLOTTING (DAYS)   :.1

PLOT IS FROM 1.0E-10 TO 1.0E+01
DO YOU WISH TO ALTER THE RANGE? (Y/N)   :Y

MINIMUM VALUE   :1.E-4

MAXIMUM VALUE   :10.

ANOTHER GRAPH? (Y/N)   :N
STOP

FIGURE 7.6.   CODE GENERATED DISPLAY AND ILLUSTRATIVE INPUT FOR THE
              CODE GRAPH

7.3   The code GRAPH

      This code enables the results from a run of MOSAIC which were stored on a disk file to be output graphically on a line printer. To run the code, the user types GRAPH<CR> from the CP/M prompt (A>). The code is interactive and the various prompts and required inputs are summarised below (see also Fig. 7.6).

- The code asks for the name of the file in which the results are stored. This should be input as in Section 7.2.1. The device on which the disk containing this file is situated is also required.

- A flag in the first record of the file tells the code the format of the data in the file. A message is displayed informing the user of the options available. The user then enters the number of lines to be plotted. Each line is then defined by entering the label (either the compartment number or the relevant tissue index).

- There is an option to alter the time range of the plot. If this option is selected, the code prompts the user for the new time range.

- The time step is requested. This defines the number of points on the x-axis. A maximum of 200 points can be accomodated by the code and an error flag is set if this value is exceeded.

- The code calculates the values to be plotted and displays its progress.

- The range of the calculated values is displayed and the user is given the option of changing the range. If this option is taken, the code prompts the user for the new limits of the range.

- The graph is now printed (see Fig. 7.7).

- The code gives the user the option of listing the value of each point plotted (output on the line printer).

- The option of plotting another graph is offered.

7.4   References

ICRP, 1975.   Report of the Task Group on Reference Man, Pergamon Press, Oxford.

ICRP, 1981.   Limits for Intakes of Radionuclides by Workers, ICRP Publication 30, Part 1.   Annals of the ICRP, 6, No.2/3.

Jacquez, J.A., 1972.   Compartmental Analysis in Biology and Medicine, Elsevier, Amsterdam.

Microsoft FORTRAN-80 Manual, 1979.

Thorne, M.C. and Jackson, D.   Models for the Metabolism of Chemical Carcinogens in Man.   ANS Report No.347, September 1983.

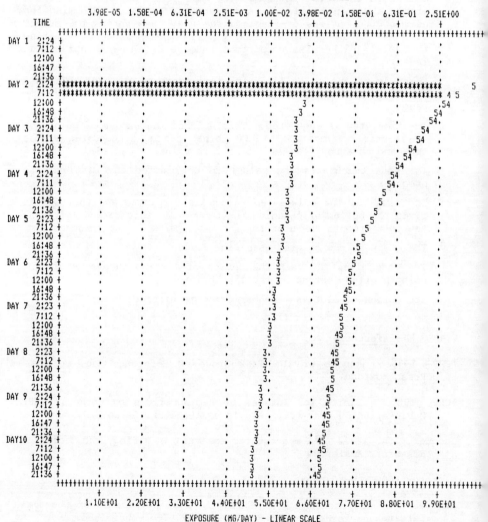

FIGURE 7.7. GRAPHICAL OUTPUT OF A LINE PRINTER PRODUCED BY THE CODE GRAPH

8
Implications of different regions of exposure

To illustrate the operation of the code, simulations of the main exposure regimes were performed for each carcinogen model. Each exposure was by inhalation, and the ICRP lung model was used. A normal dietary intake rate was assumed.

8.1   Description of exposure regimes

Chronic exposure

These are simulations of continuous exposure to the relevant carcinogen at the air concentrations listed in Table 8.1.

Acute exposure

These simulations are of an acute exposure to a high concentration of the substance in air, over the period 1.0 to 1.1 days into the simulation. The distribution of the carcinogen in the body is followed for a further nine days. The air concentrations used are given in Table 8.1 and the total amount of substance inhaled can be calculated by assuming that the "subject" inhales at a constant rate of 20 m^3 of air per day.

Shift exposure

This regime enables the changes in organ concentrations of the relevant carcinogen to be calculated, for a typical working exposure pattern. The "workday" modelled is

-     morning shift from 9.00 to 12.30
-     afternoon shift from 13.30 to 17.00

This regime is followed for five days and is followed by two days of no exposure from air, thus simulating the "working week". The

Carcinogen	Inhalation class	Dietary intake ($\mu g/d$)	Air concentration during chronic exposure ($\mu g/m^3$)	Air concentration between T= 1.0 and T= 1.1 days for acute exposure ($\mu g/m^3$)	Air concentration between 9.00 and 12.30 and 13.30 and 17.00 on workdays, for shift exposure ($\mu g/m^3$)
Arsenic	W	150	1	5000	50
Beryllium	W	20	1	500	2
Cadmium	W	150	1	5000	50
Lead	D	300	5	5000	50
Nickel	D	400	1	5000	1000
Chromium	D	75	1	500	50
Asbestos		0	1	5000	
Benzene		150	1	5000	3500
VCM		10	1	5000	2800
Benzidine		0	1	5000	24
Carbon Tetrachloride		10	1	5000	65000
Methyl Iodide		300	1	5000	28000

accumulation of the material in the body is followed for four weeks of this work pattern. Air concentrations during work exposure are the threshold limit values (TLV) recommended by the Health and Safety Executive (1978) and are shown in Table 8.1.

8.2   Discussion of Results

Each run of the code generates a histogram of urinary and of faecal excretion and also a graph of the time-dependence of tissue concentrations of the substance. These have been plotted using an in-house graphics plotter and software package. This graphical output for each simulation is included in Appendix B, and the following discussion should be read with reference to the appropriate figures in that appendix.

8.2.1   Simulations of shift working patterns

Due to limitations in the graphics software, only 20 days of the excretion patterns during the simulation could be plotted as histograms. All 30 days of the simulation are plotted on the graphs.
In this section, recent exposure refers to exposure over the previous 3 days.

Arsenic

Less than a 10% change in urine arsenic concentration is seen between pre- and post-shift urine samples (Fig. B.1). A slightly larger variation is seen in the faecal excretion of arsenic (Fig. B.2) over the working week. Neither sample would seem to be useful for monitoring purposes. With respect to time concentrations, all tissues showed a slight increase in arsenic concentration over the exposure period (Fig. B.3), but only blood and lung concentrations showed variations between pre- and post-shift levels. In blood, these changes were too small for blood to be considered a useful monitoring substance for occupational exposure levels up to the present TLV. The model calculations support the conclusions of Schrenk and Schreiber (1958) that no correlation exists between occupational exposure to and urinary concentration of arsenic, since the difference in excretion calculated by the model would be difficult to detect in a monitoring situation.

Beryllium

The urinary concentration of beryllium shows marked changes both pre- and post-shift and between occupational exposure periods and "weekend" periods (Fig. B.4) and thus seems to be an ideal monitoring substance for beryllium exposure. Faecal excretion of beryllium shows very little change throughout the simulation (Fig. B.5). Most tissues show very little change in beryllium concentrations (Fig. B.6), but lung, being the organ of intake, shows more variation with exposure.

Cadmium

Urinary cadmium is a good monitor of recent exposure (Fig. B.7), but as pre-shift urine concentrations are higher than midday urine concentrations, it may not be useful for day-to-day monitoring. Faecal excretion (Fig. B.8) does not vary sufficiently with inhalation exposure levels to be useful as a monitoring substance for occupational exposure. Tissue concentrations show a slight increase not evident on the graph (Fig. B.9).

Comparing blood levels during the working week and at weekends suggest that cadmium in blood is an indicator of recent cadmium exposure, in agreement with the findings of Roels et al. (1981). Kidney cadmium concentrations do not change very much and remains at 24 ppm, much below the "critical" concentration of 200 ppm.

Lead

Neither urine (Fig. B.10) nor faecal (Fig. B.11) excretion of lead are ideal monitors of recent lead exposure. Only lung shows any dramatic change in lead concentration (Fig. B.12), but a noticeable increase in blood and kidney lead concentrations was observed, suggesting that blood level may be a useful index of exposure.

Nickel

Urinary excretion of nickel reflects recent exposure (Fig. B.13). It is interesting to note that the urinary nickel concentrations predicted by the model ($\sim$1 µg/l) are far in excess of those observed in exposed individuals ($\sim$10 µg/l; Grandjean et al., 1980). This is probably because nickel-in-air concentrations in the working environment do not approach the TLV of 1 mg/m^3. Nickel levels in faeces are also elevated, since the amount of nickel inhaled and hence cleared to the gastrointestinal tract is of the same magnitude as the dietary intake of nickel (Fig. B.14). Tissue levels of nickel are all determined by recent exposure (Fig. B.15) except the concentration in "OTHER TISSUES" which shows a continuing accumulation.

Chromium

Urinary excretion is a good index of both shift exposure and of recent exposure (Fig. B.16). Faecal excretion shows a gradual increase from Monday to Friday (Fig. B.17) and reflects recent exposure. The urinary chromium concentrations calculated by the model ($\sim$35 µg/l) are in good agreement with literature values (Tossavainen et al., 1980). Tissue concentrations show a continuing increase (Fig. B.18) except blood and lung which reflect recent exposure.

Asbestos

Faecal excretion of asbestos is closely related to the early clearance of asbestos from the lung (see Section 4.7). Thus, faecal excretion of asbestos is a good index of recent exposure (Fig. B.19). However, the gradual accumulation of asbestos in the lung (Fig. B.20) is of more concern, since it is this material which is thought to give rise to toxic effects. Assay of accumulated asbestos burdens by faecal monitoring is not likely to be possible.

Benzene

Urinary excretion of benzene is a very good indicator of benzene exposure during the previous 24 h (Fig. B.21). Urinary phenol concentrations calculated by the model are similar to reported values in occupationally exposed subjects (Braier et al., 1981). Post shift urine gives a good indication of exposure levels during the shift. Tissue concentrations of benzene reflect the rapid metabolism of this compound, with only adipose tissue showing retention in the long-term (Fig. B.22).

Vinyl chloride

Results are similar to those for benzene, in that both urinary (Fig. B.23) and faecal (Fig. B.24) excretion patterns reflect exposure during the previous 24 h, with post-shift urine giving a good indication of total exposure during the shift. Tissue levels (Fig. B.25) reflect the very rapid metabolism of this compound.

Benzidine

No TLV is given for benzidine and the air concentration of 28 $\mu g/m^3$ was chosen so that model results could be compared with monitoring data (Meigs et al., 1984). Urinary excretion reflects exposure during the previous few hours (Fig. B.26) and the maximum calculated urinary concentration of ∿110 $\mu g/l$ is very near the mean values obtained by Meigs et al. of 150 $\mu g/l$ in occupationally exposed employees. Faecal excretion is also an indication of recent exposure (Fig. B.27). Tissue concentration (Fig. B.28) show no indication of accumulation of metabolites.

Carbon tetrachloride

Urinary excretion (Fig. B.29) is a good indicator of recent high levels of exposure, but the calculated differences between pre- and post-shift urine levels indicate it may not be a useful indicator of shift exposure. Faecal excretion is also a good indicator of recent exposure (Fig. B.30). Tissue concentrations show a gradual accumulation of the material in adipose tissue (Fig. B.31) and a slow decrease in the concentration of carbon tetrachloride metabolites in the body.

Methyl iodide

Urinary and faecal excretion of iodide both reflect recent exposure to methyl iodide (Figs. B.32 and B.33 respectively). Iodine concentrations in the blood and diffusion compartments reflect recent exposure, with thyroid and organic iodine concentrations showing a gradual increase (Fig. B.34).

8.2.2   Simulations of acute exposure

The graphical output from these simulations is given in Appendix B (Figs. B.35 to B.68). In general, faecal excretion reflects intake during the previous 3 or 4 days. This is to be expected because of the transit time through the gastrointestinal tract. Urinary excretion usually reflects exposure on the previous day, an important exception being lead. The main points to note from the graphs of tissue concentrations are in which tissues the substance accumulates, and the rate of clearance of the substance from the tissues.

8.2.3   Simulations of chronic exposure

Graphical output is given in Appendix B (Figs. B.69 to B.102). In general, the organic carcinogens considered reach equilibrium conditions far more quickly than the metalloids.

8.2.4   Simulations with the new lung model

To compare the new lung model with the ICRP lung model, the code was run under identical conditions with the relevant lung model used to calculate lung deposition and retention.

An acute inhalation of cadmium at a concentration of 5 mg/m³ over the period 1.0 to 1.1 days into the simulation was used as the exposure regime. The concentration of cadmium in the lung was followed for a further nine days. Two mean particle diameters were used, 0.2 and 9.0 µm, as these values are at the limits of the range for which the ICRP model can calculate the deposition and retention in the lung accurately. A comparison of the effects of nose and mouth breathing was also made, when using the new model. The results are represented graphically in Fig. B.103 in which the lung concentration of cadmium is plotted as a function of time for each simulation. The symbol for each line represents the simulation as defined below.

A   =   ICRP model, 0.2 µm particles

B   =   ICRP model, 9.0 µm particles

C   =   New model, 0.2 µm particles, nose breathing

D   =   New model, 9.0 µm particles, nose breathing

E   =   New model, 0.2 µm particles, mouth breathing

F   =   New model, 0.2 µm particles, mouth breathing

With both models, small (0.2 µm) particles are deposited more in the respiratory region of the lung, whereas large (9.0 µm) particles are deposited more in the upper respiratory tract, and cleared rapidly via the mucociliary escalator.

From Fig. B.103 it can be seen that the clearance of cadmium from the lung as calculated by the new model is identical for nose and mouth breathing of small particles. This is because small particles are not deposited in the nasal region.   By comparison, there is a marked difference in the deposition of large particles between nose and mouth breathing patterns, due to the efficiency of the nasal region at trapping particles of this size.   This aspect of deposition is not adequately covered by the ICRP model.

The initial rate of clearance of material from the lung is more rapid with the ICRP model.   This highlights one of the inadequacies of the ICRP model, in that early clearance from the respiratory region of the lung is not considered in detail.   This reflects a lack of good quantitative data on the dynamics of early clearance when the ICRP lung model was formulated.

8.3   REFERENCES

Braier, L., Levy, A., Dror, K. and Pardo, A., 1981.   Benzene in blood and phenol in urine in monitoring benzene exposure in industry. Am. J. Indust. Med., 2, 119-123.

Grandjean, P., Selikoff, I.J., Shen, S.K. and Sunderman, F.W., 1980. Nickel concentrations in plasma and urine of shipyard workers. Am. J. Indust. Med., 1, 181-189.

Health and Safety Executive, 1978.   Threshold limit values for 1978. Guidance note EH15/78 from the H & S.

Meigs, J.W., Sciarini, L.J., and Van Sandt, W.A., 1954.   Skin penetration by diamines of the benzidine group.   Arch. Ind. Hyg., 9, 122-132.

Roels, H.A., Lauwerys, R.R., Buchet, J-P., Bernard, A., Chettle, D.R., Harvey, T.C. and Al-Haddad, I.K., 1981.   In vivo measurement of liver and kidney cadmium in workers exposed to this metal: its significance with respect to cadmium in blood and urine. Environ. Res., 26, 217-240.

Schrenk, H.H. and Schreibeis, L., 1958.   Urinary arsenic levels as an index of industrial exposure.   J. Am. Ind. Hyg. Assoc., 19, 225-228.

Tossavainen, A., Nurminen, M., Mutanen, P. and Tola, S., 1980. Application of mathematical modelling for assessing the biological half-times of chromium and nickel in field studies.   Br. J. Indust. Med., 37, 285-291.

9
Conclusions and recommendations

By a comprehensive review of the published literature it has proved possible to develop pharmacokinetic models for all the materials included in this study. It has also been possible to implement these models on a micro-computer based system and to simulate a wide range of types of exposure. The existence of this model means that it is now straightforward to investigate other proposed exposure regimes and comment upon them in respect of changes in tissue levels, or in respect of appropriate monitoring programmes. It is clear that this programme of review and modelling could be extended to many other toxic, and, in particular, carcinogenic, materials.

A review of data relevant to movement through, and uptake from, the gastrointestinal tract has demonstrated that the model used by the International Commission on Radiological Protection (ICRP) which was developed nearly twenty years ago, is consistent with more recent data and is still generally applicable. In contrast, a large number of studies have revealed limitations and deficiencies in the ICRP lung model and a new model has been proposed. There is a need to subject this new model to critical review and it is recommended that the relevant sections of this report be made available to experts in this topic. It is recognised that many individuals and groups will wish to continue to use the ICRP lung model, if only for comparative purposes. For this reason, both models have been implemented and results for both have been presented.

The implementation of the models have been fully documented, both at a user and at a programmer level. Except in the graphics facilities, implementation is in standard FORTRAN, so the implementation of the models on computer systems other than those used by ANS should be a straightforward undertaking.

Examination of model results indicates, as expected, that urinary monitoring is generally an appropriate technique for assessing recent exposures, but that it may need to be supplemented by faecal monitoring for some substances. Assaying accumulated exposure is a more intractable problem and further work is required on this topic, both in respect of physiological indicators and in respect of non-invasive assays of tissue contents or concentrations.

10
Acknowledgements

We would like to thank the large number of individuals who have contributed to this study. In particular, out typists G. Tiplady, M. Barrett, P. Skam and M. Razzell for coping with our very variable manuscripts; our librarian M. Metcalf for handling the tide of literature; and our technical assistants R. Baker, L. Charlwood, D. Hannant and R. Hicks for support in all areas, especially computing. Thanks must also go to W. Hunter of DG(V) of the CEC and to the ANS Management, in particular D. Read, A. Martin and B.C. Woodfine for their support of this study. In respect to the lung review, special thanks are due to M. Bailey of the National Radiological Protection Board who made available his very extensive bibliography of relevant publications.

Appendix A

Computer programs for evaluating the implications of different exposure regions

Program listing of the computer code MOSAIC

```
      PROGRAM MOSAIC
C
C     DYNAMIC MODEL FOR METABOLISM OF CARCINOGENS
C
      DIMENSION Y(40),A(80),ITO(80),IFROM(80),AIN(40),
     1 TMAT(30),POL(10),TFLAG(120),ESP(5,60),GUT(2,12),B(8),YN(2),
     2 CL(3),URINE(200),FAECES(200),CARC(5,12)
      LOGICAL*1 FNAME(11),GNAME(11)
      DATA CL/'D  ','W  ','Y  '/,YN/'Y  ','N  '/
      DATA GUT/0.8,0.15,0.005,0.02,0.05,0.15,0.15,0.3,0.05,0.4,0.01,
     1 0.075,0.1,0.0,1.0,0.15,1.0,0.08,1.0,0.0,1.0,0.01,1.0,0.3/
      DATA CARC/'ARSE','NIC ','   ','   ','   ','BERY','LLIU',
     1 'M   ','   ','   ','CADM','IUM ','   ','   ','   ','LEAD',
     2 '   ','   ','   ','NICK','EL  ','   ','   ','   ',
     3 'CHRO','MIUM','   ','   ','ASBE','STOS','   ','   ','   ',
     4 '   ','BENZ','ENE ','   ','   ','   ','VINY','L CH','LORI',
     5 'DE  ','   ','BENZ','IDIN','E   ','   ','   ','CARB','ON T',
     6 'ETRA','CHLO','RIDE','METH','YL I','ODID','E   ','   '/
C          SELECT CARCINOGEN TO BE MODELLED
    2 WRITE (1,3)
    3 FORMAT (23(/),30X,'ARSENIC =  1'/28X,'BERYLLIUM =  2'/30X,
     1 'CADMIUM =  3'/33X,'LEAD =  4'/31X,'NICKEL =  5'/29X,'CHROMIUM',
     2 ' =  6'/29X,'ASBESTOS =  7'/30X,'BENZENE =  8'/23X,'VINYL CHLO',
     3 'RIDE =  9'/28X,'BENZIDINE = 10'/17X,'CARBON TETRACHLORIDE = 1',
     4 '1'/24X,'METHYL IODIDE = 12'/34X,'END = 13',6(/),5X,'WHICH CAR',
     5 'CINOGEN?   :')
      READ (1,5) ICARC
    5 FORMAT (I2)
      IF (ICARC.GT.0.AND.ICARC.LT.13) GO TO 7
      IF (ICARC.EQ.13) GO TO 400
      WRITE (1,6)
    6 FORMAT(5X,'THIS CARCINOGEN MODEL IS NOT AVAILABLE'/)
      GO TO 2
C          DEFINE RUNNING MODE OF CODE
    7 DO 10 I=1,11
      FNAME(I)=' '
   10 GNAME(I)=' '
      WRITE (1,15)
   15 FORMAT (23(/),20X,'THE MODEL CAN BE RUN IN THREE MODES',//,10X,
     1 'FULL DEBUGGING OUTPUT (PRINTS RESULTS AT EACH ITERATION)',
     2 /10X,'STORE ORGAN CONCENTRATIONS ON FILE',/10X,'STORE ALL ',
     3 'COMPARTMENTAL CONTENTS ON FILE'//20X,'ALL THREE MODES CAN ',
     4 'BE RUN SIMULTANEOUSLY'/)
      IOUT=0
      MODA=0
      MODB=0
      IDEV=0
      JDEV=0
      WRITE (1,20)
   20 FORMAT (5(/),5X,'DO YOU REQUIRE FULL DEBUGGING MODE? (Y/N)   :')
      READ (1,70) ANS
      IF (ANS.EQ.YN(1)) IOUT=1
      WRITE (1,25)
   25 FORMAT (23(/),5X,'DO YOU WISH TO SAVE ORGAN CONCENTRATIONS?',
     1 ' (Y/N)   :')
      READ (1,70) ANS
      IF (ANS.EQ.YN(2)) GO TO 40
      MODA=1
      WRITE (1,30)
   30 FORMAT (5(/),5X,'IN WHICH FILE ARE ORGAN CONCENTRATIONS TO BE',
     1 ' STORED?   :')
      READ (1,35) FNAME
   35 FORMAT (11A1)
      FNAME(9)='D'
      FNAME(10)='A'
      FNAME(11)='T'
      WRITE (1,36)
   36 FORMAT (//5X,'ON WHICH DISK DRIVE IS THIS FILE LOCATED?'/5X,
     1 'PRESENT DRIVE = 1  EXPANSION DRIVE = 2   :')
```

```
          READ (1,5) IDEV
    40    WRITE (1,45)
    45    FORMAT (23(/),5X,'DO YOU WISH TO SAVE ALL COMPARTMENTAL',
       1  ' CONTENTS? (Y/N)  :')
          READ (1,70) ANS
          IF (ANS.EQ.YN(2)) GO TO 49
          MODB=1
          WRITE (1,47)
    47    FORMAT (5(/),5X,'IN WHICH FILE ARE COMPARTMENTAL CONTENTS TO',
       1  ' BE STORED?  :')
          READ (1,35) GNAME
          GNAME(9)='D'
          GNAME(10)='A'
          GNAME(11)='T'
          WRITE (1,36)
          READ (1,5) JDEV
C             SET COMPARTMENT LABELS TO ZERO INITIALLY
    49    IBL=0
          IST=0
          IC1=0
          IC2=0
          IC3=0
          IC4=0
          IURINE=0
          IFECES=0
          ITYPE=0
          IEXT=0
          NESP=0
          N2=0
          LMOD=0
          NM=0
          AIRC=0.0
          FDEX=0.0
          SKIN=0.0
          XA=0.0
          XB=0.0
          FIN=0.0
          GREX=0.0
C             SET CONTENTS OF ARRAYS TO ZERO
          DO 50 I=1,40
          Y(I)=0.0
    50    AIN(I)=0.0
          DO 51 I=1,80
          ITO(I)=0
          IFROM(I)=0
    51    A(I)=0.0
          DO 52 I=1,10
    52    POL(I)=0.0
          DO 53 I=1,30
    53    TMAT(I)=0.0
          DO 54 I=1,60
          DO 54 J=1,5
    54    ESP(J,I)=0.0
          DO 55 I=1,120
    55    TFLAG(I)=0.0
          DO 56 I=1,200
          URINE(I)=0.0
    56    FAECES(I)=0.0
          DO 57 I=1,8
    57    B(I)=0.0
C             SET UP LUNG MODEL PARAMETERS (AMAD,CLASS)
          IF (ICARC.GT.6) GO TO 86
          WRITE (1,58)
    58    FORMAT (23(/),25X,'INHALATION PARAMETERS'//)
    59    WRITE (1,60)
    60    FORMAT (5X,'ENTER MEAN PARTICLE DIAMETER (MICRONS)   :')
          READ (1,110) AMAD
          IF (AMAD.GE.0.1.AND.AMAD.LE.10.0) GO TO 71
          WRITE (1,65)
    65    FORMAT (10X,'AMAD OUTSIDE AVAILABLE RANGE'/)
          GO TO 59
```

```
      70   FORMAT (A4)
      71   WRITE (1,72)
      72   FORMAT (23(/),5X,'WHICH LUNG MODEL IS TO BE USED? ICRP = 0',
          1 ' NEW MODEL = 1    :')
           READ (1,5) LMOD
           IF (LMOD.EQ.1) GO TO 82
           WRITE (1,75)
      75   FORMAT (//5X,'INPUT INHALATION CLASS (D,W,Y)  :')
           READ (1,70) CLAS
           ICLA=0
           DO 80 I=1,3
      80   IF (CLAS.EQ.CL(I)) ICLA=I
           IF (ICLA.NE.0) GO TO 85
           WRITE (1,81)
      81   FORMAT (10X,'INVALID INHALATION CLASS'/)
           GO TO 71
      82   WRITE (1,83)
      83   FORMAT (23(/),5X,'WHICH BREATHING PATTERN? NOSE = 0 ',
          1 'MOUTH = 1  :')
           READ (1,5) NM
      85   CALL LUNG1(A,ITO,IFROM,MM,B,AMAD,ICLA,N,IBL,IST,LUNG,NM,LMOD,
          1 ICARC)
C              SET FRACTIONAL ABSORPTION FROM GI TRACT
      86   WRITE (1,87)
      87   FORMAT (23(/),25X,'DIETARY PARAMETERS'//)
           IF (ICARC.EQ.7) GO TO 93
           WRITE (1,88) GUT(1,ICARC)
      88   FORMAT (5X,'THE PRESENT VALUE OF F1 =',1PE11.4/
          1 5X,'DO YOU WISH TO CHANGE THIS? (Y/N)   :')
           READ (1,70) ANS1
           IF (ANS1.EQ.YN(2)) GO TO 92
      89   WRITE (1,90)
      90   FORMAT (5X,'ENTER NEW VALUE OF F1   :')
           READ (1,110) FA
           IF (FA.GE.0.0.AND.FA.LE.1.0) GO TO 93
           WRITE (1,91)
      91   FORMAT (5X,'F1 MUST BE A DECIMAL FRACTION OF 1.0'/)
           GO TO 89
      92   FA=GUT(1,ICARC)
C              SET DIETARY INTAKE
      93   WRITE (1,94) GUT(2,ICARC)
      94   FORMAT (5X,'THE PRESENT DIETARY INTAKE =',1PE11.4,' MG/DAY'/
          1 5X,'DO YOU WISH TO CHANGE THIS? (Y/N)   :')
           READ (1,70) ANS2
           IF (ANS2.EQ.YN(2)) GO TO 98
      95   WRITE (1,96)
      96   FORMAT (5X,'ENTER NEW DIETARY INTAKE (MG/DAY)   :')
           READ (1,110) FOOD
           IF (FOOD.GE.0.0.AND.FOOD.LT.1E3) GO TO 99
           WRITE (1,97)
      97   FORMAT (5X,'THIS DIETARY INTAKE IS UNREALISTIC'/)
           GO TO 95
      98   FOOD=GUT(2,ICARC)
      99   IF (ICARC.GT.6) GO TO 100
           CALL GUT1(A,ITO,IFROM,MM,FA,N,IBL,IST,IFECES)
     100   CALL MOD1(Y,A,ITO,IFROM,MM,N,IBL,IC1,IC2,IC3,IC4,IURINE,IFECES,
          1 XA,XB,ICARC,FIN,B,LUNG)
C              SET STEP SIZE,VENTILATION RATE AND ERROR LIMIT
           VENT=20.0
           H1=1.0E-06
           ESCAL=1.0E-06
C              EDIT THE MODEL IF NESSARY
           WRITE (1,105)
     105   FORMAT (23(/),5X,'DO TOU WISH TO EDIT THE MODEL? (Y/N)   :')
           READ (1,70) ANS8
           IF (ANS8.EQ.YN(2)) GO TO 112
           CALL MODED(N,MM,Y,AIN,FIN,A,ITO,IFROM,ICARC,YN,ESCAL,H1,VENT,
          1 CARC)
     110   FORMAT (E12.4)
     112   WRITE (1,115)
     115   FORMAT (23(/),30X,'EVALUATION TIMES'///20X,'ORGAN',
```

```
     1 ' CONCENTRATIONS AT THESE TIMES ARE',//20X,'TABULATED AT THE',
     2 ' END OF THE SIMULTION',10(/),5X,'HOW MANY EVALUATION TIMES ',
     3 'DO YOU REQUIRE?    :')
   116 READ (1,5) M
       IF (M.GT.0.OR.M.LE.30) GO TO 118
       WRITE (1,117)
   117 FORMAT (23(/),5X,'A MAXIMUM OF 30 EVALUATION TIMES ARE ALLOWED',
     1 5(/),5X,'ENTER VALID NUMBER OF EVALUATION TIMES    :')
       GO TO 116
   118 WRITE (1,119)
   119 FORMAT (23(/))
       DO 125 I=1,M
   120 WRITE (1,121) I
   121 FORMAT (//5X,'ENTER EVALUATION TIME',I3,' (DAYS)    :')
       READ (1,110) T
       IF (T.GT.0.0) GO TO 123
       WRITE (1,122)
   122 FORMAT (//5X,'TIMES MUST BE GREATER THAN ZERO'/)
       GO TO 120
   123 IF (I.EQ.1) GO TO 125
       J=I-1
       IF (T.GT.TMAT(J)) GO TO 125
       WRITE (1,124)
   124 FORMAT (//5X,'TIMES MUST BE GREATER THAN THE PREVIOUS VALUE'//)
       GO TO 120
   125 TMAT(I)=T
       TMAX=TMAT(M)
C           DEFINE EXPOSURE REGIME AND BRANCH ACCORDINGLY
   130 WRITE (1,140)
   140 FORMAT (23(/),10X,'WHICH EXPOSURE REGIME? CHRONIC=0 ACUTE=1  :')
       READ (1,5) IESP
       IF (IESP) 130,145,170
C           ENTER INPUTS FOR CHRONIC EXPOSURE
   145 WRITE (1,149)
   149 FORMAT (23(/),25X,'CHRONIC EXPOSURE',//)
       WRITE (1,150)
   150 FORMAT (/5X,'ENTER AIR CONCENTRATION (MG/M3)  :')
       READ (1,110) AIRC
       WRITE (1,154)
   154 FORMAT (/5X,'ENTER ADDITIONAL INPUT TO TO GI TRACT(MG/DAY)  :')
       READ (1,110) FDEX
       IF (ICARC.NE.8.AND.ICARC.NE.10.AND.ICARC.NE.11) GO TO 158
       WRITE (1,156)
   156 FORMAT (/5X,'ENTER INPUT TO SKIN (MG/DAY)   :')
       READ (1,110) SKIN
C           SET INPUTS TO VARIOUS COMPARTMENTS
   158 IF (ICARC.GT.7) GO TO 163
       DO 161 I=1,8
   161 AIN(I)=B(I)*AIRC*VENT
       AIN(IST)=FOOD+FDEX
       IF (ICARC.EQ.7) GO TO 164
       IF (LMOD.NE.1.AND.NM.NE.1) GO TO 164
       AIN(IST)=AIN(IST)+AIN(1)+AIN(2)
       AIN(1)=0.0
       AIN(2)=0.0
       GO TO 164
   163 GREX=FA*(FOOD+FDEX)+VENT*AIRC*FIN+SKIN
       AIN(IBL)=GREX
C           SET TIME-DEPENDENCE OF CHRONIC EXPOSURE IF NECESSARY
   164 WRITE (1,165)
   165 FORMAT (/10X,'IS THE EXPOSURE TIME-DEPENDENT? (Y/N)   :')
       READ (1,70) ANSC
       IF (ANSC.EQ.YN(2)) GO TO 180
       IEXT=1
       WRITE (1,166)
   166 FORMAT (5X,'THE INITIAL EXPOSURE IS TIME-DEPENDENT AND WILL'/
     1 5X,'BE SCALED ACCORDING TO THE POLYNOMIAL :-'/5X,
     2 'EXPOSURE(T)=EXPOSURE(0)*(K1+K2*T+K3*T**2...ETC)'/)
       WRITE (1,167)
   167 FORMAT (5X,'ENTER ORDER OF POLYNOMIAL    :')
       READ (1,5) ITYPE
```

```
          DO 169 I=1,ITYPE
          WRITE (1,168) I
  168     FORMAT (5X,'ENTER K',I1,'   :')
  169     READ (1,110) POL(I)
          GO TO 180
C              CALL ROUTINE FOR ENTERING ACUTE EXPOSURES
  170     IF (IESP.NE.1) GO TO 130
          WRITE (1,175)
  175     FORMAT (23(/),25X,'ACUTE EXPOSURE',//)
          CALL ENTERE(TFLAG,ESP,NESP,N2,YN,ICARC)
C              CALL URINE AND FECAL SAMPLING ROUTINES
  180     IF (ICARC.EQ.7) GO TO 194
          WRITE (1,185)
  185     FORMAT (23(/),25X,'URINE SAMPLING TIMES',//)
          WRITE (1,187)
  187     FORMAT (//10X,'COLLECTION OF EXCRETION SAMPLES IS SIMULATED AT',
         1 //10X,'THESE TIMES EACH DAY THROUGHOUT THE SIMULATION',10(/))
          WRITE (1,190)
  190     FORMAT (5X,'HOW MANY URINE SAMPLES PER DAY?   :')
          READ (1,5) NU
          CALL SAMPLE(URINE,TMAX,JU,NU)
  194     IF (ICARC.EQ.8) GO TO 210
          WRITE (1,195)
  195     FORMAT (23(/),25X,'FAECAL SAMPLING TIMES',//)
          WRITE (1,187)
          WRITE (1,200)
  200     FORMAT (5X,'HOW MANY FAECAL SAMPLES PER DAY   :')
          READ (1,5) NF
          CALL SAMPLE(FAECES,TMAX,JF,NF)
  210     CALL LOSS(A,ITO,IFROM,MM,N)
          IF (ICARC.GT.7.OR.IESP.EQ.1) GO TO 279
          DO 275 I=1,N
  275     GREX=GREX+AIN(I)
  279     IED=0
          CALL OUT1(H1,ESCAL,VENT,N,Y,AIN,FIN,MM,ITO,IFROM,A,ICARC,IED,
         1 CARC,TMAT,M,ESP,IESP,IEXT,POL,ITYPE,NESP,FNAME,IDEV,AMAD,ICLA,
         2 CL,FOOD,FA,AIRC,SKIN,GNAME,JDEV,MODA,MODB,LMOD,NM)
          IF (IOUT.EQ.0) GO TO 305
          WRITE (2,285)
  285     FORMAT (///20X,'TABLE OF COMPARTMENTAL CONTENTS (MG) AT TIME',
         1 ' (T)'/)
  305     WRITE (1,310)
  310     FORMAT (12(/),20X,'PARAMETERS ARE BEING WRITTEN TO FILE',12(/))
          CALL WRITE(IESP,ITYPE,IEXT,IOUT,ICARC,IDEV,N,M,IFECES,
         1 IBL,IC1,IC2,IC3,IC4,IURINE,IST,MM,NESP,N2,JF,JU,ITO,IFROM,
         2 H1,ESCAL,FOOD,VENT,GREX,AIRC,FDEX,FNAME,Y,A,AIN,TMAT,POL,TFLAG,
         3 ESP,B,URINE,FAECES,FIN,SKIN,FA,XA,XB,LUNG,GNAME,JDEV,MODA,MODB,
         4 LMOD,NM)
          CALL FCHAIN ('TOXIC2  COM',0)
  400     STOP
          END
C
C===================================================================
C
          SUBROUTINE TIME(T)
C
C         ROUTINE TO CONVERT A 24HR TIME TO ITS DECIMAL EQUIVALENT
C
          TT=0.0
          IF (T.LT.1.0) GO TO 2
    1     T=T-1.0
          TT=TT+1.0
          IF (T.GE.1.0) GO TO 1
    2     T=T*5.0/3.0
          T=TT+T
          T=T/24.0
          RETURN
          END
C
C===================================================================
C
```

```
      SUBROUTINE MODED(N,MM,Y,AIN,FIN,A,ITO,IFROM,ICARC,YN,ESCAL,H1,
     1 VENT,CARC)
C
C         ROUTINE TO EDIT MODEL PARAMETERS
C
      DIMENSION Y(40),A(80),ITO(80),IFROM(80),AIN(40),YN(2),ITEM(20),
     1 CARC(5,12)
C         PRINT A SUMMARY OF PARAMETERS IF NECESSARY
      WRITE (1,5)
    5 FORMAT (23(/),5X,'DO YOU REQUIRE A SUMMARY OF MODEL',
     1 ' PARAMETERS? (Y/N)   :')
      READ (1,160) ANSA
      IF (ANSA.EQ.YN(2)) GO TO 10
      IED=1
      CALL OUT1(H1,ESCAL,VENT,N,Y,AIN,FIN,MM,ITO,IFROM,A,ICARC,IED,
     1 CARC)
C         CHOOSE PARAMETERS TO BE EDITED
   10 WRITE (1,15)
   15 FORMAT (23(/))
      WRITE (1,20)
   20 FORMAT (23(/),11X,'CHANGE EXISTING MODEL PARAMETERS = 1'/19X,
     1 'ADD NEW MODEL PARAMETERS = 2'/37X,'RETURN = 3',10(/),
     2 5X,'WHICH OPTION?   :')
      READ (1,30) IOPT
   30 FORMAT (I3)
      WRITE (1,15)
      IF (IOPT-2) 100,500,900
C         EDIT EXISTING MODEL PARAMETERS
  100 WRITE (1,101)
  101 FORMAT (3(/),21X,'EDIT INITIAL TIME STEP = 1'/18X,'EDIT ',
     1 'VALUE OF ERROR LIMIT = 2'/22X,'EDIT VENTILATION RATE = 3')
      NI=4
      IF (ICARC.LT.8) GO TO 1010
      WRITE (1,1000)
 1000 FORMAT (21X,'EDIT FRACTIONAL UPTAKE = 4')
      NI=5
 1010 WRITE (1,1011) NI
 1011 FORMAT (35X,'CONTINUE =',I2,10(/),5X,'WHICH OPTION?   :')
      READ (1,30) LOPT
      IF (ICARC.LT.8.AND.LOPT.EQ.4) LOPT=5
      WRITE (1,15)
      IF (LOPT-2) 102,107,110
  102 WRITE (1,103) H1
  103 FORMAT (3(/),5X,'THE INITIAL STEPSIZE =',1PE12.4,' DAYS'/
     1 /5X,'ENTER NEW VALUE FOR STEP SIZE (IN DAYS)   :')
      READ (1,180) X
      IF (X.LE.0.0.OR.X.GT.1.0E-3) GO TO 105
      H1=X
      GO TO 100
  105 WRITE (1,104)
  104 FORMAT (//5X,'THIS VALUE WILL GIVE AN INACCURATE SOLUTION')
      GO TO 102
C         EDIT ERROR LIMIT
  107 WRITE (1,108) ESCAL
  108 FORMAT (3(/),5X,'THE PRESENT ERROR LIMIT =',1PE12.4//
     1 5X,'ENTER NEW VALUE FOR ERROR LIMIT   :')
      READ (1,180) X
      IF (X.LE.0.0.OR.X.GT.1.0E-3) GO TO 109
      ESCAL=X
      GO TO 100
  109 WRITE (1,104)
      GO TO 107
C         EDIT VENTILATION RATE
  110 IF (LOPT-4) 111,2000,118
  111 WRITE (1,112) VENT
  112 FORMAT (3(/),5X,'THE PRESENT VENTILATION RATE =',1PE12.4,' ',
     1 'M3/DAY'//5X,'ENTER NEW VALUE FOR VENTILATION RATE (M3/DAY)  :')
      READ (1,180) X
      IF (X.LE.0.0.OR.X.GT.50.0) GO TO 117
      VENT=X
      GO TO 100
```

```
      117  WRITE (1,114)
      114  FORMAT (//5X,'ONLY CROSS-COUNTRY SKIERS CAN ACHIEVE THIS RATE!')
           GO TO 111
C            EDIT FRACTIONAL UPTAKE (FOR GASES ONLY)
     2000  WRITE (1,2002) FIN
     2002  FORMAT (///,5X,'PRESENT FRACTIONAL INTAKE =',1PE12.4//5X,
         1  'ENTER NEW VALUE FOR FRACTIONAL INTAKE    :')
           READ (1,180) X
           IF (X.LT.0.0.OR.X.GT.1.0) GO TO 2005
           FIN=X
           GO TO 100
     2005  WRITE (1,2006)
     2006  FORMAT (/5X,'FRACTIONAL INTAKES MUST BE BETWEEN 0.0 AND 1.0')
           GO TO 2000
      118  WRITE (1,119)
      119  FORMAT (23(/),15X,'EDIT COMPARMENTAL CONTENTS = 1'/21X,
         1  'EDIT RATE PARAMETERS = 2'/37X,'EXIT = 3',10(/),5X,
         2  'WHICH OPTION?   :')
           READ (1,30) JOPT
           WRITE (1,15)
           IF (JOPT-2) 120,300,10
C            EDIT COMPARMENTAL PARAMETERS
      120  WRITE (1,130) N
      130  FORMAT (3(/),5X,'THERE ARE',I3,' COMPARTMENTS. WHICH DO YOU',
         1  ' WANT TO EDIT?   :')
           READ (1,30) IC
           IF (IC.GT.0.AND.IC.LE.N) GO TO 137
           WRITE (1,135) N
      135  FORMAT (/5X,'THERE ARE ONLY',I3,' COMPARTMENTS')
           GO TO 120
      137  DO 290 I=1,N
           IF (I.NE.IC) GO TO 290
           WRITE (1,140) Y(I)
      140  FORMAT (23(/),5X,'PRESENT COMPARTMENTAL CONTENTS =',1PE12.4,
         1  ' MG')
           WRITE (1,150)
      150  FORMAT (/5X,'DO YOU WISH TO CHANGE THIS? (Y/N)   :')
           READ (1,160) ANS1
      160  FORMAT (A4)
           IF (ANS1.EQ.YN(2)) GO TO 190
           WRITE (1,170)
      170  FORMAT (/5X,'ENTER NEW COMPARTMENTAL CONTENTS (MG)   :')
           READ (1,180) Y(I)
      180  FORMAT (E12.4)
C            EDIT INTAKE RATES
      190  WRITE (1,200) AIN(I)
      200  FORMAT (//5X,'PRESENT INTAKE RATE =',1PE12.4,' MG/DAY')
           WRITE (1,150)
           READ (1,160) ANS2
           IF (ANS2.EQ.YN(2)) GO TO 290
           WRITE (1,210)
      210  FORMAT (/5X,'ENTER NEW INTAKE RATE (MG/DAY)   :')
           READ (1,180) AIN(I)
      290  CONTINUE
           GO TO 118
C            EDIT TRANSFER PARAMETERS
      300  WRITE (1,310) N
      310  FORMAT (3(/),30X,'THERE ARE',I3,' COMPARTMENTS'//5X,
         1  'FROM WHICH COMPARTMENT DOES THIS TRANSFER ORIGINATE?   :')
           READ (1,30) IF
           IF (IF.GT.0.AND.IF.LE.N) GO TO 315
           WRITE (1,135) N
           GO TO 300
      315  J=0
           DO 320 I=1,MM
           IF (IFROM(I).NE.IF) GO TO 320
           J=J+1
           ITEM(J)=ITO(I)
      320  CONTINUE
           IF (J.GT.0) GO TO 325
           WRITE (1,321)
```

```
321   FORMAT (///5X,'THERE ARE NO TRANSFERS FROM THIS COMPARTMENT'//)
      GO TO 300
325   WRITE (1,330) IF,(ITEM(I),I=1,J)
330   FORMAT (//5X,'TRANSFERS ARE FROM COMPARTMENT',I3,' TO THE',
     1 ' FOLLOWING COMPARTMENTS :-',//,20X,15I3)
      WRITE (1,331)
331   FORMAT (//5X,'TO WHICH COMPARTMENT IS THE TRANSFER YOU ',
     1 'WISH TO EDIT?    :')
      READ (1,30) IT
      IF (IT.GT.0.AND.IT.LE.N) GO TO 335
      WRITE (1,135) N
      GO TO 325
335   DO 470 I=1,MM
      IF (IFROM(I).EQ.IF.AND.ITO(I).EQ.IT) GO TO 340
      GO TO 470
340   WRITE (1,350) IFROM(I)
350   FORMAT (///5X,'TRANSFER IS FROM COMPARTMENT',I3)
      WRITE (1,150)
      READ (1,160) ANS4
      IF (ANS4.EQ.YN(2)) GO TO 390
360   WRITE (1,370)
370   FORMAT (/5X,'ENTER NEW VALUE FOR COMPARTMENT (FROM)    :')
      READ (1,30) ITEMP
      IF (ITEMP.GT.0.AND.ITEMP.LE.N) GO TO 380
      WRITE (1,135) N
      GO TO 360
380   IFROM(I)=ITEMP
390   WRITE (1,400) ITO(I)
400   FORMAT (///5X,'TRANSFER IS TO COMPARTMENT',I3)
      WRITE (1,150)
      READ (1,160) ANS5
      IF (ANS5.EQ.YN(2)) GO TO 440
410   WRITE (1,420)
420   FORMAT (/5X,'ENTER NEW VALUE FOR COMPARTTMENT (TO)   :')
      READ (1,30) ITEMP
      IF (ITEMP.GT.0.AND.ITEMP.LE.N) GO TO 430
      WRITE (1,135) N
      GO TO 410
430   ITO(I)=ITEMP
C         EDIT TRANSFER COEFFICIENT
440   WRITE (1,450) A(I)
450   FORMAT (///5X,'TRANSFER COEFFICIENT =',1PE12.4,' (1/DAYS)')
      WRITE (1,150)
      READ (1,160) ANS6
      IF (ANS6.EQ.YN(2)) GO TO 470
      WRITE (1,460)
460   FORMAT (/5X,'ENTER NEW VALUE FOR TRANSFER COEFFICIENT (1/DAYS)',
     1 '    :')
      READ (1,180) A(I)
470   CONTINUE
      GO TO 118
C         ADD NEW MODEL PARAMETERS
500   WRITE (1,510)
510   FORMAT (23(/),15X,'ADD ANOTHER COMPARTMENT = 1'/18X,
     1 'ADD ANOTHER TRANSFER = 2'/34X,'EXIT = 3',10(/),5X,
     2 'WHICH OPTION?    :')
      READ (1,30) KOPT
      WRITE (1,15)
      IF (KOPT-2) 520,600,10
520   N=N+1
      WRITE (1,530) N
530   FORMAT (5X,'ENTER INITIAL CONTENTS OF COMPARTMENT',I3,
     1 ' (MG)    :')
      READ (1,180) Y(N)
      WRITE (1,540) N
540   FORMAT (//5X,'ENTER RATE OF INTAKE OF COMPARTMENT',I3,
     1 ' (MG/DAY)   :')
      READ (1,180) AIN(N)
      GO TO 500
C         ADD A NEW TRANSFER
600   MM=MM+1
```

```
      610   WRITE (1,620)
      620   FORMAT (3(/),5X,'ENTER NUMBER OF COMPARTMENT TRANSFER IS FROM',
           1 '    :')
            READ (1,30) ITEMP
            IF (ITEMP.GT.0.AND.ITEMP.LE.N) GO TO 630
            WRITE (1,135) N
            GO TO 610
      630   IFROM(MM)=ITEMP
      640   WRITE (1,650)
      650   FORMAT (//,5X,'ENTER NUMBER OF COMPARTMENT TRANSFER IS TO   :')
            READ (1,30) ITEMP
            IF (ITEMP.GT.0.AND.ITEMP.LE.N) GO TO 660
            WRITE (1,135) N
            GO TO 640
      660   ITO(MM)=ITEMP
            WRITE (1,670)
      670   FORMAT (//5X,'ENTER VALUE OF TRANSFER COEFFICIENT (1/DAYS)   :')
            READ (1,180) A(MM)
            GO TO 500
      900   CONTINUE
            RETURN
            END
C
C================================================================
C
            SUBROUTINE SAMPLE(X,TMAX,JE,NE)
C
C            ROUTINE TO SET TIMES OF EXCRETA SAMPLING
C
            DIMENSION X(200)
C            ENTER EXCRETA SAMPLING REGIMEN
            DO 3 I=1,NE
            WRITE (1,1) I
        1   FORMAT (/5X,'AT WHAT TIME IS SAMPLE',I2,
           1 ' VOIDED? (24-HR CLOCK)   :')
            READ (1,2) T
        2   FORMAT (E12.4)
            CALL TIME(T)
        3   X(I)=T
C            SET UP EXCRETA SAMPLING TIMES FOR REST OF TIME
            TE=0.0
            KE=0
            JE=NE
        4   TE=TE+1.0
            KE=KE+NE
            DO 5 I=1,NE
            Y=X(I)+TE
            IF (Y.GE.TMAX) GO TO 5
            JE=KE+I
            X(JE)=Y
        5   CONTINUE
            IF (Y.LT.TMAX) GO TO 4
            RETURN
            END
C
C================================================================
C
            SUBROUTINE ENTERE(TFLAG,ESP,NESP,N2,YN,ICARC)
C
C            ROUTINE TO ENTER ACUTE EXPOSURES TO A MATRIX
C
            DIMENSION TFLAG(120),ESP(5,60),YN(2)
            K=0
            T=0.0
            WRITE (1,5)
        5   FORMAT (5X,'WHICH ACUTE EXPOSURE PATTERN? SHIFT=0 SPIKE=1   :')
            READ (1,30) ITP
            IF (ITP.EQ.1) GO TO 300
            WRITE (1,9)
        9   FORMAT (23(/),30X,'SHIFT EXPOSURE',5(/),10X,'THIS OPTION SETS ',
           1 'UP A DEFINED DIURNAL EXPOSURE REGIMEN'//10X,'FOR A SPECIFIED ',
```

```
    2  'NUMBER OF DAYS'///5X,'THE CODE CANNOT CALCULATE OVERNIGHT',
    3  'SHIFT EXPOSURES',//5X'IF THIS FACILITY IS REQUIRED,ENTER THE',
    4  ' EXPOSURE PATTERN AS AN EXPOSURE UP',//,5X,' TO 23.59 AND AN',
    5  '   EXPOSURE FROM 00.00 THE NEXT DAY'//////)
   10  WRITE (1,20)
   20  FORMAT (5X,'HOW MANY DAYS DOES THIS EXPOSURE PATTERN LAST?  :')
       READ (1,30) NDAY
   30  FORMAT (I2)
       WRITE (1,40)
   40  FORMAT (5X,'HOW MANY EXPOSURES PER DAY ARE THERE?  :')
       READ (1,30) JESP
       MESP=NESP+1
       KESP=NESP+JESP
       DO 220 I=1,JESP
       WRITE (1,100)
  100  FORMAT (23(/))
       NESP=NESP+1
  110  FORMAT (E12.4)
  150  WRITE (1,200) I
  200  FORMAT (/5X,'ENTER TIME EXPOSURE',I2,' BEGINS (24-HOUR CLOCK)',
      1  '  :')
       READ (1,110) TB
       CALL TIME(TB)
       IF (TB.GE.0.0) GO TO 203
       WRITE (1,202)
  202  FORMAT (//10X,'TIMES MUST NOT BE LESS THAN THAN ZERO'//)
       GO TO 150
  203  TB=TB+T
       IF (NESP.EQ.1) GO TO 210
       J=NESP-1
       IF (TB.GT.ESP(2,J)) GO TO 210
       WRITE (1,205)
  205  FORMAT (//10X,'TIMES MUST BE GREATER THAN PREVIOUS VALUE'//)
       GO TO 150
  210  ESP(1,NESP)=TB
  211  WRITE (1,212) I
  212  FORMAT (/5X,'ENTER TIME EXPOSURE',I2,' ENDS (24-HOUR CLOCK)  :')
       READ (1,110) TE
       CALL TIME(TE)
       IF (TE.GE.0.0) GO TO 213
       WRITE (1,202)
       GO TO 211
  213  TE=TE+T
       IF (TE.GT.ESP(1,NESP)) GO TO 214
       WRITE (1,205)
       GO TO 211
  214  ESP(2,NESP)=TE
       WRITE (1,215)
  215  FORMAT (/5X,'ENTER AIR CONCENTRATION (MG/M3)  :')
       READ (1,110) ESP(3,NESP)
       WRITE (1,216)
  216  FORMAT (/5X,'ENTER INPUT TO TO GI TRACT (MG)  :')
       READ (1,110) X
       Y=ESP(2,NESP)-ESP(1,NESP)
       ESP(4,NESP)=X/Y
       IF (ICARC.NE.8.AND.ICARC.NE.10.AND.ICARC.NE.11) GO TO 220
       WRITE (1,218)
  218  FORMAT (/5X,'ENTER INPUT TO SKIN (MG)   :')
       READ (1,110) X
       ESP(5,NESP)=X/Y
  220  CONTINUE
       T=T+1.0
       TA=1.0
       NN=1
  230  IF (NDAY.EQ.NN) GO TO 265
       DO 250 I=MESP,KESP
       NESP=NESP+1
       DO 240 N=1,2
  240  ESP(N,NESP)=ESP(N,I)+TA
       DO 250 N=3,5
  250  ESP(N,NESP)=ESP(N,I)
```

```
          T=T+1.0
          TA=TA+1.0
          NN=NN+1
          GO TO 230
  265     WRITE (1,100)
          WRITE (1,270)
  270     FORMAT (5X,'ANOTHER EXPOSURE PATTERN? (Y/N)   :')
          READ (1,280) ANS
  280     FORMAT (A4)
          IF (ANS.EQ.YN(1)) GO TO 10
          GO TO 400
  300     WRITE (1,301)
  301     FORMAT (23(/),30X,'SPIKE EXPOSURE',5(/),15X,'THIS OPTION SETS ',
        1 'UP A DEFINED EXPOSURE REGIMEN'//15X,'FOR A SPECIFIED NUMBER ',
        2 'OF EXPOSURES',8(/),5X,'HOW MANY EXPOSURES ARE THERE?  :')
          READ (1,30) NESP
          DO 370 I=1,NESP
          WRITE (1,100)
  308     WRITE (1,310) I
  310     FORMAT (5X,'ENTER TIME EXPOSURE',I2,' BEGINS (DAYS)   :')
          READ (1,110) TB
          IF (TB.GE.0.0) GO TO 311
          WRITE (1,202)
          GO TO 308
  311     IF (I.EQ.1) GO TO 315
          J=I-1
          IF (TB.GT.ESP(2,J)) GO TO 315
          WRITE (1,205)
          GO TO 308
  315     ESP(1,I)=TB
  318     WRITE (1,320) I
  320     FORMAT (5X,'ENTER TIME EXPOSURE',I2,' ENDS (DAYS)   :')
          READ (1,110) TE
          IF (TE.GE.0.0) GO TO 325
          WRITE (1,202)
          GO TO 318
  325     IF (TE.GT.ESP(1,I)) GO TO 327
          WRITE (1,205)
          GO TO 318
  327     ESP(2,I)=TE
          WRITE (1,330)
  330     FORMAT (5X,'ENTER AIR CONCENTRATION (MG/M3)   :')
          READ (1,110) ESP(3,I)
          WRITE (1,340)
  340     FORMAT (5X,'ENTER EXTRA INPUT TO GI TRACT (MG/DAY)   :')
          READ (1,110) ESP(4,I)
          IF (ICARC.NE.8.AND.ICARC.NE.10.AND.ICARC.NE.11) GO TO 370
          WRITE (1,360)
  360     FORMAT (5X,'ENTER INPUT TO SKIN (MG/DAY)   :')
          READ (1,110) ESP(5,I)
  370     CONTINUE
  400     DO 410 I=1,NESP
          K=K+1
          TFLAG(K)=ESP(1,I)
          K=K+1
  410     TFLAG(K)=ESP(2,I)
          N2=K
          RETURN
          END
C
C=================================================================
C
          SUBROUTINE OUT1(H1,ESCAL,VENT,N,Y,AIN,FIN,MM,ITO,IFROM,A,ICARC,
        1 IED,CARC,TMAT,M,ESP,IESP,IEXT,POL,ITYPE,NESP,FNAME,IDEV,AMAD,
        2 ICLA,CL,FOOD,FA,AIRC,SKIN,GNAME,JDEV,MODA,MODB,LMOD,NM)
C
C         ROUTINE TO PRINT A SUMMARY OF INITIAL MODEL
C         PARAMETERS ON A PRINTER.
C
          DIMENSION Y(N),A(MM),ITO(MM),IFROM(MM),AIN(N),TMAT(M),
        1 POL(ITYPE),ESP(5,NESP),CL(3),CARC(5,12),ST(2),BR(2,2)
```

```
          LOGICAL*1 FNAME(11),GNAME(11)
          DATA ST/'ICRP',' NEW'/,BR/'      ','NOSE','   M','OUTH'/
          WRITE (2,10) (CARC(I,ICARC),I=1,5)
   10     FORMAT (//20X,'SUMMARY OF MODEL PARAMETERS FOR ',5A4)
          WRITE (2,20) H1,ESCAL,N
   20     FORMAT (//5X,'FIRST STEP =',1PE12.4,' DAYS'//5X,'ERROR LIMIT =',
         1 1PE12.4,//5X,'NUMBER OF COMPARTMENTS =',I3)
          WRITE (2,21)
   21     FORMAT (//20X,'INHALATION PARAMETERS'/)
          IF (ICARC.GT.7.OR.IED.EQ.1) GO TO 24
          J=LMOD+1
          WRITE (2,1020) ST(J)
 1020     FORMAT (/5X,'THE ',A4,' LUNG MODEL IS IMPLEMENTED FOR THIS',
         1 ' SIMULATION'/)
          WRITE (2,22) AMAD
   22     FORMAT (5X,'MEAN PARTICLE DIAMETER =',1PE9.2,' MICRONS'/)
          IF (LMOD.EQ.1) GO TO 1030
          WRITE (2,23) CL(ICLA)
   23     FORMAT (5X,'INHALATION CLASS = ',4A1)
          GO TO 24
 1030     J=NM+1
          WRITE (2,1040) (BR(I,J),I=1,2)
 1040     FORMAT (2X,2A4,' BREATHING IS MODELLED FOR THIS SIMULATION')
   24     WRITE (2,25) VENT
   25     FORMAT (/5X,'VENTILATION RATE =',1PE9.2,' M3/DAY'/)
          IF (ICARC.LT.8) GO TO 1010
          WRITE (2,1000) FIN
 1000     FORMAT (5X,'FRACTIONAL UPTAKE =',1PE9.2/)
 1010     IF (IED.EQ.1) GO TO 29
          WRITE (2,26)
   26     FORMAT (//20X,'DIETARY PARAMETERS'/)
          WRITE (2,27) FOOD
   27     FORMAT (5X,'DAILY DIETARY INTAKE =',1PE10.3,' MG'/)
          WRITE (2,28) FA
   28     FORMAT (5X,'F1 =',1PE9.2//)
   29     WRITE (2,30)
   30     FORMAT(/20X,'INITIAL CONTENTS (MG) AND RATES OF INTAKE (MG/DAY)'
         1 //3(5X,'COMPARTMENT',2X,'CONTENT',5X,'RATE OF ENTRY')/)
          AP=N/3
          MP=AP
          MQ=N-3*MP
          IF (MP.EQ.0) GO TO 40
          DO 35 I=1,MP
          I1=3*(I-1)+1
          I2=I1+1
          I3=I1+2
   35     WRITE (2,50) I1,Y(I1),AIN(I1),I2,Y(I2),AIN(I2),I3,Y(I3),AIN(I3)
C             PRINT RESIDUAL COMPARTMENTAL CONTENTS AND INPUTS
   40     IF (MQ.EQ.0) GO TO 59
          MP=N-MQ+1
          IF (MQ.EQ.1) WRITE (2,50) MP,Y(MP),AIN(MP)
          IF (MQ.EQ.2) WRITE (2,50) MP,Y(MP),AIN(MP),N,Y(N),AIN(N)
   50     FORMAT (3(8X,I3,4X,1PE12.4,2X,1PE12.4,2X))
   59     WRITE (2,60)
   60     FORMAT (//20X,'TRANSFER RATES (1/DAYS)'//4(5X,'TO',2X,'FROM',7X,
         1 'RATE',4X)/)
C             CALCULATE NO. OF SETS OF 4 & REMAINDER FOR TRANSFER RATES
          AP=MM/4
          MP=AP
          MQ=MM-4*MP
C          PRINT SETS OF 4 AS NECESSARY
          IF (MP.EQ.0) GO TO 70
          DO 65 I=1,MP
          I1=4*(I-1)+1
          I2=I1+1
          I3=I1+2
          I4=I1+3
   65     WRITE (2,85) ITO(I1),IFROM(I1),A(I1),ITO(I2),IFROM(I2),A(I2),
         1 ITO(I3),IFROM(I3),A(I3),ITO(I4),IFROM(I4),A(I4)
C          PRINT RESIDUAL TRANSFER RATES AS NECESSARY
   70     IF (MQ.EQ.0) GO TO 80
```

```
       MP=MM-MQ+1
       MP1=MP+1
       IF (MQ.EQ.1) WRITE (2,85) ITO(MP),IFROM(MP),A(MP)
       IF (MQ.EQ.2) WRITE (2,85) ITO(MP),IFROM(MP),A(MP),ITO(MP1),
     1 IFROM(MP1),A(MP1)
       IF (MQ.EQ.3) WRITE (2,85) ITO(MP),IFROM(MP),A(MP),ITO(MP1),
     1 IFROM(MP1),A(MP1),ITO(MM),IFROM(MM),A(MM)
    85 FORMAT (4(4X,I3,3X,I3,3X,1PE12.4))
C          PRINT TIMES OF EVALUATION
    80 IF (IED.EQ.1) GO TO 350
       WRITE (2,90)
    90 FORMAT (//20X,'TIMES OF EVALUATION (DAYS)'/)
       WRITE (2,100) (TMAT(I),I=1,M)
   100 FORMAT (1P10E12.4)
C          DESCRIBE EXPOSURE REGIME USED
       IF (IESP.EQ.1) GO TO 200
       IF (IEXT.EQ.1) GO TO 130
       WRITE (2,110)
   110 FORMAT (//1X,'THIS IS A SIMULATION OF CHRONIC EXPOSURE.'/
     1 1X,'THE EXPOSURES DURING THE SIMULATION ARE AS FOLLOWS:-'/)
       WRITE (2,120) AIRC,AIN(12)
   120 FORMAT (5X,'AIR CONCENTRATION =',1PE11.4,' MG/M3'//5X,
     1 'INPUT VIA GI TRACT =',1PE11.4,' MG/DAY'/)
       IF (ICARC.NE.8.AND.ICARC.NE.10.AND.ICARC.NE.11) GO TO 250
       WRITE (2,122) SKIN
   122 FORMAT (/5X'INPUT VIA SKIN =',1PE12.4,' MG/DAY'/)
       GO TO 250
   130 WRITE (2,140)
   140 FORMAT (//1X,'THIS IS A SIMULATION OF TIME-DEPENDENT CHRONIC
     1 EXPOSURE'/1X,'THE EXPOSURES AT THE BEGINNING OF THE SIMULATION
     2 ARE AS FOLLOWS:-'/)
       WRITE (2,120) AIRC,AIN(12)
       IF (ICARC.NE.8.AND.ICARC.NE.10.AND.ICARC.NE.11) GO TO 149
       WRITE (2,122) SKIN
   149 WRITE (2,150)
   150 FORMAT (/1X,'THESE ARE SCALED USING THE POLYNOMIAL:-'/5X,
     1 'EXPOSURE(T)=EXPOSURE(0)*(K1+K2*T+K3*T**2...ETC)'/)
       WRITE (2,170)
   170 FORMAT (5X,'POWER',5X,'COEFFICIENT (K)'/)
       DO 180 I=1,ITYPE
       J=I-1
   180 WRITE (2,190) J,POL(I)
   190 FORMAT (5X,I3,7X,1PE12.4)
       GO TO 250
   200 WRITE (2,210)
   210 FORMAT (//1X,'THIS IS A SIMULATION OF ACUTE EXPOSURE'/1X,
     1 'THE EXPOSURE PATTERN IS AS FOLLOWS:-'/)
       WRITE (2,220)
   220 FORMAT (7X,'T(START)',5X,'T(STOP)',6X,'AIR CONC ',2X,
     1 'EXP(GI TRACT)',1X,'SKIN EXPOSURE')
       WRITE (2,225)
   225 FORMAT (8X,'(DAYS)',6X,'(DAYS)',8X,'(MG/M3)',5X,'(MG/DAY)',5X,
     1 '(MG/DAY)'/)
       DO 230 I=1,NESP
   230 WRITE (2,240) (ESP(J,I),J=1,5)
   240 FORMAT (3X,1P5E13.4)
   250 IF (MODA.NE.1) GO TO 310
       WRITE (2,260) FNAME
   260 FORMAT (//10X,'ORGAN CONCENTRATIONS ARE STORED IN FILE ',11A1)
       IF (IDEV-1) 270,270,290
   270 WRITE (2,280)
   280 FORMAT (10X,'THIS FILE IS ON THIS DISK'/)
       GO TO 310
   290 WRITE (2,300)
   300 FORMAT (10X,'THIS FILE IS ON THE DISK IN THE EXPANSION DRIVE'/)
   310 IF (MODB.NE.1) GO TO 350
       WRITE (2,320) GNAME
   320 FORMAT (//10X,'COMPARTMENTAL CONTENTS ARE STORED IN FILE ',11A1)
       IF (JDEV-1) 330,330,340
   330 WRITE (2,280)
       GO TO 350
```

```
  340   WRITE (2,300)
  350   RETURN
        END
C
C===================================================================
C
        SUBROUTINE LOSS(A,ITO,IFROM,MM,N)
C
C           ROUTINE TO CALCULATE TOTAL COMPARTMENTAL LOSSES
C
        DIMENSION A(80),ITO(80),IFROM(80),ALOS(40)
C           SET TOTAL LOSS RATE COEFFICIENT TO ZERO
        DO 1 I=1,N
    1   ALOS(I)=0.0
C           CALCULATE TOTAL LOSS RATE COEFFICIENT
        DO 3 I=1,N
        DO 3 J=1,MM
        IF (IFROM(J).NE.I) GO TO 3
        IF (IFROM(J).NE.ITO(J)) GO TO 2
        ALOS(I)=ALOS(I)+A(J)
        GO TO 3
    2   ALOS(I)=ALOS(I)-A(J)
    3   CONTINUE
C           INCORPORATE LOSS RATES INTO MODEL
        MX=MM+1
        MM=MM+N
        J=0
        DO 4 I=MX,MM
        J=J+1
        ITO(I)=J
        IFROM(I)=J
    4   A(I)=ALOS(J)
        RETURN
        END
C
C===================================================================
C
        SUBROUTINE WRITE(IESP,ITYPE,IEXT,IOUT,ICARC,IDEV,N,M,IFECES,
    1   IBL,IC1,IC2,IC3,IC4,IURINE,IST,MM,NESP,N2,JF,JU,ITO,IFROM,H1,
    2   ESCAL,FOOD,VENT,GREX,AIRC,FDEX,FNAME,Y,A,AIN,TMAT,POL,TFLAG,ESP,
    3   B,URINE,FAECES,FIN,SKIN,FA,XA,XB,LUNG,GNAME,JDEV,MODA,MODB,LMOD,
    4   NM)
C
C           ROUTINE TO WRITE VARIABLES INTO RAM FILE FOR FCHAINING
C
        DIMENSION Y(N),A(MM),ITO(MM),IFROM(MM),AIN(N),TMAT(M),
    1   POL(ITYPE),TFLAG(N2),ESP(5,NESP),B(8),URINE(JU),FAECES(JF)
        LOGICAL*1 FNAME(11),GNAME(11)
C           OPEN STORAGE FILE
        CALL OPEN (3,'DATASAVEDAT',0)
C           SET RECORD FLAG TO ZERO
        NREC=0
C           WRITE INTEGER VALUES TO FILE
        NREC=NREC+1
        WRITE (3,10,REC=NREC) IESP,ITYPE,IEXT,IOUT,ICARC,IDEV,N,M,
    1   IFECES,IBL,IC1,IC2,IC3,IC4,IURINE,IST,MM,NESP,N2,JF,JU,LUNG,
    2   JDEV,MODA,MODB,LMOD,NM
   10   FORMAT (30I4)
C           WRITE REAL CONSTANTS TO FILE
        NREC=NREC+1
        WRITE (3,70,REC=NREC) H1,ESCAL,FOOD,VENT,GREX,AIRC,FDEX,XA,XB
        NREC=NREC+1
        WRITE (3,70,REC=NREC) FA,SKIN,FIN
C           WRITE TRANSFER ROUTES TO FILE
        MC=23
        MB=1
   30   IF (MC.LT.MM) GO TO 40
        NREC=NREC+1
        WRITE (3,10,REC=NREC) (ITO(I),I=MB,MM)
        NREC=NREC+1
        WRITE (3,10,REC=NREC) (IFROM(I),I=MB,MM)
```

```
            GO TO 50
     40     NREC=NREC+1
            WRITE (3,10,REC=NREC) (ITO(I),I=MB,MC)
            NREC=NREC+1
            WRITE (3,10,REC=NREC) (IFROM(I),I=MB,MC)
            MB=MB+23
            MC=MC+23
            GO TO 30
C               WRITE TRANSFER COEFFICIENTS TO FILE
     50     MC=10
            MB=1
     60     IF (MC.LT.MM) GO TO 80
            NREC=NREC+1
            WRITE (3,70,REC=NREC) (A(I),I=MB,MM)
     70     FORMAT (1P10E12.4)
            GO TO 90
     80     NREC=NREC+1
            WRITE (3,70,REC=NREC) (A(I),I=MB,MC)
            MB=MB+10
            MC=MC+10
            GO TO 60
C               WRITE INITIAL CONTENTS AND INPUTS TO FILE
     90     MB=1
            MC=10
    100     IF (MC.LT.N) GO TO 110
            NREC=NREC+1
            WRITE (3,70,REC=NREC) (Y(I),I=MB,N)
            NREC=NREC+1
            WRITE (3,70,REC=NREC) (AIN(I),I=MB,N)
            GO TO 120
    110     NREC=NREC+1
            WRITE (3,70,REC=NREC) (Y(I),I=MB,MC)
            NREC=NREC+1
            WRITE (3,70,REC=NREC) (AIN(I),I=MB,MC)
            MB=MB+10
            MC=MC+10
            GO TO 100
C               WRITE POLYNOMIAL COEFFICIENTS TO FILE
    120     IF (IEXT.EQ.0) GO TO 125
            NREC=NREC+1
            WRITE (3,70,REC=NREC) (POL(I),I=1,ITYPE)
C               WRITE EVALUATION TIMES TO FILE
    125     MB=1
            MC=10
    130     IF (MC.LT.M) GO TO 140
            NREC=NREC+1
            WRITE (3,70,REC=NREC) (TMAT(I),I=MB,M)
            GO TO 150
    140     NREC=NREC+1
            WRITE (3,70,REC=NREC) (TMAT(I),I=MB,MC)
            MB=MB+10
            MC=MC+10
            GO TO 130
C               WRITE ACUTE EXPOSURE PATTERN TO FILE
    150     IF (IESP.EQ.0) GO TO 190
            DO 160 I=1,NESP
            NREC=NREC+1
    160     WRITE (3,70,REC=NREC) (ESP(J,I),J=1,5)
C               WRITE ACUTE EXPOSURE FLAG TIMES TO FILE
            MC=10
            MB=1
    170     IF (MC.LT.N2) GO TO 180
            NREC=NREC+1
            WRITE (3,70,REC=NREC) (TFLAG(I),I=MB,N2)
            GO TO 190
    180     NREC=NREC+1
            WRITE (3,70,REC=NREC) (TFLAG(I),I=MB,MC)
            MB=MB+10
            MC=MC+10
            GO TO 170
C               WRITE LUNG INPUT PARAMETERS TO FILE
```

```
  190   IF (ICARC.GT.7) GO TO 195
        NREC=NREC+1
        WRITE (3,70,REC=NREC) (B(I),I=1,8)
C             WRITE URINE SAMPLING TIMES TO FILE
  195   MC=10
        MB=1
  200   IF (MC.LT.JU) GO TO 210
        NREC=NREC+1
        WRITE (3,70,REC=NREC) (URINE(I),I=MB,JU)
        GO TO 220
  210   NREC=NREC+1
        WRITE (3,70,REC=NREC) (URINE(I),I=MB,MC)
        MB=MB+10
        MC=MC+10
        GO TO 200
C             WRITE FAECAL SAMPLING TIMES TO FILE
  220   MC=10
        MB=1
  230   IF (MC.LT.JF) GO TO 240
        NREC=NREC+1
        WRITE (3,70,REC=NREC) (FAECES(I),I=MB,JF)
        GO TO 250
  240   NREC=NREC+1
        WRITE (3,70,REC=NREC) (FAECES(I),I=MB,MC)
        MB=MB+10
        MC=MC+10
        GO TO 230
C             WRITE STORAGE FILENAMES TO FILE
  250   NREC=NREC+1
        WRITE (3,260,REC=NREC) FNAME,GNAME
  260   FORMAT (22A1)
        ENDFILE 3
        RETURN
        END
C
C=====================================================================
C
        SUBROUTINE GUT1(A,ITO,IFROM,MM,FA,N,IBL,IST,IFECES)
C
C          ROUTINE TO SET UP ICRP GUT MODEL FOR MAN
C
        DIMENSION A(80),ITO(80),IFROM(80)
C          SET UP TRANSFER OF FOOD THROUGH GUT
        MM=MM+1
        KK=N+1
        ITO(MM)=KK
        IFROM(MM)=IST
        A(MM)=24.0
        N=N+1
        MM=MM+1
        K=N+1
        ITO(MM)=K
        IFROM(MM)=N
        A(MM)=6.0
        N=N+1
        MM=MM+1
        K=N+1
        ITO(MM)=K
        IFROM(MM)=N
        A(MM)=1.8
        N=N+1
        MM=MM+1
        IFECES=N+1
        ITO(MM)=IFECES
        IFROM(MM)=N
        A(MM)=1.0
        N=N+1
C          SET UP TRANSFER FROM GUT TO BLOOD
        MM=MM+1
        ITO(MM)=IBL
        IFROM(MM)=KK
```

```
              IF (FA.EQ.1.0) GO TO 10
              A(MM)=6*FA/(1-FA)
              GO TO 20
        10    A(MM)=24.0
        20    CONTINUE
              RETURN
              END
C
C==================================================================
C
              SUBROUTINE MOD1(Y,A,ITO,IFROM,MM,N,IBL,IC1,IC2,IC3,IC4,IURINE,
            1 IFECES,XA,XB,ICARC,FIN,B,LUNG)
C
C             ROUTINE TO SET UP GENERAL BODY MODEL
C
              DIMENSION Y(40),A(80),ITO(80),IFROM(80),ASBE(6,2),CD(6),PB(10),
            1 AN(5),CR(8),ASB(4),BZEN(7),VC(7),BZID(8),CT(10),AM(6),
            2 CONT(5,12),B(8),DEP(3,2)
              DATA ASBE/18.48,9.24,0.336,0.012,9.24,0.0,0.32,0.88,0.046,
            1 0.00046,0.66,0.22/,CD/1.0E-5,2.0,3.2,0.8,0.2/,PB/0.04,0.18,0.02,
            2 0.01,0.015,
            3 0.693,0.0015,0.0000866,0.03,0.003/,AN/1.05,0.45,0.00052,6.0,
            4 0.000058/,CR/0.34,0.5,0.07,0.053,0.0035,0.0000693,0.36,0.1/,
            5 ASB/0.693,0.0693,0.00347,0.333/,BZEN/100.0,12.0,0.5,0.5,12.0,
            6 108.0,2.4/,VC/91.6,50.0,45.8,48.7,0.3,1.3,0.1/,BZID/20.0,10.0,
            7 50.0,1.4,0.25,2.8,1.0,0.4/,CT/0.15,0.5,2.4,0.5,1.2,10.0,
            8 14.2,0.4,0.1,0.005/,AM/48.0,6.9,18.7,0.0525,0.00583,0.00875/
              DATA CONT/0.714,9.988,2*0.0,0.013,7.905E-4,0.217,2*0.0,1.136E-4,
            1 0.0025,26.1,4.14,7.13,0.0011,3.11,0.3,15.31,128.5,1.18,0.00241,
            2 10.71,0.0,0.0,0.01375,0.01045,0.242,1.65,0.0,0.00163,25*0.0,0.3,
            3 10.0,1.2,0.0,0.3/
              DATA DEP/0.925,0.05,0.025,0.85,0.05,0.1/
C             LABEL EACH COMPARTMENT
              J=0
              IF (ICARC.GT.6) MM=0
              IF (ICARC.GT.7) IBL=1
              IF (ICARC.GT.7) N=IBL
              IF (ICARC.EQ.7) N=0
              IC1=N+1
              IC2=N+2
              IC3=N+3
              IC4=N+4
C             INITIALISE COMPARTMENTAL CONTENTS
              Y(IC1)=CONT(1,ICARC)
              Y(IC2)=CONT(2,ICARC)
              Y(IC3)=CONT(3,ICARC)
              Y(IC4)=CONT(4,ICARC)
              IF (ICARC.EQ.7) GO TO 10
              Y(IBL)=CONT(5,ICARC)
C             BRANCH TO APPROPRIATE CARCINOGEN MODEL
        10    GO TO (100,100,200,250,300,350,400,450,500,550,600,650),ICARC
C             ROUTINE TO SET UP MODEL FOR ARSENIC OR BERYLLIUM METABOLISM
       100    CONTINUE
C             SET UP REVERSIBLE TRANSFERS FROM BLOOD TO TISSUES
              N=N+3
              DO 110 I=IC1,IC2
              MM=MM+1
              J=J+1
              ITO(MM)=I
              IFROM(MM)=IBL
       110    A(MM)=ASBE(J,ICARC)
              DO 120 I=IC1,IC2
              J=J+1
              MM=MM+1
              ITO(MM)=IBL
              IFROM(MM)=I
       120    A(MM)=ASBE(J,ICARC)
C             SET UP EXCRETION IN URINE
              IURINE=N
              MM=MM+1
              J=J+1
```

```
         ITO(MM)=IURINE
         IFROM(MM)=IBL
         A(MM)=ASBE(J,ICARC)
C            SET UP FAECAL EXCRETION
         IF (ICARC.EQ.1) GO TO 900
         MM=MM+1
         J=J+1
         ITO(MM)=IFECES
         IFROM(MM)=IBL
         A(MM)=ASBE(J,ICARC)
         GO TO 900
C
C            ROUTINE TO SET UP GENERAL BODY MODEL FOR CADMIUM
C
   200   CONTINUE
         N=N+5
C            SET UP TRANSFERS BETWEEN BLOOD AND TISSUES
         J=J+1
         DO 210 I=IC2,IC4
         MM=MM+1
         ITO(MM)=IBL
         IFROM(MM)=I
   210   A(MM)=CD(J)
         DO 220 I=IC3,IC4
         MM=MM+1
         ITO(MM)=IC1
         IFROM(MM)=I
   220   A(MM)=CD(J)
         J=J+1
         DO 230 I=IC1,IC3,2
         MM=MM+1
         ITO(MM)=I
         IFROM(MM)=IBL
   230   A(MM)=CD(J)
         MM=MM+1
         J=J+1
         ITO(MM)=IC2
         IFROM(MM)=IBL
         A(MM)=CD(J)
         J=J+1
         MM=MM+1
         ITO(MM)=IC4
         IFROM(MM)=IC1
         A(MM)=CD(J)
C            SET UP EXCRETION IN URINE
         J=J+1
         IURINE=N
         MM=MM+1
         ITO(MM)=IURINE
         IFROM(MM)=IC1
         A(MM)=CD(J)
C            SET UP ENDOGENOUS FAECAL EXCRETION
         MM=MM+1
         ITO(MM)=IFECES
         IFROM(MM)=IBL
         A(MM)=CD(J)
         J=J+1
         MM=MM+1
         ITO(MM)=IFECES
         IFROM(MM)=IC3
         A(MM)=CD(1)
         GO TO 900
C
C            ROUTINE TO SET UP GENERAL BODY MODEL FOR LEAD
C
   250   CONTINUE
C            SET UP REVERSIBLE TRANSFER FROM BLOOD TO TISSUES
         DO 260 I=IC1,IC4
         MM=MM+1
         J=J+1
         ITO(MM)=I
```

```
          IFROM(MM)=IBL
   260    A(MM)=PB(J)
          DO 270 I=IC1,IC4
          J=J+1
          MM=MM+1
          ITO(MM)=IBL
          IFROM(MM)=I
   270    A(MM)=PB(J)
          N=N+5
C              SET UP EXCRETION IN URINE
          IURINE=N
          J=J+1
          MM=MM+1
          ITO(MM)=N
          IFROM(MM)=IBL
          A(MM)=PB(J)
C              SET UP ENDOGENOUS FAECAL EXCRETION
          J=J+1
          MM=MM+1
          ITO(MM)=IFECES
          IFROM(MM)=IC1
          A(MM)=PB(J)
          GO TO 900
C
C              ROUTINE TO SET UP GENERAL BODY MODEL FOR NICKEL
C
   300    CONTINUE
          N=N+3
          IURINE=N
C              SET UP REVERSIBLE TRANSFERS FROM BLOOD TO TISSUES
          DO 310 I=IC1,IC2
          MM=MM+1
          J=J+1
          ITO(MM)=I
          IFROM(MM)=IBL
   310    A(MM)=AN(J)
          MM=MM+1
          J=J+1
          ITO(MM)=IBL
          IFROM(MM)=IC2
          A(MM)=AN(J)
C              SET UP EXCRETION IN URINE
          MM=MM+1
          J=J+1
          ITO(MM)=IURINE
          IFROM(MM)=IC1
          A(MM)=AN(J)
C              SET UP ENDOGENOUS FAECAL EXCRETION
          MM=MM+1
          J=J+1
          ITO(MM)=IFECES
          IFROM(MM)=IBL
          A(MM)=AN(J)
          GO TO 900
C
C              ROUTINE TO SET UP GENERAL BODY MODEL FOR CHROMIUM
C
   350    CONTINUE
          N=N+4
C              SET UP REVERSIBLE TRANSFERS FROM BLOOD TO TISSUES
          DO 360 I=IC1,IC3
          MM=MM+1
          J=J+1
          ITO(MM)=I
          IFROM(MM)=IBL
   360    A(MM)=CR(J)
          DO 370 I=IC1,IC3
          J=J+1
          MM=MM+1
          ITO(MM)=IBL
          IFROM(MM)=I
```

```
  370   A(MM)=CR(J)
C               SET UP EXCRETION IN URINE
        IURINE=N
        J=J+1
        MM=MM+1
        ITO(MM)=IURINE
        IFROM(MM)=IBL
        A(MM)=CR(J)
C               SET UP ENDOGENOUS FAECAL EXCRETION
        J=J+1
        MM=MM+1
        ITO(MM)=IFECES
        IFROM(MM)=IBL
        A(MM)=CR(J)
        GO TO 900
C
C               ROUTINE TO SET UP GENERAL BODY MODEL FOR ASBESTOS
C
  400   CONTINUE
        LUNG=3
        IST=4
        IFECES=5
        WRITE (1,410)
  410   FORMAT (23(/),5X,'WHICH TYPE OF ASBESTOS? CHRYSOTILE = 1',
      1 '  AMPHIBOLE = 2    :')
        READ (1,420) IASB
  420   FORMAT (I2)
        DO 430 I=1,3
        B(I)=DEP(I,IASB)
        MM=MM+1
        ITO(MM)=IST
        IFROM(MM)=I
  430   A(MM)=ASB(MM)
        MM=MM+1
        ITO(MM)=IFECES
        IFROM(MM)=IST
        A(MM)=ASB(MM)
        N=5
        GO TO 900
C
C               ROUTINE TO SET UP MODEL FOR BENZENE ELIMINATION
C
  450   CONTINUE
C               SET UP NUMBER OF COMPARTMENTS
        N=6
C               SET UP TRANSFERS
        DO 460 I=IC1,IC2
        MM=MM+1
        J=J+1
        ITO(MM)=I
        IFROM(MM)=IBL
        A(MM)=BZEN(J)
        MM=MM+1
        J=J+1
        ITO(MM)=IBL
        IFROM(MM)=I
  460   A(MM)=BZEN(J)
        J=J+1
        DO 470 I=IBL,IC1
        MM=MM+1
        ITO(MM)=IC3
        IFROM(MM)=I
  470   A(MM)=BZEN(J)
        MM=MM+1
        J=J+1
        ITO(MM)=IC4
        IFROM(MM)=IBL
        A(MM)=BZEN(J)
C               LABEL EXCRETA COMPARTMENTS
        IURINE=6
        IFECES=7
```

```
C          SET UP URINARY EXCRETION OF METABOLITES
        MM=MM+1
        J=J+1
        ITO(MM)=IURINE
        IFROM(MM)=IC3
        A(MM)=BZEN(J)
C          SET UP FRACTIONAL INTAKE
        FIN=0.5
        GO TO 900
C
C          ROUTINE TO SET UP MODEL FOR VINYL CHLORIDE ELIMINATION
C
  500   CONTINUE
C          SET UP NUMBER OF COMPARTMENTS
        N=7
C          SET UP FRACTIONAL INTAKE
        FIN=0.5
C          LABEL EXCRETA COMPARTMENTS
        IURINE=5
        IFECES=6
C          SET UP TRANSFERS
        DO 510 I=IC1,7,5
        MM=MM+1
        ITO(MM)=I
        IFROM(MM)=IBL
  510   A(MM)=VC(MM)
        MM=MM+1
        ITO(MM)=IBL
        IFROM(MM)=IC1
        A(MM)=VC(MM)
        MM=MM+1
        ITO(MM)=IC2
        IFROM(MM)=IC1
        A(MM)=VC(MM)
        DO 520 I=4,IFECES
        MM=MM+1
        ITO(MM)=I
        IFROM(MM)=IC2
  520   A(MM)=VC(MM)
        GO TO 900
C
C          ROUTINE TO SET UP MODEL FOR BENZIDINE ELIMINATION
C
  550   CONTINUE
C          SET UP NUMBER OF COMPARTMENTS
        N=7
C          SET UP TRANSFERS
        MM=MM+1
        ITO(MM)=IC1
        IFROM(MM)=IBL
        A(MM)=BZID(MM)
        MM=MM+1
        ITO(MM)=IC2
        IFROM(MM)=IBL
        A(MM)=BZID(MM)
C          CALCULATE METABOLISM
        MM=MM+1
        ITO(MM)=IC2
        IFROM(MM)=IC1
        A(MM)=BZID(MM)
C          SET UP REVERSIBLE TRANSFER TO 'BOUND METABOLITES' COMP
        MM=MM+1
        ITO(MM)=IC4
        IFROM(MM)=IC2
        A(MM)=BZID(MM)
        MM=MM+1
        ITO(MM)=IC2
        IFROM(MM)=IC4
        A(MM)=BZID(MM)
C          SET UP BILIARY EXCRETION
        J=MM+1
```

```
         DO 560 I=IC1,IC2
         MM=MM+1
         ITO(MM)=IC3
         IFROM(MM)=I
   560   A(MM)=BZID(J)
C              LABEL EXCRETA COMPARTMENTS
         IURINE=6
         IFECES=7
C              SET UP EXCRETION IN URINE & FAECES
         DO 570 I=IBL,IC2,2
         MM=MM+1
         ITO(MM)=IURINE
         IFROM(MM)=I
   570   A(MM)=BZID(J)
         MM=MM+1
         J=J+1
         ITO(MM)=IFECES
         IFROM(MM)=IC3
         A(MM)=BZID(J)
C              SET UP REFLUX TERM
         MM=MM+1
         J=J+1
         ITO(MM)=IC2
         IFROM(MM)=IC3
         A(MM)=BZID(J)
C              SET UP FRACTIONAL INTAKE
         FIN=1.0
         GO TO 900
C
C              ROUTINE TO SET UP MODEL FOR CCL4 ELIMINATION
C
   600   CONTINUE
C              SET UP NUMBER OF COMPARTMENTS
         N=8
C              SET UP TRANSFERS
         DO 610 I=IC1,IC2
         J=J+1
         MM=MM+1
         ITO(MM)=IBL
         IFROM(MM)=I
   610   A(MM)=CT(J)
         DO 620 I=IC1,IC2
         J=J+1
         MM=MM+1
         ITO(MM)=I
         IFROM(MM)=IBL
   620   A(MM)=CT(J)
         DO 630 I=IBL,IC2,2
         MM=MM+1
         J=J+1
         ITO(MM)=IC3
         IFROM(MM)=I
   630   A(MM)=CT(J)
         MM=MM+1
         J=J+1
         ITO(MM)=8
         IFROM(MM)=IBL
         A(MM)=CT(J)
C              LABEL EXCRETA COMPARTMENTS
         IURINE=6
         IFECES=7
C              SET UP EXCRETION OF METABOLITES
         DO 640 I=IC4,IFECES
         MM=MM+1
         J=J+1
         ITO(MM)=I
         IFROM(MM)=IC3
   640   A(MM)=CT(J)
C              SET UP FRACTIONAL INTAKE
         FIN=0.3
         GO TO 900
```

```
C
C                ROUTINE TO SET UP MODEL FOR METHYL IODIDE ELIMINATION
C
  650    CONTINUE
C                SET UP NUMBER OF COMPARTMENTS
         N=6
C                SET UP TRANSFERS
         DO 660 I=2,6,4
         MM=MM+1
         ITO(MM)=I
         IFROM(MM)=1
  660    A(MM)=AM(MM)
         MM=MM+1
         ITO(MM)=1
         IFROM(MM)=2
         A(MM)=AM(MM)
         DO 670 I=2,5,3
         MM=MM+1
         ITO(MM)=I
         IFROM(MM)=4
  670    A(MM)=AM(MM)
         MM=MM+1
         ITO(MM)=4
         IFROM(MM)=3
         A(MM)=AM(MM)
C                LABEL EXCRETA COMPARTMENTS
         IURINE=5
         IFECES=6
C                SET UP FRACTIONAL INTAKE
         FIN=0.75
C                TRANSFER CONSTANTS TO CALCULATE THYROID UPTAKE
         XA=(AM(4)+AM(5))*AM(2)
         XB=AM(5)
  900    CONTINUE
         RETURN
         END
C
C=====================================================================
C
         SUBROUTINE LUNG1(A,ITO,IFROM,MM,B,AMAD,ICLA,N,IBL,IST,LUNG,NM,
        1 LMOD,ICARC)
C
C                ROUTINE TO SET UP ICRP LUNG MODEL FOR MAN
C
         DIMENSION A(80),ITO(80),IFROM(80),B(8),AMV(6),ANP(6),AP(6),
        1 FP(10,3),TP(10,3),SOL(7),FMV(7),GNM(7,2),GTB(7,2),GA(7,2),
        2 RATE(9)
         DATA AMV/0.2,0.5,1.0,2.0,5.0,10.01/
         DATA ANP/0.05,0.17,0.3,0.47,0.7,0.85/
         DATA AP/0.5,0.35,0.25,0.18,0.09,0.05/
         DATA FP/0.5,0.5,0.95,0.05,0.8,0.0,0.0,0.2,1.0,0.0,
        1 0.1,0.9,0.5,0.5,0.15,0.4,0.4,0.05,1.0,0.0,
        2 0.01,0.99,0.01,0.99,0.05,0.4,0.4,0.15,0.9,0.1/
         DATA TP/69.3,69.3,69.3,3.47,1.39,0.0,0.0,1.39,1.39,0.0,
        1 69.3,1.73,69.3,3.47,0.0139,0.693,0.0139,0.0139,0.0139,0.0,
        2 69.3,1.73,69.3,3.47,0.00139,0.693,0.00139,0.00139,0.000693,
        3 0.000693/
         DATA FMV/0.1,0.3,0.7,1.0,2.0,5.0,10.01/
         DATA GNM/4*0.0,0.33,0.85,1.0,4*0.0,0.03,0.19,0.31/
         DATA GTB/2*0.04,0.05,0.06,0.09,0.1,0.0,2*0.04,0.05,0.06,0.13,
        1 0.53,0.64/
         DATA GA/2*0.16,0.15,0.14,0.17,0.03,0.0,2*0.16,0.15,0.14,0.24,
        1 0.18,0.0/,SOL/0.07,0.005,0.0009,1.4,1.4,1.4,0.001/
         DATA RATE/100.0,25.0,3.0,0.046,0.025,0.0016,0.0012,0.00017,1.5/
         IF (LMOD.EQ.1) GO TO 100
C                LABEL COMPARTMENT NUMBERS
         LUNG=10
         IBL=LUNG+1
         IST=LUNG+2
C                CALCULATE DEPOSITIONS IN REGIONS OF LUNG
         DTB=0.08
```

```
      IFA=0
      DO 10 I=1,5
      J=I+1
 10   IF (AMAD.GE.AMV(I).AND.AMAD.LT.AMV(J)) IFA=I
      J=IFA+1
      R=(AMAD-AMV(IFA))/(AMV(J)-AMV(IFA))
      DNP=ANP(IFA)+R*(ANP(J)-ANP(IFA))
      DP=AP(IFA)+R*(AP(J)-AP(IFA))
C        CALCULATE FRACTIONAL INPUTS TO VARIOUS REGIONS OF LUNG
      B(1)=DNP*FP(1,ICLA)
      B(2)=DNP*FP(2,ICLA)
      B(3)=DTB*FP(3,ICLA)
      B(4)=DTB*FP(4,ICLA)
      B(5)=DP*FP(5,ICLA)
      B(6)=DP*FP(6,ICLA)
      B(7)=DP*FP(7,ICLA)
      B(8)=DP*FP(8,ICLA)
C        SET UP TRANSFER FROM LUNGS TO BLOOD
      MM=0
      DO 20 I=1,5,2
      MM=MM+1
      ITO(MM)=IBL
      IFROM(MM)=I
 20   A(MM)=TP(I,ICLA)
C        SET UP TRANSFER FROM LUNGS TO GI TRACT
      DO 30 I=2,4,2
      MM=MM+1
      ITO(MM)=IST
      IFROM(MM)=I
 30   A(MM)=TP(I,ICLA)
C        SET UP INTERNAL LUNG TRANSFERS
      DO 40 I=6,7
      MM=MM+1
      ITO(MM)=4
      IFROM(MM)=I
 40   A(MM)=TP(I,ICLA)
C        SET UP TRANSFER FROM LUNGS TO PULMONARY LYMPH NODES
      DO 50 I=9,10
      MM=MM+1
      ITO(MM)=I
      IFROM(MM)=8
 50   A(MM)=TP(8,ICLA)*FP(I,ICLA)
C        SET UP TRANSFER FROM LYMPH NODES TO BLOOD
      MM=MM+1
      ITO(MM)=IBL
      IFROM(MM)=9
      A(MM)=TP(9,ICLA)
C        SET NO OF COMPARTMENTS
      N=LUNG+2
      GO TO 200
 100  LUNG=8
      IBL=LUNG+2
      IST=LUNG+3
      N=11
      INM=NM+1
      IFA=0
      DO 110 I=1,6
      J=I+1
 110  IF (AMAD.GE.FMV(I).AND.AMAD.LT.FMV(J)) IFA=I
      J=IFA+1
      R=(AMAD-FMV(IFA))/(FMV(J)-FMV(IFA))
      DNM=GNM(IFA,INM)+R*(GNM(J,INM)-GNM(IFA,INM))
      DTB=GTB(IFA,INM)+R*(GTB(J,INM)-GTB(IFA,INM))
      DA=GA(IFA,INM)+R*(GA(J,INM)-GA(IFA,INM))
      B(1)=DNM*0.45
      B(2)=DNM*0.55
      B(3)=DTB*0.4
      B(4)=DTB*0.6
      B(6)=DA*0.1
      B(7)=DA*0.9
      B(5)=0.0
```

```
          B(8)=0.0
          MM=0
          DO 120 I=1,8
          MM=MM+1
          ITO(MM)=IBL
          IFROM(MM)=I
  120     A(MM)=SOL(ICARC)
          J=0
          DO 130 I=2,5
          MM=MM+1
          J=J+1
          ITO(MM)=IST
          IFROM(MM)=I
  130     A(MM)=RATE(J)
          DO 140 I=6,7
          DO 140 K=5,8,3
          J=J+1
          MM=MM+1
          ITO(MM)=K
          IFROM(MM)=I
  140     A(MM)=RATE(J)
          MM=MM+1
          J=J+1
          ITO(MM)=9
          IFROM(MM)=1
          A(MM)=RATE(J)
  200     RETURN
          END
C
C================================================================
C
          PROGRAM TOXIC2
C
C             PROCESSER STAGE OF MOSAIC CALLED BY FCHAINING FROM MOSAIC
C
          DIMENSION Y(40),YA(40),YB(40),YC(40),YD(40),YE(40),F1(40),
        1 F2(40),A(80),ITO(80),IFROM(80),AIN(40),TMAT(30),VAL(30,10),
        2 POL(10),TFLAG(120),ESP(5,60),B(8),URINE(2,200),FAECES(2,200),
        3 HEADER(30)
          LOGICAL*1 FNAME(11),GNAME(11)
C             SET ALL ARRAYS TO ZERO
          CALL ZERO(Y,YA,YB,YC,YD,YE,F1,F2,A,AIN,TMAT,VAL,POL,TFLAG,ESP,
        1 B,URINE,FAECES,ITO,IFROM)
C             READ VARIABLES FROM MOSAIC (STORED IN FILE DATASAVEDAT)
          CALL VALUES(IESP,ITYPE,IEXT,IOUT,ICARC,IDEV,N,M,IFECES,
        1 IBL,IC1,IC2,IC3,IC4,IURINE,IST,MM,NESP,N2,JF,JU,ITO,IFROM,
        2 H1,ESCAL,FOOD,VENT,GREX,AIRC,FDEX,FNAME,Y,A,AIN,TMAT,POL,TFLAG,
        3 ESP,B,URINE,FAECES,FIN,SKIN,FA,XA,XB,LUNG,GNAME,JDEV,MODA,MODB,
        4 LMOD,NM)
C             DEFINE NUMBER OF COLUMNS IN TABLES
          GO TO (1,2,1,2,3,4,6,3,5,3,3,3),ICARC
        1 NCOL=8
          GO TO 7
        2 NCOL=9
          GO TO 7
        3 NCOL=7
          GO TO 7
        4 NCOL=10
          GO TO 7
        5 NCOL=6
          GO TO 7
        6 NCOL=4
C             SET UP COLUMN HEADINGS
        7 CALL LABEL(HEADER,ICARC)
C             CALL DIFFERENTIAL EQUATION SOLVING ROUTINE
          CALL CALC(Y,YA,YB,YC,YD,YE,F1,F2,A,ITO,IFROM,MM,AIN,TMAT,VAL,H1,
        1 N,M,IESP,POL,ITYPE,TFLAG,NESP,ESP,N2,IEXT,ESCAL,IC1,IC2,IC3,IC4,
        2 B,FOOD,VENT,IOUT,GREX,ICARC,AIRC,FDEX,SKIN,FNAME,IDEV,IFECES,
        3 IURINE,URINE,FAECES,IST,JU,JF,FIN,FA,XA,XB,HEADER,LUNG,NCOL,IBL,
        4 GNAME,JDEV,MODA,MODB,LMOD,NM)
          CALL OUT2(TMAT,VAL,M,NCOL,HEADER)
          IL=1
```

```
      CALL HIST(URINE,JU,IL)
      IL=IL+1
      CALL HIST(FAECES,JF,IL)
      STOP
      END
C
C======================================================================
C
      SUBROUTINE CALC(Y,YA,YB,YC,YD,YE,F1,F2,A,ITO,IFROM,MM,AIN,TMAT,
     1 VAL,H1,N,M,IESP,POL,ITYPE,TFLAG,NESP,ESP,N2,1EXT,ESCAL,IC1,IC2,
     2 IC3,IC4,B,FOOD,VENT,IOUT,GREX,ICARC,AIRC,FDEX,SKIN,FNAME,IDEV,
     3 IFECES,IURINE,URINE,FAECES,IST,JU,JF,FIN,FA,XA,XB,HEADER,LUNG,
     4 NCOL,IBL,GNAME,JDEV,MODA,MODB,LMOD,NM)
C
C          ROUTINE TO CALCULATE TIME-DEPENDENT CHANGES
C          IN COMPARTMENTAL CONTENTS.
C
      DIMENSION Y(N),YA(N),YB(N),YC(N),YD(N),YE(N),F1(N),F2(N),A(MM),
     1 ITO(MM),IFROM(MM),AIN(N),TMAT(M),VAL(M,NCOL),
     2 POL(ITYPE),TFLAG(N2),ESP(5,NESP),B(8),URINE(2,JU),
     3 FAECES(2,JF),HEADER(30),ORIG(40),TMET(2,200),C(10)
      LOGICAL*1 FNAME(11),GNAME(11)
      COMMON/PASS/ESCAL1
      ESCAL1=ESCAL
      GREX1=GREX
      NREC=0
      IREC=0
      SUMU=0.0
      SUMF=0.0
      WU=1.4
      WF=0.13
      IF (IEXT.EQ.0) GO TO 2
      DO 1 I=1,N
    1 ORIG(I)=AIN(I)
    2 IF (ICARC.NE.12) GO TO 3
      MET1=MM+1
      MET2=MM+2
      MM=MM+2
      ITO(MET1)=3
      IFROM(MET1)=1
      ITO(MET2)=1
      IFROM(MET2)=1
    3 IMET=0
      NE=1
      T=0.0
C        SET URINE,FECAL & EXPOSURE FLAGS
      IU=1
      IF=1
      NN=1
      NAA=4
      SAA=4.0
      IF (IESP.EQ.1) CALL EXTYPE(AIN,POL,ESP,N,NESP,NN,T,B,VENT,GREX,
     1 ICARC,ITYPE,GREX1,IESP,FOOD,AIRC,FDEX,IST,FIN,FA,ORIG,LMOD,NM)
C        WRITE WARNING MESSAGE ON SCREEN
      WRITE (1,4)
    4 FORMAT (15(/),25X,'PLEASE LEAVE - PROGRAM RUNNING',13(/))
      IF (IOUT.EQ.0) GO TO 6
      WRITE (2,5) T,GREX
    5 FORMAT (10X,'TIME =',1PE12.4,' DAYS',10X,'EXPOSURE =',1PE12.4,
     1 ' MG/DAY')
      WRITE (2,120) Y
    6 IF (MODA.NE.1) GO TO 9
      CALL OPEN (5,FNAME,IDEV)
      NREC=NREC+1
      ID=0
      WRITE (5,7,REC=NREC) NCOL,IEXT,ID
    7 FORMAT (3I5)
      NREC=NREC+1
      WRITE (5,8,REC=NREC) HEADER
    8 FORMAT (30A4)
      CALL ORGAN(Y,T,GREX,ICARC,N,LUNG,IBL,IC1,IC2,IC3,IC4,C)
```

```
         NREC=NREC+1
         WRITE (5,120,REC=NREC) (C(I),I=1,NCOL)
      9  IF (MODB.NE.1) GO TO 10
         CALL OPEN (4,GNAME,JDEV)
         IREC=IREC+1
         WRITE (4,7,REC=IREC) N,IEXT,MODB
         CALL CONSAV(N,Y,IREC,T,GREX)
     10  TA=T+H1
         INDEX=0
         JINDEX=0
         IF (IESP.EQ.0) GO TO 12
         DO 11 I=1,N2
         IF (T.LT.TFLAG(I).AND.TA.GE.TFLAG(I)) JINDEX=I
         IF (JINDEX.GT.0) GO TO 12
     11  CONTINUE
     12  HR=H1
         DO 15 I=1,N
     15  YE(I)=Y(I)
         IF (JINDEX.NE.0) H1=TFLAG(JINDEX)-T
         TB=T+H1
         DO 20 I=1,M
         IF (T.LT.TMAT(I).AND.TB.GE.TMAT(I)) INDEX=I
         IF (INDEX.NE.0) GO TO 25
     20  CONTINUE
     25  IF (INDEX.NE.0) H1=TMAT(INDEX)-T
         IF (H1.LE.1.0E-30) GO TO 65
         IF (T.GE.ESP(2,NN)) NN=NN+1
         IF (IESP.EQ.1.OR.IEXT.EQ.1) CALL EXTYPE(AIN,POL,ESP,N,NESP,NN,T,
        1 B,VENT,GREX,ICARC,ITYPE,GREX1,IESP,FOOD,AIRC,FDEX,IST,FIN,FA,
        2 ORIG,LMOD,NM)
         H2=H1/SAA
C            STORE FECAL & URINE CONTENTS
         BU=Y(IURINE)
         BF=Y(IFECES)
C            CALCULATE THYROID UPTAKE FOR METHYL IODIDE
         IF (ICARC.EQ.12.AND.IMET.EQ.0) CALL UPTAKE(TMET,NE,T,AIN,XA,XB,
        1 Y,MET1,MET2,A)
         IMET=0
         CALL RUNKA1(H2,Y,YA,YB,YC,YD,F1,F2,N,A,ITO,IFROM,MM,AIN)
         DO 35 J=1,N
         YA(J)=YB(J)
     35  Y(J)=YE(J)
         IFFL=0
         DO 40 I=2,NAA
         CALL PRCOR(H2,Y,YA,YB,YC,YD,F1,F2,N,A,ITO,IFROM,MM,AIN,ISTP)
         IF (ISTP.EQ.-1) IFFL=1
     40  CONTINUE
         DO 45 I=1,N
     45  Y(I)=YA(I)
         DO 50 I=1,N
         IF (YE(I).LT.1.0E-20) GO TO 50
         AFFL=Y(I)/YE(I)
         IF (AFFL.GE.0.0.AND.AFFL.LT.10.0) GO TO 50
         IFFL=1
     50  CONTINUE
         IF (IFFL.EQ.0) GO TO 65
         H1=H1/2.0
         DO 55 I=1,N
     55  Y(I)=YE(I)
         IF (H1.LE.1.0E-15) GO TO 58
         IMET=1
         GO TO 10
     58  WRITE (1,60)
         WRITE (2,60)
     60  FORMAT (/10X,'ERROR - DIFEQ - RUNGE-KUTTA UNSTABLE'/)
         GO TO 230
     65  TT=T
         T=T+H1
         SMCH=0.0
         DO 70 I=1,N
         IF (Y(I).LT.0.0) Y(I)=0.0
```

```
   70    SMCH=SMCH+Y(I)
         SMCH=SMCH*1.0E-15
         DO 80 I=1,N
   80    IF (Y(I).LT.SMCH) Y(I)=0.0
C              UPDATE THYROID UPTAKE FOR METHYL IODIDE
         IF (ICARC.NE.12) GO TO 83
         TMET(1,NE)=T
         TMET(2,NE)=AIN(1)*H1
C              STORE NEW CONTENTS OF FAECES & URINE
   83    AU=Y(IURINE)
         AF=Y(IFECES)
C              IF AN EXCRETA SAMPLING TIME IS CROSSED CALL SAMPLING ROUTINE
         IF (T.GT.URINE(1,IU).AND.TT.LE.URINE(1,IU)) CALL EXCRET(TT,T,IU,
        1 AU,BU,URINE,JU,SUMU,WU)
         IF (T.GT.FAECES(1,IF).AND.TT.LE.FAECES(1,IF)) CALL EXCRET(TT,T,
        1 IF,AF,BF,FAECES,JF,SUMF,WF)
         CALL ORGAN(Y,T,GREX,ICARC,N,LUNG,IBL,IC1,IC2,IC3,IC4,C)
         IF (INDEX.EQ.0) GO TO 110
         DO 85 I=3,NCOL
         J=I-2
   85    VAL(INDEX,J)=C(I)
         WRITE (1,90)
   90    FORMAT (10(/),25X,'PLEASE LEAVE - PROGRAM RUNNING'//////)
         WRITE (1,95) TMAT(INDEX)
   95    FORMAT (/20X,'TIME=',1PE12.4,' DAYS')
         WRITE (1,100)
  100    FORMAT (/10X,'COMPARTMENTAL CONTENTS (MG)')
         WRITE (1,105) Y
  105    FORMAT (1P5E16.3)
         WRITE (1,106)
  106    FORMAT (/)
  110    IF (IOUT.EQ.0) GO TO 122
         WRITE (2,5) T,GREX
         WRITE (2,120) Y
  120    FORMAT (1P10E12.4)
  122    IF (MODA.NE.1) GO TO 123
         NREC=NREC+1
         WRITE (5,120,REC=NREC) (C(I),I=1,NCOL)
  123    IF (MODB.EQ.1) CALL CONSAV(N,Y,IREC,T,GREX)
         WRITE (1,125) T
  125    FORMAT ('+',50X,1PE12.4,' DAYS')
         IF (T.GE.TMAT(M)) GO TO 230
         H1=HR
         IF (INDEX.NE.0.OR.JINDEX.NE.0) GO TO 10
         INDEX=0
         JINDEX=0
         TA=T+H1
         IF (IESP.EQ.0) GO TO 132
         DO 130 I=1,N2
         IF (T.LT.TFLAG(I).AND.TA.GE.TFLAG(I)) JINDEX=I
         IF (JINDEX.GT.0) GO TO 132
  130    CONTINUE
  132    IF (JINDEX.NE.0) GO TO 12
         DO 140 I=1,M
         IF (T.LT.TMAT(I).AND.TA.GE.TMAT(I)) INDEX=I
         IF (INDEX.GT.0) GO TO 142
  140    CONTINUE
  142    IF (INDEX.EQ.0) GO TO 150
         HR=H1
         DO 145 I=1,N
  145    YE(I)=Y(I)
         GO TO 25
  150    DO 152 I=1,N
         YA(I)=Y(I)
  152    Y(I)=YE(I)
  153    IF (T.GE.ESP(2,NN)) NN=NN+1
         IF (IESP.EQ.1.OR.IEXT.EQ.1) CALL EXTYPE(AIN,POL,ESP,N,NESP,NN,T,
        1 B,VENT,GREX,ICARC,ITYPE,GREX1,IESP,FOOD,AIRC,FDEX,IST,FIN,FA,
        2 ORIG,LMOD,NM)
C              STORE FAECAL & URINE CONTENTS
         BU=YA(IURINE)
```

```
      BF=YA(IFECES)
C         CALCULATE THYROID UPTAKE FOR METHYL IODIDE
      IF (ICARC.EQ.12) CALL UPTAKE(TMET,NE,T,AIN,XA,XB,YA,MET1,MET2,A)
      CALL PRCOR(H1,Y,YA,YB,YC,YD,F1,F2,N,A,ITO,IFROM,MM,AIN,ISTP)
      IF (ISTP.EQ.-1) GO TO 165
      TT=T
      T=T+H1
      SMCH=0.0
      DO 155 I=1,N
      IF (YA(I).LT.0.0) YA(I)=0.0
  155 SMCH=SMCH+YA(I)
      SMCH=SMCH*1.0E-15
      DO 157 I=1,N
  157 IF (YA(I).LT.SMCH) YA(I)=0.0
C         UPDATE THYROID INTAKE ARRAY
      IF (ICARC.NE.12) GO TO 158
      TMET(1,NE)=T
      TMET(2,NE)=AIN(1)*H1
C         STORE NEW CONTENTS OF FAECES AND URINE
  158 AU=YA(IURINE)
      AF=YA(IFECES)
C         IF AN EXCRETA SAMPLING TIME IS CROSSED CALL SAMPLING ROUTINE
      IF (T.GT.URINE(1,IU).AND.TT.LE.URINE(1,IU)) CALL EXCRET(TT,T,IU,
     1 AU,BU,URINE,JU,SUMU,WU)
      IF (T.GT.FAECES(1,IF).AND.TT.LE.FAECES(1,IF)) CALL EXCRET(TT,T,
     1 IF,AF,BF,FAECES,JF,SUMF,WF)
      IF (IOUT.EQ.0) GO TO 160
      WRITE (2,5) T,GREX
      WRITE (2,120) YA
  160 IF (MODA.NE.1) GO TO 162
      CALL ORGAN(YA,T,GREX,ICARC,N,LUNG,IBL,IC1,IC2,IC3,IC4,C)
      NREC=NREC+1
      WRITE (5,120,REC=NREC) (C(I),I=1,NCOL)
  162 IF (MODB.EQ.1) CALL CONSAV(N,YA,IREC,T,GREX)
      WRITE (1,125) T
      IF (T.GE.TMAT(M)) GO TO 230
      IF (ISTP.EQ.0) GO TO 180
  165 IF (ISTP.NE.-1) GO TO 166
      H1=H1/2.0
      IMET=1
      GO TO 168
  166 IF (H1.GE.0.1) GO TO 180
      IF (ISTP.GT.0) H1=H1*2.0
  168 DO 170 I=1,N
  170 Y(I)=YA(I)
      GO TO 10
  180 INDEX=0
      JINDEX=0
      TA=T+H1
      IF (IESP.EQ.0) GO TO 192
      DO 190 I=1,N2
      IF (T.LT.TFLAG(I).AND.TA.GE.TFLAG(I)) JINDEX=I
      IF (JINDEX.GT.0) GO TO 192
  190 CONTINUE
  192 IF (JINDEX.EQ.0) GO TO 200
      DO 195 I=1,N
  195 Y(I)=YA(I)
      GO TO 12
  200 DO 210 I=1,M
      IF (T.LT.TMAT(I).AND.TA.GE.TMAT(I)) INDEX=I
      IF (INDEX.GT.0) GO TO 215
  210 CONTINUE
  215 IF (INDEX.EQ.0) GO TO 153
      HR=H1
      DO 220 I=1,N
      Y(I)=YA(I)
  220 YE(I)=Y(I)
      GO TO 25
  230 DO 240 I=1,N
  240 YD(I)=-10.0
      IF (MODA.NE.1) GO TO 250
```

```
            NREC=NREC+1
            WRITE (5,120,REC=NREC) (YD(I),I=1,10)
      250   IF (MODB.NE.1) GO TO 260
            T=-10.0
            GREX=-10.0
            CALL CONSAV(N,YD,IREC,T,GREX)
      260   ENDFILE 5
            ENDFILE 4
            RETURN
            END
C
C=================================================================
C
C
            SUBROUTINE EXCRET(TT,T,IE,AE,BE,X,NE,SUM,WT)
C
C           ROUTINE TO CALCULATE EXCRETA CONTENTS AT SAMPLING TIME
C
            DIMENSION X(2,NE)
C           SET UP SCALING FACTOR
            R=(X(1,IE)-TT)/(T-TT)
C           CALCULATE TIME SINCE LAST SAMPLE
            J=IE-1
            DT=X(1,IE)-X(1,J)
            IF (IE.EQ.1) DT=X(1,IE)
C           CALCULATE EXCRETA COMPARTMENT CONTENTS
            X(2,IE)=BE+R*(AE-BE)-SUM
C           INCREASE TOTAL EXCRETA OUTPUT
            SUM=SUM+X(2,IE)
C           CONVERT URINE CONTENTS INTO AN OUTPUT RATE
            IF (DT.EQ.0.0) GO TO 1
            X(2,IE)=X(2,IE)/(WT*DT)
C           INCREMENT  SAMPLE FLAG BY 1
        1   IE=IE+1
            RETURN
            END
C
C=================================================================
C
            SUBROUTINE VALUES(IESP,ITYPE,IEXT,IOUT,ICARC,IDEV,N,M,IFECES,
       1    IBL,IC1,IC2,IC3,IC4,IURINE,IST,MM,NESP,N2,JF,JU,ITO,IFROM,H1,
       2    ESCAL,FOOD,VENT,GREX,AIRC,FDEX,FNAME,Y,A,AIN,TMAT,POL,TFLAG,
       3    ESP,B,URINE,FAECES,FIN,SKIN,FA,XA,XB,LUNG,GNAME,JDEV,MODA,MODB,
       4    LMOD,NM)
C
C           ROUTINE TO READ VARIABLES FROM RAM FILE FOR FCHAINING
C
            DIMENSION Y(40),A(80),ITO(80),IFROM(80),AIN(40),TMAT(30),
       1    POL(10),TFLAG(120),ESP(5,60),B(8),URINE(2,200),FAECES(2,200)
            LOGICAL*1 FNAME(11),GNAME(11)
C           OPEN STORAGE FILE
            CALL OPEN (3,'DATASAVEDAT',0)
C           SET RECORD FLAG TO ZERO
            NREC=0
C           READ INTEGER VALUES FROM FILE
            NREC=NREC+1
            READ (3,10,REC=NREC) IESP,ITYPE,IEXT,IOUT,ICARC,IDEV,N,M,
       1    IFECES,IBL,IC1,IC2,IC3,IC4,IURINE,IST,MM,NESP,N2,JF,JU,LUNG,
       2    JDEV,MODA,MODB,LMOD,NM
       10   FORMAT (30I4)
C           READ REAL CONSTANTS FROM FILE
            NREC=NREC+1
            READ (3,70,REC=NREC) H1,ESCAL,FOOD,VENT,GREX,AIRC,FDEX,XA,XB
            NREC=NREC+1
            READ (3,70,REC=NREC) FA,SKIN,FIN
C           READ TRANSFER ROUTES FROM FILE
            MC=23
            MB=1
       30   IF (MC.LT.MM) GO TO 40
            NREC=NREC+1
            READ (3,10,REC=NREC) (ITO(I),I=MB,MM)
```

```
          NREC=NREC+1
          READ (3,10,REC=NREC) (IFROM(I),I=MB,MM)
          GO TO 50
     40   NREC=NREC+1
          READ (3,10,REC=NREC) (ITO(I),I=MB,MC)
          NREC=NREC+1
          READ (3,10,REC=NREC) (IFROM(I),I=MB,MC)
          MB=MB+23
          MC=MC+23
          GO TO 30
C              READ TRANSFER COEFFICIENTS FROM FILE
     50   MC=10
          MB=1
     60   IF (MC.LT.MM) GO TO 80
          NREC=NREC+1
          READ (3,70,REC=NREC) (A(I),I=MB,MM)
     70   FORMAT (1P10E12.4)
          GO TO 90
     80   NREC=NREC+1
          READ (3,70,REC=NREC) (A(I),I=MB,MC)
          MB=MB+10
          MC=MC+10
          GO TO 60
C              READ INITIAL CONTENTS AND INPUTS FROM FILE
     90   MB=1
          MC=10
    100   IF (MC.LT.N) GO TO 110
          NREC=NREC+1
          READ (3,70,REC=NREC) (Y(I),I=MB,N)
          NREC=NREC+1
          READ (3,70,REC=NREC) (AIN(I),I=MB,N)
          GO TO 120
    110   NREC=NREC+1
          READ (3,70,REC=NREC) (Y(I),I=MB,MC)
          NREC=NREC+1
          READ (3,70,REC=NREC) (AIN(I),I=MB,MC)
          MB=MB+10
          MC=MC+10
          GO TO 100
C              READ POLYNOMIAL COEFFICIENTS FROM FILE
    120   IF (IEXT.EQ.0) GO TO 125
          NREC=NREC+1
          READ (3,70,REC=NREC) (POL(I),I=1,ITYPE)
C              READ EVALUATION TIMES FROM FILE
    125   MB=1
          MC=10
    130   IF (MC.LT.M) GO TO 140
          NREC=NREC+1
          READ (3,70,REC=NREC) (TMAT(I),I=MB,M)
          GO TO 150
    140   NREC=NREC+1
          READ (3,70,REC=NREC) (TMAT(I),I=MB,MC)
          MB=MB+10
          MC=MC+10
          GO TO 130
C              READ ACUTE EXPOSURE PATTERN FROM FILE
    150   IF (IESP.EQ.0) GO TO 190
          DO 160 I=1,NESP
          NREC=NREC+1
    160   READ (3,70,REC=NREC) (ESP(J,I),J=1,4)
C              READ ACUTE EXPOSURE FLAG TIMES FROM FILE
          MC=10
          MB=1
    170   IF (MC.LT.N2) GO TO 180
          NREC=NREC+1
          READ (3,70,REC=NREC) (TFLAG(I),I=MB,N2)
          GO TO 190
    180   NREC=NREC+1
          READ (3,70,REC=NREC) (TFLAG(I),I=MB,MC)
          MB=MB+10
          MC=MC+10
```

```
              GO TO 170
C             READ LUNG INPUT PARAMETERS FROM FILE
      190 IF (ICARC.GT.7) GO TO 195
              NREC=NREC+1
              READ (3,70,REC=NREC) (B(I),I=1,8)
C             READ URINE SAMPLING TIMES FROM FILE
      195 MC=10
              MB=1
      200 IF (MC.LT.JU) GO TO 210
              NREC=NREC+1
              READ (3,70,REC=NREC) (URINE(1,I),I=MB,JU)
              GO TO 220
      210 NREC=NREC+1
              READ (3,70,REC=NREC) (URINE(1,I),I=MB,MC)
              MB=MB+10
              MC=MC+10
              GO TO 200
C             READ FAECAL SAMPLING TIMES FROM FILE
      220 MC=10
              MB=1
      230 IF (MC.LT.JF) GO TO 240
              NREC=NREC+1
              READ (3,70,REC=NREC) (FAECES(1,I),I=MB,JF)
              GO TO 250
      240 NREC=NREC+1
              READ (3,70,REC=NREC) (FAECES(1,I),I=MB,MC)
              MB=MB+10
              MC=MC+10
              GO TO 230
C             READ STORAGE FILENAMES FROM FILE
      250 NREC=NREC+1
              READ (3,260,REC=NREC) FNAME,GNAME
      260 FORMAT (22A1)
              ENDFILE 3
              RETURN
              END
C
C==================================================================
C
          SUBROUTINE OUT2(TMAT,VAL,M,NCOL,HEADER)
C
C             ROUTINE TO PRINT CONTENTS AT SPECIFIED TIMES.
C
          DIMENSION TMAT(M),VAL(M,NCOL),HEADER(30)
          MCOL=NCOL-2
          WRITE (2,1)
      1 FORMAT (///20X,'RESULTS AT SPECIFIED TIMES'/)
          WRITE (2,2)
      2 FORMAT (20X,'COMPARTMENTAL CONCENTRATIONS IN PPM')
          DO 3 I=4,27
          J=I+3
      3 HEADER(I)=HEADER(J)
          DO 4 I=28,30
      4 HEADER(I)='       '
          WRITE (2,5) HEADER
      5 FORMAT (3X,30A4)
          DO 6 I=1,M
      6 WRITE (2,7) TMAT(I),(VAL(I,J),J=1,MCOL)
      7 FORMAT (3X,1P10E12.4)
          RETURN
          END
C
C==================================================================
C
          SUBROUTINE ZERO(Y,YA,YB,YC,YD,YE,F1,F2,A,AIN,TMAT,VAL,POL,TFLAG,
      1 ESP,B,URINE,FAECES,ITO,IFROM)
C
C             ROUTINE TO SET ALL ARRAY VALUES TO ZERO
C
          DIMENSION Y(40),YA(40),YB(40),YC(40),YD(40),YE(40),F1(40),
      1 F2(40),A(80),ITO(80),IFROM(80),AIN(40),TMAT(30),VAL(30,10),
```

```
      2 POL(10),TFLAG(120),ESP(5,60),B(8),URINE(2,200),FAECES(2,200)
        DO 1 I=1,40
        Y(I)=0.0
        YA(I)=0.0
        YB(I)=0.0
        YC(I)=0.0
        YD(I)=0.0
        YE(I)=0.0
        F1(I)=0.0
        F2(I)=0.0
      1 AIN(I)=0.0
        DO 2 J=1,5
        DO 2 I=1,60
      2 ESP(J,I)=0.0
        DO 3 I=1,80
        A(I)=0.0
        ITO(I)=0
      3 IFROM(I)=0
        DO 4 I=1,30
        TMAT(I)=0.0
        DO 4 J=1,10
        VAL(I,J)=0.0
      4 POL(J)=0.0
        DO 5 I=1,120
      5 TFLAG(I)=0.0
        DO 6 I=1,200
        DO 6 J=1,2
        URINE(J,I)=0.0
      6 FAECES(J,I)=0.0
        DO 7 I=1,8
      7 B(I)=0.0
        RETURN
        END
C
C=====================================================================
C
        SUBROUTINE HIST(X,NE,IL)
C
C          ROUTINE TO PRINT OUT HISTOGRAM OF EXCRETION
C
        DIMENSION X(2,NE),D(2),E(2,2)
        LOGICAL*1 P(52),C(4)
        DATA C/' ','+','X','.'/,D/'MG/L',' PPM'/,E/' URI','NARY',' FAE',
      1 'CAL '/
C          FIND MAXIMUM VALUE OF X
        XMAX=-1.E25
        DO 10 I=1,NE
        XVAL=X(2,I)
     10 IF (XVAL.GT.XMAX) XMAX=XVAL
        IF (XMAX.LE.0.0) RETURN
C          PRINT TITLE OF HISTOGRAM
        WRITE (2,15) (E(I,IL),I=1,2)
     15 FORMAT (10(/),20X,'HISTOGRAM OF',2A4,' EXCRETION'//)
C          PRINT SURROUND TO HISTOGRAM
        DO 20 I=1,52
     20 P(I)=C(2)
        WRITE (2,30) P,D(IL)
     30 FORMAT (7X,'TIME',2X,52A1,2X,'OUTPUT(',A4,')')
C          CALCULATE EACH ELEMENT OF HISTOGRAM
        MDAY=0
        DO 170 I=1,NE
        DO 40 J=2,51
     40 P(J)=C(1)
        V=(X(2,I)*50.0/XMAX)+1.5
        IV=V
        IF (IV.LT.2) GO TO 60
        DO 50 J=2,IV
     50 P(J)=C(3)
     60 DO 70 J=6,46,5
     70 P(J)=C(4)
        TA=X(1,I)
```

```
      CALL EMIT(TA,ND,IH,MINS)
C         PRINT LINE
      IF (ND.GT.MDAY) GO TO 110
      IF (MINS.LT.10) GO TO 90
      WRITE (2,80) IH,MINS,P,X(2,I)
   80 FORMAT (7X,I2,':',I2,1X,52A1,1PE10.3)
      GO TO 170
   90 WRITE (2,100) IH,MINS,P,X(2,I)
  100 FORMAT (7X,I2,':0',I1,1X,52A1,1PE10.3)
      GO TO 170
  110 IF (MINS.LT.10) GO TO 130
      WRITE (2,120) ND,IH,MINS,P,X(2,I)
  120 FORMAT (1X,'DAY',I2,I3,':',I2,1X,52A1,1PE10.3)
      MDAY=MDAY+1
      GO TO 170
  130 WRITE (2,140) ND,IH,MINS,P,X(2,I)
  140 FORMAT (1X,'DAY',I2,I3,':0',I1,1X,52A1,1PE10.3)
      MDAY=MDAY+1
  170 CONTINUE
C         FINISH OFF BORDER
      DO 180 I=1,52
  180 P(I)=C(2)
      WRITE (2,190) P
  190 FORMAT (13X,52A1)
      RETURN
      END
C
C================================================================
C
      SUBROUTINE EMIT(T,ND,IH,MINS)
C
C         ROUTINE TO CONVERT A DECIMAL TIME INTO A 24 HOUR TIME
C
C         CALCULATE NUMBER OF DAYS
      ND=1
      IF (T.LT.1.0) GO TO 2
    1 T=T-1.0
      ND=ND+1
      IF (T.GE.1.0) GO TO 1
C         CALCULATE NUMBER OF HOURS
    2 T=T*24.0
      IH=0
      IF (T.LT.1.0) GO TO 4
    3 T=T-1.0
      IH=IH+1
      IF (T.GE.1.0) GO TO 3
C         CALCULATE NUMBER OF MINUTES
    4 T=T*3.0/5.0
      MINS=T*100
      RETURN
      END
C
C================================================================
C
      SUBROUTINE UPTAKE(TMET,NE,T,AIN,XA,XB,YD,MET1,MET2,A)
C
C         ROUTINE TO CALCULATE THYROID UPTAKE
C
      DIMENSION YD(40),A(80),AIN(40),TMET(2,200)
      J=NE+1
      TMET(2,J)=-10.0
C         BRANCH IF T<0.25 DAYS
      IF (T.LT.0.25) GO TO 5
      I=1
C         CALCULATE NO OF ARRAY ELEMENTS TO BE DISCARDED
    1 IF (T-TMET(1,I).LE.0.25) GO TO 2
      I=I+1
      GO TO 1
C         DISCARD UNNECESSARY ELEMENTS FROM ARRAY
    2 J=1
    3 DO 4 M=1,2
```

```
      4 TMET(M,J)=TMET(M,I)
        IF (TMET(2,J).LT.0.0) GO TO 5
        J=J+1
        I=I+1
        GO TO 3
C           CALCULATE SUM OF ARRAY COLUMN 2
      5 SUM=0.0
        NE=J-1
        DO 6 I=1,NE
      6 SUM=SUM+TMET(2,I)
C           CALCULATE TIME STEP
        IF (T.GT.0.25) GO TO 7
        T1=0.25-T
        SUM=SUM+0.3*T1
        DT=0.25
        GO TO 8
      7 DT=TMET(1,NE)-TMET(1,1)
      8 AVER=SUM/DT
C           CALCULATE THYROID UPTAKE
        UP=XA*YD(4)/(AVER-XB*YD(4))
        IF ((AVER-XB*YD(4)).LE.0.0) UP=XA*YD(4)
C          UPDATE TRANSFER COEFFICIENTS
        A(MET1)=UP
        A(MET2)=-UP
C         INCREASE ELEMENT NUMBER FOR NEXT TIME
        NE=NE+1
        RETURN
        END
C
C======================================================================
C
        SUBROUTINE EXTYPE (AIN,POL,ESP,N,NESP,NN,T,B,VENT,GREX,ICARC,
      1 ITYPE,GREX1,IESP,FOOD,AIRC,FDEX,IST,FIN,FA,ORIG,LMOD,NM)
C
C       ROUTINE TO CALCULATE EXTRA INPUT TO LUNGS GI TRACT & SKIN
C       AT A GIVEN TIME.
C
        DIMENSION AIN(N),POL(ITYPE),ESP(5,NESP),B(8),ORIG(N),BACK(12)
        DATA BACK/0.0,0.0,0.0,0.0,0.0,0.0,0.0,0.0,0.0,0.0,0.0,0.0/
C          IF EXPOSURE IS ACUTE GO TO APPROPRIATE SECTION
        IF (IESP.EQ.1) GO TO 22
C           CALCULATE SCALING FACTOR FOR TIME DEPENDENCE
        SF=POL(1)
        DO 10 I=2,ITYPE
        J=I-1
     10 SF=SF+POL(I)*T**J
C           CALCULATE NEW COMPARTMENTAL INPUTS
        DO 20 I=1,N
     20 AIN(I)=SF*ORIG(I)
C           CALCULATE SCALED EXPOSURE PARAMETERS
        GREX=SF*GREX1
        GO TO 40
     22 IF (NN.GT.NESP) GO TO 25
        IF (T.GE.ESP(1,NN).AND.T.LT.ESP(2,NN)) GO TO 32
     25 IF (ICARC.GT.7) GO TO 30
        DO 26 I=1,8
     26 AIN(I)=B(I)*BACK(ICARC)*VENT
        AIN(IST)=FOOD
        IF (ICARC.EQ.7) GO TO 28
        IF (LMOD.NE.1.AND.NM.NE.1) GO TO 28
        AIN(IST)=AIN(IST)+AIN(1)+AIN(2)
        AIN(1)=0.0
        AIN(2)=0.0
C         CALCULATE TOTAL EXPOSURE (FOR GRAPH1)
     28 GREX=0.0
        DO 29 I=1,N
     29 GREX=GREX+AIN(I)
        GO TO 40
     30 GREX=BACK(ICARC)*VENT*FIN+FA*FOOD
        AIN(1)=GREX
        GO TO 40
```

```
  32   IF (ICARC.GT.7) GO TO 38
       DO 35 I=1,8
  35   AIN(I)=ESP(3,NN)*VENT*B(I)
       AIN(IST)=ESP(4,NN)+FOOD
       IF (ICARC.EQ.7) GO TO 36
       IF (LMOD.NE.1.AND.NM.NE.1) GO TO 36
       AIN(IST)=AIN(IST)+AIN(1)+AIN(2)
       AIN(1)=0.0
       AIN(2)=0.0
  36   GREX=0.0
       DO 37 I=1,N
  37   GREX=GREX+AIN(I)
       GO TO 40
  38   GREX=ESP(3,NN)*VENT*FIN+FA*(ESP(4,NN)+FOOD)+ESP(5,NN)
       AIN(1)=GREX
  40   RETURN
       END
C
C=====================================================================
C
       SUBROUTINE RUNKA1(H,Y,YA,YB,YC,YD,F1,F2,N,A,ITO,IFROM,MM,AIN)
       DIMENSION Y(N),YA(N),YB(N),YC(N),YD(N),F1(N),F2(N),A(MM),
     1 ITO(MM),IFROM(MM),AIN(N)
       H2=H/2.0
       H6=H/6.0
       CALL DFDT(Y,F1,N,A,ITO,IFROM,MM,AIN)
       DO 1 I=1,N
  1    YB(I)=Y(I)+H2*F1(I)
       CALL DFDT(YB,F2,N,A,ITO,IFROM,MM,AIN)
       DO 2 I=1,N
  2    YB(I)=Y(I)+H2*F2(I)
       CALL DFDT(YB,YC,N,A,ITO,IFROM,MM,AIN)
       DO 3 I=1,N
  3    YB(I)=Y(I)+H*YC(I)
       CALL DFDT(YB,YD,N,A,ITO,IFROM,MM,AIN)
       DO 4 I=1,N
  4    YB(I)=Y(I)+H6*(F1(I)+2.0*F2(I)+2.0*YC(I)+YD(I))
       RETURN
       END
C
C=====================================================================
C
       SUBROUTINE DFDT(Y,F,N,A,ITO,IFROM,MM,AIN)
       DIMENSION Y(N),F(N),A(MM),ITO(MM),IFROM(MM),AIN(N)
       DO 1 I=1,N
  1    F(I)=AIN(I)
       DO 2 II=1,MM
       I=ITO(II)
       J=IFROM(II)
  2    F(I)=F(I)+A(II)*Y(J)
       RETURN
       END
C
C=====================================================================
C
       SUBROUTINE PRCOR(H,Y,YA,YB,YC,YD,F1,F2,N,A,ITO,IFROM,MM,
     1 AIN,ISTP)
       DIMENSION Y(N),YA(N),YB(N),YC(N),YD(N),F1(N),F2(N),A(MM),
     1 ITO(MM),IFROM(MM),AIN(N)
       COMMON/PASS/ESCAL
       YMAX=0.0
       DO 1 I=1,N
  1    IF (YA(I).GT.YMAX) YMAX=YA(I)
       EPA=ESCAL*YMAX+1.E-10
       CALL DFDT(YA,F1,N,A,ITO,IFROM,MM,AIN)
       DO 2 I=1,N
  2    YB(I)=Y(I)+2.0*H*F1(I)
       ILP=0
  3    ILP=ILP+1
       CALL DFDT(YB,F2,N,A,ITO,IFROM,MM,AIN)
       DO 4 I=1,N
```

```
      4  YC(I)=YA(I)+0.5*H*(F1(I)+F2(I))
         IF (ILP.NE.1 ) GO TO 6
         DO 5 I=1,N
      5  YD(I)=YC(I)
      6  IFL=0
         DO 7 I=1,N
         D=ABS(YC(I)-YB(I))
      7  IF (D.GT.EPA) IFL=1
         IF (IFL.EQ.0) GO TO 9
         IF (ILP.GT.16) GO TO 9
         DO 8 I=1,N
      8  YB(I)=YC(I)
         GO TO 3
      9  ISTP=0
         IF (ILP.LE.3) ISTP=1
         IF (ILP.GT.6) ISTP=-1
         IF (ISTP.EQ.-1) RETURN
         DO 10 I=1,N
         YB(I)=YC(I)
         Y(I)=YA(I)
     10  YA(I)=YB(I)
         RETURN
         END
C
C=================================================================
C
         SUBROUTINE ORGAN(YD,T,GREX,ICARC,N,LUNG,IBL,IC1,IC2,IC3,IC4,C)
C
C          ROUTINE TO CALCULATE INDIVIDUAL ORGAN CONTENTS
C
         DIMENSION YD(N),C(10)
C          ZERO OUTPUT ARRAY
         DO 10 I=1,10
     10  C(I)=0.0
C          ALLOCATE TIME AND EXPOSURE VALUES
         C(1)=T
         C(2)=GREX
         TOT=0.0
C          CALCULATE LUNG CONTENTS IF NECESSARY
         IF (ICARC.GT.7) GO TO 30
         DO 20 I=1,LUNG
     20  TOT=TOT+YD(I)
         C(4)=TOT/1.0
C          CALCULATE TOTAL AMOUNT OF SUBSTANCE IN BODY
     30  TOT=TOT+YD(IBL)+YD(IC1)+YD(IC2)
         IF (ICARC.LT.3.OR.ICARC.EQ.5.OR.ICARC.EQ.9) GO TO 35
         TOT=TOT+YD(IC3)
         IF (ICARC.GT.4) GO TO 35
         TOT=TOT+YD(IC4)
     35  GO TO (40,50,60,70,80,90,100,110,120,130,140,150),ICARC
C          ARSENIC
     40  C(3)=0.24*YD(IBL)*1.6/5.5
         C(6)=(0.64*YD(IBL)+0.05*YD(IC1)+0.052*YD(IC2))/0.31
         C(5)=(0.12*YD(IBL)+0.01*YD(IC1)+0.008*YD(IC2))/1.8
         C(7)=0.94*(YD(IC1)+YD(IC2))/61.39
         C(8)=TOT
         GO TO 160
C          BERYLLIUM
     50  C(6)=(0.025*YD(IBL)+0.19*YD(IC1)+0.02*YD(IC2))/1.8
         C(5)=(0.005*YD(IBL)+0.19*YD(IC1)+0.02*YD(IC2))/0.31
         C(3)=(0.4*YD(IBL)+0.12*YD(IC1)+0.06*YD(IC2))/28.0
         C(7)=(0.075*YD(IBL)+0.795*YD(IC2))/10.0
         C(8)=(0.495*YD(IBL)+0.5*YD(IC1)+0.105*YD(IC2))/28.89
         C(9)=TOT
         GO TO 160
C          CADMIUM
     60  C(3)=(YD(IBL)+YD(IC1))/5.5
         C(6)=YD(IC3)/1.8
         C(5)=YD(IC4)/0.31
         C(7)=YD(IC2)/61.39
         C(8)=TOT
```

```
            GO TO 160
C               LEAD
     70  C(3)=YD(IBL)/5.5
         C(6)=YD(IC1)/1.8
         C(5)=YD(IC2)/0.31
         C(7)=YD(IC4)/10.0
         C(8)=YD(IC3)/51.39
         C(9)=TOT
            GO TO 160
C               NICKEL
     80  C(3)=(YD(IBL)+0.003*YD(IC2))/5.5
         C(5)=(YD(IC1)+0.004*YD(IC2))/0.31
         C(6)=0.993*YD(IC2)/63.19
         C(7)=TOT
            GO TO 160
C               CHROMIUM
     90  C(3)=YD(IBL)/5.5
         AMOUNT=YD(IC1)+YD(IC2)
         C(6)=0.02*AMOUNT/1.8
         C(5)=0.01*AMOUNT/0.31
         C(8)=0.002*AMOUNT/0.18
         C(9)=0.968*AMOUNT/51.21
         C(7)=YD(IC3)/10.0
         C(10)=TOT
            GO TO 160
C               ASBESTOS
    100  C(3)=TOT/1.0
         C(4)=TOT
            GO TO 160
C               BENZENE
    110  C(3)=YD(IBL)/5.5
         C(5)=YD(IC1)/10.0
         C(4)=YD(IC2)/15.0
         C(6)=YD(IC3)/70.0
         C(7)=TOT
            GO TO 160
C               VINYL CHLORIDE
    120  C(3)=YD(IBL)/5.5
         C(4)=YD(IC1)/64.5
         C(5)=YD(IC2)/70.0
         C(6)=TOT
            GO TO 160
C               BENZIDINE
    130  C(3)=YD(IBL)/5.5
         C(4)=YD(IC1)/1.8
         C(5)=(YD(IC2)+YD(IC4))/70.0
         C(6)=YD(IC3)/0.75
         C(7)=TOT
            GO TO 160
C               CARBON TETRACHLORIDE
    140  C(3)=YD(IBL)/5.5
         C(4)=YD(IC1)/15.0
         C(5)=YD(IC2)/1.8
         C(6)=YD(IC3)/70.0
         C(7)=TOT
            GO TO 160
C               METHYL IODIDE
    150  C(3)=YD(IBL)/5.5
         C(4)=YD(IC1)/9.0
         C(5)=YD(IC2)/0.02
         C(6)=YD(IC3)/70.0
         C(7)=TOT
    160  RETURN
         END
C
C================================================================
```

```
C
      SUBROUTINE CONSAV(N,YD,IREC,T,GREX)
C
C         ROUTINE TO STORE ALL COMPARTMENTAL CONTENTS ON FILE
C
      DIMENSION YD(N)
      MA=1
      MB=8
      IF (MB.LT.N) GO TO 20
      IREC=IREC+1
      WRITE (4,10,REC=IREC) T,GREX,(YD(I),I=MA,N)
   10 FORMAT (1P10E12.4)
      GO TO 70
   20 IREC=IREC+1
      WRITE (4,10,REC=IREC) T,GREX,(YD(I),I=MA,MB)
   30 MA=MA+8
      MB=MB+10
      IF (MB.LT.N) GO TO 40
      IREC=IREC+1
      WRITE (4,10,REC=IREC) (YD(I),I=MA,N)
      GO TO 70
   40 IREC=IREC+1
      WRITE (4,10,REC=IREC) (YD(I),I=MA,MB)
   50 MA=MA+10
      MB=MB+10
      IF (MB.LT.N) GO TO 60
      IREC=IREC+1
      WRITE (4,10,REC=IREC) (YD(I),I=MA,N)
      GO TO 70
   60 IREC=IREC+1
      WRITE (4,10,REC=IREC) (YD(I),I=MA,MB)
      GO TO 50
   70 RETURN
      END
C
C======================================================================
C
      SUBROUTINE LABEL(HEADER,ICARC)
C
C         ROUTINE TO GENERATE COLUMN HEADINGS
C
      DIMENSION HEADER(30),BLOCK(3,17)
      DATA BLOCK/'    ','TIME','    ','    E','XPOS','URE ','    ',
     1 'BLOO','D   ','    ','    ','LUNG','    ','    ','    ','KIDN','EY  ','    ',
     2 'LIVE','R   ','    ','    ','BONE','    ','    ','    ','SPLE','EN  ','    ',
     3 'OTHE','RS  ','    ','    ','MUSC','LE  ','    ','MET ','ABOL','ITES','    ',
     4 ' FAT','    ','    ','  DI','FFUS','ION ','    ','  T ','HYRO','ID  ','  OR',
     5 'GANI','C I ','    ','  TO','TAL ','(MG)','    ','  GI ','CONT','ENTS'/
      DO 5 I=1,30
    5 HEADER(I)='    '
      IH=0
      DO 10 I=1,2
      DO 10 J=1,3
      IH=IH+1
   10 HEADER(IH)=BLOCK(J,I)
      IF (ICARC.NE.7) GO TO 13
      DO 11 I=1,3
      IH=IH+1
   11 HEADER(IH)=BLOCK(I,4)
      GO TO 220
   13 IF (ICARC.EQ.2) GO TO 30
      DO 20 I=1,3
      IH=IH+1
   20 HEADER(IH)=BLOCK(I,3)
      GO TO 50
   30 DO 40 I=1,3
      IH=IH+1
   40 HEADER(IH)=BLOCK(I,10)
   50 IF (ICARC.GT.7) GO TO 120
      DO 60 I=4,5
```

```
          DO 60 J=1,3
          IH=IH+1
   60     HEADER(IH)=BLOCK(J,I)
          IF (ICARC.EQ.5) GO TO 100
          DO 70 I=1,3
          IH=IH+1
   70     HEADER(IH)=BLOCK(I,6)
          IF (ICARC.EQ.3.OR.ICARC.EQ.1) GO TO 100
          DO 80 I=1,3
          IH=IH+1
   80     HEADER(IH)=BLOCK(I,7)
          IF (ICARC.NE.6) GO TO 100
          DO 90 I=1,3
          IH=IH+1
   90     HEADER(IH)=BLOCK(I,8)
  100     DO 110 I=1,3
          IH=IH+1
  110     HEADER(IH)=BLOCK(I,9)
          GO TO 220
  120     IF (ICARC.NE.8.AND.ICARC.NE.11) GO TO 140
          DO 130 I=1,3
          IH=IH+1
  130     HEADER(IH)=BLOCK(I,12)
  140     IF (ICARC.NE.10.AND.ICARC.NE.11) GO TO 160
          DO 150 I=1,3
          IH=IH+1
  150     HEADER(IH)=BLOCK(I,6)
  160     IF (ICARC.NE.8) GO TO 180
          DO 170 I=1,3
          IH=IH+1
  170     HEADER(IH)=BLOCK(I,7)
  180     IF (ICARC.NE.9) GO TO 185
          DO 183 I=1,3
          IH=IH+1
  183     HEADER(IH)=BLOCK(I,9)
  185     IF (ICARC.EQ.12) GO TO 200
          DO 190 I=1,3
          IH=IH+1
  190     HEADER(IH)=BLOCK(I,11)
          IF (ICARC.NE.10) GO TO 220
          DO 195 J=1,3
          IH=IH+1
  195     HEADER(IH)=BLOCK(J,17)
          GO TO 220
  200     DO 210 I=13,15
          DO 210 J=1,3
          IH=IH+1
  210     HEADER(IH)=BLOCK(J,I)
  220     DO 230 J=1,3
          IH=IH+1
  230     HEADER(IH)=BLOCK(J,16)
          RETURN
          END
C
C==================================================================
```

Program listing of the computer code GRAPH

```
      PROGRAM GRAPH
C
C         MAIN PROGRAM FOR CARCINOGENS GRAPH PLOTTING ROUTINE
C
      DIMENSION YN(2),JCOM(8),HEADER(30),BLOCK(3,10)
      LOGICAL*1 FNAME(11)
      DATA YN/'Y    ','N    '/
C         CLEAR THE SCREEN
    1 WRITE (1,3)
    3 FORMAT (23(/),25X,'GRAPH PLOTTER',12(/))
C         OPEN DATA FILE FOR READING DATA
      WRITE (1,5)
    5 FORMAT (5X,'FILE NAME ON WHICH RESULTS ARE STORED   :')
      READ (1,6) FNAME
    6 FORMAT (11A1)
      FNAME(9)='D'
      FNAME(10)='A'
      FNAME(11)='T'
      WRITE (1,7)
    7 FORMAT (5X,'ON WHICH DISK DRIVE IS THIS FILE LOCATED?'/
    2 5X,'PRESENT DRIVE = 1 EXPANSION DRIVE = 2   :')
      READ (1,15) IDEV
      CALL OPEN (5,FNAME,IDEV)
C         DEFINE WHICH COMPARTMENTS ARE TO BE PLOTTED
      NREC=1
      READ (5,14,REC=NREC) N,IE,IDAT
   14 FORMAT (3I5)
   15 FORMAT (I5)
      IF (IDAT.EQ.0) GO TO 19
      WRITE (1,17) N
   17 FORMAT (23(/),5X,'THIS FILE CONTAINS THE CONTENTS OF ALL',I3,
    1 ' COMPARTMENTS'//)
      GO TO 38
C         READ COLUMN LABELS FROM FILE
   19 NREC=NREC+1
      READ (5,20,REC=NREC) HEADER
   20 FORMAT (30A4)
      I=0
      DO 25 J=1,N
      DO 25 K=1,3
      I=I+1
   25 BLOCK(K,J)=HEADER(I)
      WRITE (1,30)
   30 FORMAT (23(/),5X,'THIS FILE CONTAINS THE CONTENTS OF THE',
    1 ' FOLLOWING TISSUES :-',////)
      DO 35 I=3,N
      K=I-2
   35 WRITE (1,37) (BLOCK(J,I),J=1,3),K
   37 FORMAT (30X,3A4,' (',I1,')')
   38 WRITE (1,40)
   40 FORMAT (/5X,'HOW MANY LINES DO YOU WANT TO PLOT? (MAX = 8)   :')
      READ (1,15) ICOM
      IF (ICOM.GT.8) GO TO 38
      DO 70 I=1,ICOM
      WRITE (1,60) I
   60 FORMAT (//5X,'ENTER NUMBER OF REQUIRED PARAMETER FOR LINE',I3,
    1 //5X,'(COMPARTMENT NUMBER OR ORGAN LABEL)   :')
   70 READ (1,15) JCOM(I)
      CALL SORT(ICOM,JCOM)
C         SET FLAG TO SAY WHETHER EXPOSURE IS TO BE PLOTTED
      NGEX=0
      WRITE (1,80)
   80 FORMAT (/5X,'DO YOU WANT EXPOSURE PLOTTING? (Y/N)   :')
      READ (1,85) ANS1
   85 FORMAT (A4)
      IF (ANS1.EQ.YN(1)) NGEX=1
C         DEFINE RANGE OF TIME AXIS
```

```
          TS=0.0
          TF=1.0E+10
          WRITE (1,86)
    86    FORMAT (23(/),5X,'DO YOU WISH TO CHANGE TIME RANGE? (Y/N)  :')
          READ (1,85) ANS1
          IF (ANS1.EQ.YN(2)) GO TO 90
          WRITE (1,87)
    87    FORMAT (/5X,'ENTER START TIME  :')
          READ (1,110) TS
          WRITE (1,88)
    88    FORMAT (/5X,'ENTER STOP TIME  :')
          READ (1,110) TF
C             SET TIME-STEP (DEFINES SPACING ON X-AXIS)
    90    WRITE (1,100)
   100    FORMAT (/5X,'ENTER TIME STEP FOR DATA PLOTTING (DAYS)   :')
          READ (1,110) DT
   110    FORMAT (E12.4)
          IF (DT.LT.0.0.OR.DT.GT.365.25) GO TO 90
C             WRITE WARNING MESSAGE ON SCREEN
          WRITE (1,117)
   117    FORMAT (12(/),25X,'PLEASE LEAVE - PROGRAM RUNNING',12(/))
C             CALL ROUTINE TO CALCULATE POINTS
          CALL POINTS(JCOM,ICOM,NGEX,NREC,DT,YN,TS,TF,BLOCK,IDAT,N,IE)
C             SET FLAG FOR ANOTHER GRAPH PLOT (1=ANOTHER PLOT)
          WRITE (1,120)
   120    FORMAT (23(/),5X,'ANOTHER GRAPH? (Y/N)   :')
          READ (1,85) ANS2
          IF (ANS2.EQ.YN(1)) GO TO 1
          STOP
          END
C
C===================================================================
C
          SUBROUTINE POINTS(JCOM,ICOM,NGEX,NREC,DT,YN,TS,TF,BLOCK,IDAT,N,
         1 IE)
C
C             ROUTINE TO CALCULATE POINTS USED BY PLOT1
C
          DIMENSION P(8),P1(8),P2(200,8),GRX(200),YN(2),JCOM(ICOM),
         1 BLOCK(3,10)
          NS=1
          TA=0.5*DT+TS
          JJ=0
          TG=0.0
          IF (IDAT.EQ.1) GO TO 15
C             READ FIRST VALUES OF T,EXPOSURE & CONTENTS
          NREC=NREC+1
          READ (5,10,REC=NREC) T,GREX,P
    10    FORMAT (1P10E12.4)
          GO TO 19
    15    CALL CONSAV(N,P,NREC,T,GREX,ICOM,JCOM)
C             EXIT IF NO TIMES ARE FOUND
    19    IF (T.LT.0.0) GO TO 70
C             READ NEXT VALUES OF TIME,EXPOSURE & CONTENTS
    20    IF (IDAT.EQ.1) GO TO 23
          NREC=NREC+1
          READ (5,10,REC=NREC) T1,GREX1,P1
          GO TO 25
    23    CALL CONSAV(N,P1,NREC,T1,GREX1,ICOM,JCOM)
C             EXIT IF NO DATA POINTS ARE FOUND
    25    IF (T1.LT.0.0.OR.T1.GE.TF) GO TO 110
C             IF START TIME IS NOT REACHED GET NEXT SET OF POINTS
          IF (T1.LT.TS) GO TO 50
C             IF A PLOTTED TIME IS NOT REACHED MOVE SECOND CONTENTS TO
C             FIRST CONTENTS BUFFER AND READ ANOTHER LINE OF DATA
    30    IF (TA.GT.T1) GO TO 50
C             IF A PLOTTED TIME IS REACHED CALCULATE PLOTTED POINTS
          R=(TA-T)/(T1-T)
          IF (IDAT.EQ.1) GO TO 46
          DO 40 K=1,ICOM
          DO 40 J=1,8
```

```
         IF (J.NE.JCOM(K)) GO TO 40
         P2(NS,K)=P(J)+R*(P1(J)-P(J))
   40    CONTINUE
         GO TO 48
   46    DO 47 I=1,ICOM
   47    P2(NS,I)=P(I)+R*(P1(I)-P(I))
   48    IF (NGEX.NE.1) GO TO 49
         IF (IE.EQ.1) GO TO 1000
         GRX(NS)=GREX1
         IF (JJ.GT.0) GRX(NS)=TG
         GO TO 49
 1000    GRX(NS)=GREX+R*(GREX1-GREX)
C           AS A PLOTTED TIME HAS BEEN REACHED UPDATE TIME AND LINE NO.
   49    TA=TA+DT
         NS=NS+1
         JJ=0
         TG=0.0
         WRITE (1,58) NS
   58    FORMAT ('+',50X,'POINT =',I4)
C           EXIT IF MORE THAN 200 LINES HAVE BEEN CALCULATED
         IF (NS.GT.200) GO TO 90
         GO TO 30
   50    T=T1
         IF (GREX1.LE.GREX) GO TO 55
         JJ=JJ+1
         IF (GREX1.GT.TG) TG=GREX1
   55    GREX=GREX1
         DO 60 I=1,8
   60    P(I)=P1(I)
         GO TO 20
C           ERROR MESSAGES
   70    WRITE (2,80)
   80    FORMAT (/5X,'ERROR - POINTS - NO TIMES FOUND'/)
         GO TO 170
   90    WRITE (2,100)
  100    FORMAT (/5X,'ERROR - POINTS - END OF RUN NOT REACHED IN 200',
        1 1X,'POINTS - TO PLOT THIS GRAPH :- INCREASE TIME STEP'/)
         GO TO 170
  110    IF (NS.GT.1) GO TO 123
         WRITE (2,120)
  120    FORMAT (/5X,'ERROR - POINTS - END OF RUN BEFORE TIME STEP',
        1 1X,'REACHED - TO PLOT THIS GRAPH :- DECREASE TIME STEP'/)
         GO TO 170
C            WRITE TITLE OF GRAPH
  123    IF (IDAT.EQ.0) GO TO 130
         WRITE (2,125)
  125    FORMAT (5(/),25X,'GRAPH OF COMPARTMENTAL CONTENTS (MG) AGAINST',
        1 ' TIME'//)
         GO TO 135
  130    WRITE (2,132)
  132    FORMAT (5(/),25X,'GRAPH OF ORGAN CONCENTRATIONS (PPM) AGAINST',
        1 ' TIME'//)
C            WRITE PLOTTING SYMBOLS AND CALL PLOTTING ROUTINE
  135    NS=NS-1
         DO 150 J=1,ICOM
         DO 150 I=1,N
         IF (I.NE.(JCOM(J)+2)) GO TO 150
         IF (IDAT.EQ.1) GO TO 140
         K=JCOM(J)+2
         WRITE (2,138) J,(BLOCK(L,K),L=1,3)
  138    FORMAT (30X,I3,' =',3A4)
         GO TO 150
  140    WRITE (2,145) J,JCOM(J)
  145    FORMAT (30X,I3,' = COMPARTMENT',I3)
  150    CONTINUE
         IF (NGEX.NE.1) GO TO 165
         WRITE (2,160)
  160    FORMAT (32X,'* =     EXPOSURE'/)
  165    CALL PLOT1(ICOM,NGEX,DT,P2,GRX,NS,YN,TS,IDAT)
  170    ENDFILE 5
         RETURN
         END
```

```
C
        SUBROUTINE PLOT1(ICOM,NGEX,DT,P2,GRX,NS,YN,TS,IDAT)
C
C          ROUTINE TO PLOT THE GRAPH
C
        DIMENSION P2(200,8),GRX(NS),YV(9),YN(2)
        LOGICAL*1 L(102),C(4),S(8)
        DATA C/' ','+',' ','*'/
        DATA S/'1','2','3','4','5','6','7','8'/
C          CALCULATE RANGE OF POINTS
        I2=0
        AMX=-60.0
        AMN=60.0
        DO 20 I=1,NS
        DO 20 J=1,ICOM
        VAX=P2(I,J)
        IF (VAX.EQ.0.0) GO TO 20
        VAL=ALOG10(VAX)
        IF (VAL.GT.AMX) AMX=VAL
        IF (VAL.LT.AMN) AMN=VAL
   20   CONTINUE
C          RETURN IF THERE IS NO SPREAD OF DATA
        IF (AMX.GT.AMN) GO TO 40
        WRITE (2,30)
   30   FORMAT (/5X,'WARNING - PLOT1 - NO SPREAD OF DATA'/)
        GO TO 270
C          CALCULATE RANGE OF EXPOSURE IF NECESSARY
   40   IF (NGEX.NE.1) GO TO 60
        EXMN=0.0
        EXMX=0.0
        DO 50 I=1,NS
   50   IF (GRX(I).GT.EXMX) EXMX=GRX(I)
        BB=EXMX/10.0
        EXMX=EXMX+BB
        EXMN=FLOAT(IFIX(EXMN))
        EXMX=FLOAT(IFIX(EXMX))
        IF (EXMX.EQ.0.0) NGEX=0
   60   IF (AMX.GT.0.0) AMX=AMX+1.0
        IF (AMN.LT.0.0) AMN=AMN-1.0
        AMN=FLOAT(IFIX(AMN))
        AMX=FLOAT(IFIX(AMX))
        BMN=10.0**AMN
        BMX=10.0**AMX
C          ADJUST RANGE OF Y-AXIS SCALE IF NECESSARY
        WRITE (1,66) BMN,BMX
   66   FORMAT (5X,'PLOT IS FROM',1PE8.1,' TO',1PE8.1/
       1 5X,'DO YOU WISH TO ALTER THE RANGE? (Y/N)   :')
        READ (1,67) ANS
   67   FORMAT (A4)
        IF (ANS.NE.YN(1)) GO TO 71
        WRITE (1,68)
   68   FORMAT (5X,'MINIMUM VALUE    :')
        READ (1,69) BMN
   69   FORMAT (E12.4)
        WRITE (1,70)
   70   FORMAT (5X,'MAXIMUM VALUE    :')
        READ (1,69) BMX
   71   WRITE (2,72) BMN,BMX
   72   FORMAT (32X,'RANGE =',1PE10.3,' TO',1PE10.3//)
C          CALCULATE AND PRINT SCALE OF CONTENT AXIS
        IF (IDAT.EQ.0) GO TO 74
        WRITE (2,73)
   73   FORMAT (43X,'COMPARTMENTAL CONTENTS (MG) - LOG SCALE'/)
        GO TO 76
   74   WRITE (2,75)
   75   FORMAT (43X,'TISSUE CONCENTRATIONS (PPM) - LOG SCALE'/)
   76   BR=ALOG(BMX/BMN)/10.0
        BR=EXP(BR)
```

```
          YV(1)=BMN*BR
          DO 78 I=2,9
          J=I-1
    78    YV(I)=YV(J)*BR
          WRITE (2,80) YV
    80    FORMAT (18X,1P9E10.2)
C             CALCULATE SCALING FACTOR
          AMN=ALOG(BMN)
          AMX=ALOG(BMX)
          ADF=AMX-AMN
C             PRINT AXIS
          DO 90 I=1,102
    90    L(I)=C(1)
          DO 100 I=11,91,10
   100    L(I)=C(2)
          WRITE (2,110) L
   110    FORMAT (7X,'TIME',2X,102A1,1X,'TIME(DAYS)')
          DO 120 I=1,102
   120    L(I)=C(2)
          WRITE (2,125) L
   125    FORMAT (13X,102A1)
C             CALCULATE POSITION OF POINTS ON EACH LINE AND PRINT LINE
          MDAY=0
          DO 170 I=1,NS
          DO 130 J=2,101
   130    L(J)=C(1)
          DO 140 J=11,91,10
   140    L(J)=C(3)
          DO 142 J=1,ICOM
          VAX=P2(I,J)
          IF (VAX.EQ.0.0) GO TO 142
          VAX=ALOG(VAX)
          IF (VAX.LT.AMN.OR.VAX.GE.AMX) GO TO 142
          FR=(VAX-AMN)/ADF
          CH=100.0*FR+1.0
          ICH=CH
          IF (ICH.EQ.1) GO TO 142
          L(ICH)=S(J)
   142    CONTINUE
C             ALLOCATE POSITION OF EXPOSURE POINT IF NECESSARY
          IF (NGEX.NE.1) GO TO 150
          I3=I2
          FRE=GRX(I)/EXMX
          CHE=100.0*FRE+1.0
          ICHE=CHE
          I2=ICHE
          IF (ICHE.LE.1) GO TO 143
          L(ICHE)=C(4)
   143    IF (I.LT.2.OR.ICHE.EQ.I3) GO TO 150
          IA=I2
          IB=I3
          EI2=FLOAT(IA)
          EI3=FLOAT(IB)
          IF (ABS(EI2-EI3).LT.(EI2/1.1)) GO TO 150
          IF (IA.GT.IB) GO TO 144
          ITEM=IA
          IA=IB
          IB=ITEM
   144    DO 146 M=IB,IA
          IF (M.LT.2) GO TO 146
          L(M)=C(4)
   146    CONTINUE
C             CALCULATE VALUE OF TIME AT THIS LINE
   150    T=I
          T=(T-0.5)*DT+TS
          TA=T
          CALL EMIT(TA,ND,IH,MINS)
          IF (ND.GT.MDAY) GO TO 158
          IF (MINS.LT.10) GO TO 156
          WRITE (2,155) IH,MINS,L,T
   155    FORMAT (7X,I2,':',I2,1X,102A1,1PE10.3)
```

```
          GO TO 170
    156   WRITE (2,157) IH,MINS,L,T
    157   FORMAT (7X,I2,':0',I1,1X,102A1,1PE10.3)
          GO TO 170
    158   IF (MINS.LT.10) GO TO 160
          WRITE (2,159) ND,IH,MINS,L,T
    159   FORMAT (1X,'DAY',I2,1X,I2,':',I2,1X,102A1,1PE10.3)
          MDAY=MDAY+1
          GO TO 170
    160   WRITE (2,161) ND,IH,MINS,L,T
    161   FORMAT (1X,'DAY',I2,1X,I2,':0',I1,1X,102A1,1PE10.3)
          MDAY=MDAY+1
    170   CONTINUE
          DO 180 I=1,102
    180   L(I)=C(2)
          WRITE (2,125) L
C             PRINT EXPOSURE AXIS AND LABEL IF NECESSARY
          IF (NGEX.NE.1) GO TO 220
          DO 190 I=1,102
    190   L(I)=C(1)
          DO 195 I=11,91,10
    195   L(I)=C(2)
          WRITE (2,125) L
          YV(1)=EXMX/10.0
          DO 200 I=2,9
          J=I-1
    200   YV(I)=YV(J)+YV(1)
          WRITE (2,80) YV
          WRITE (2,210)
    210   FORMAT (/44X,'EXPOSURE (MG/DAY) - LINEAR SCALE')
    220   WRITE (2,230)
    230   FORMAT (10(/))
          WRITE (1,240)
    240   FORMAT (5X,'DO YOU WANT POINT VALUES? (Y/N)  :')
          READ (1,67) ANS1
          IF (ANS1.EQ.YN(2)) GO TO 270
          DO 245 I=1,NS
          DO 245 J=1,ICOM
          IF (P2(I,J).LE.0.0) GO TO 245
          P2(I,J)=ALOG(P2(I,J))
    245   CONTINUE
          DO 250 I=1,NS
    250   WRITE (2,260) I,(P2(I,J),J=1,ICOM),GRX(I)
    260   FORMAT (I5,1P9E12.3)
    270   RETURN
          END
C
C=================================================================
C
          SUBROUTINE CONSAV(N,X,NREC,A,B,ICOM,JCOM)
C
C             ROUTINE TO READ COMPARTMENTAL CONTENTS FROM FILE
C
          DIMENSION X(N),JCOM(ICOM),Y(25)
          MA=1
          MB=8
          IF (MB.LT.N) GO TO 20
          NREC=NREC+1
          READ (5,10,REC=NREC) A,B,(Y(I),I=MA,N)
    10    FORMAT (1P10E12.4)
          GO TO 70
    20    NREC=NREC+1
          READ (5,10,REC=NREC) A,B,(Y(I),I=MA,MB)
    30    MA=MA+8
          MB=MB+10
          IF (MB.LT.N) GO TO 40
          NREC=NREC+1
          READ (5,10,REC=NREC) (Y(I),I=MA,N)
          GO TO 70
    40    NREC=NREC+1
          READ (5,10,REC=NREC) (Y(I),I=MA,MB)
```

```
  50    MA=MA+10
        MB=MB+10
        IF (MB.LT.N) GO TO 60
        NREC=NREC+1
        READ (5,10,REC=NREC) (Y(I),I=MA,N)
  GO TO 70
  60    NREC=NREC+1
        READ (5,10,REC=NREC) (Y(I),I=MA,MB)
        GO TO 50
  70    DO 80 I=1,N
        DO 80 J=1,ICOM
        IF (I.NE.JCOM(J)) GO TO 80
        X(J)=Y(I)
  80    CONTINUE
        RETURN
        END
C
C======================================================================
C
        SUBROUTINE EMIT(T,ND,IH,MINS)
C
C           ROUTINE TO CONVERT A DECIMAL TIME INTO A 24 HOUR TIME
C
C           CALCULATE NUMBER OF DAYS
        ND=1
        IF (T.LT.1.0) GO TO 20
  10    T=T-1.0
        ND=ND+1
        IF (T.GE.1.0) GO TO 10
C           CALCULATE NUMBER OF HOURS
  20    T=T*24.0
        IH=0
        IF (T.LT.1.0) GO TO 40
  30    T=T-1.0
        IH=IH+1
        IF (T.GE.1.0) GO TO 30
C           CALCULATE NUMBER OF MINUTES
  40    T=T*3.0/5.0
        MINS=T*100
        RETURN
        END
C
C======================================================================
C
        SUBROUTINE SORT(ICOM,JCOM)
C
C           ROUTINE TO SORT COMPONENTS OF AN ARRAY INTO ORDER
C
        DIMENSION JCOM(ICOM)
        MCOM=ICOM-1
        DO 1 I=1,MCOM
        DO 1 K=I,ICOM
        IF (JCOM(I).LE.JCOM(K)) GO TO 1
        ITEMP=JCOM(I)
        JCOM(I)=JCOM(K)
        JCOM(K)=ITEMP
  1     CONTINUE
        RETURN
        END
C
C======================================================================
C
```

Appendix B

Graphical output of simulations of the model

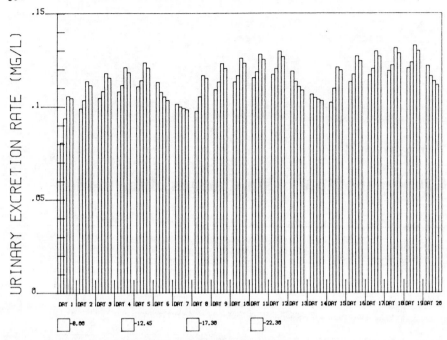

FIGURE B.1.   URINARY EXCRETION OF ARSENIC DURING SHIFT EXPOSURE

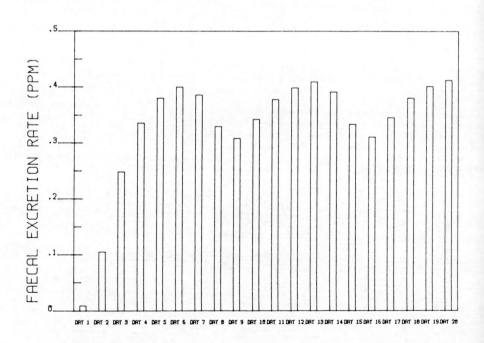

FIGURE B.2.   FAECAL EXCRETION OF ARSENIC DURING SHIFT EXPOSURE

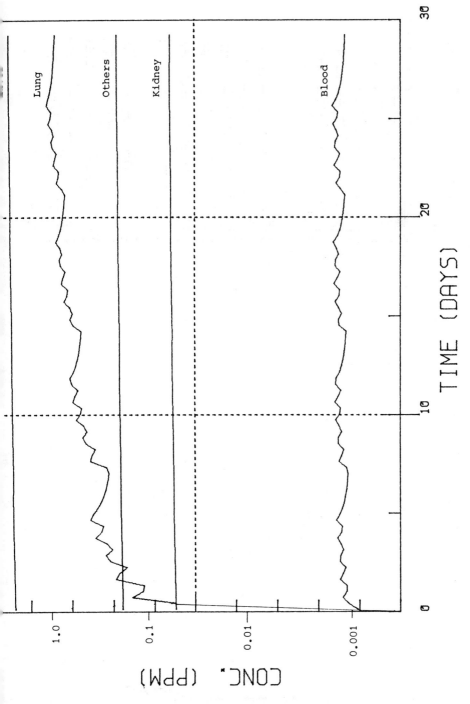

FIGURE B.3. TISSUE CONCENTRATIONS OF ARSENIC DURING SHIFT EXPOSURE

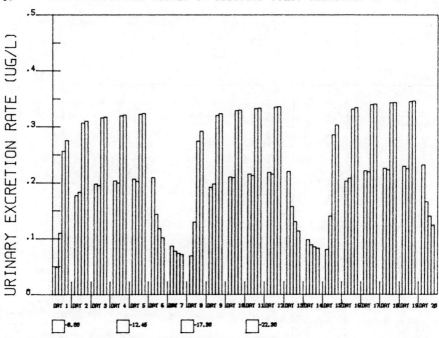

FIGURE B.4.   URINARY EXCRETION OF BERYLLIUM DURING SHIFT EXPOSURE

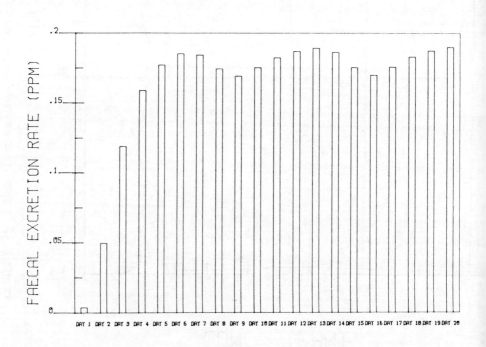

FIGURE B.5.   FAECAL EXCRETION OF BERYLLIUM DURING SHIFT EXPOSURE

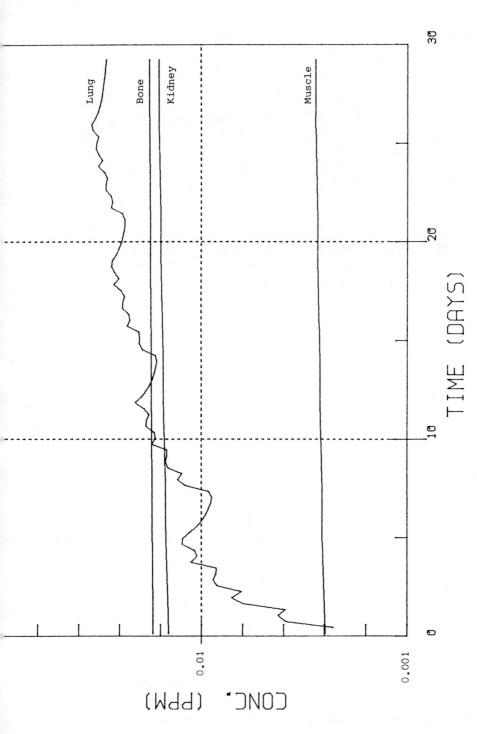

FIGURE B.6. TISSUE BERYLLIUM CONCENTRATIONS DURING SHIFT EXPOSURE

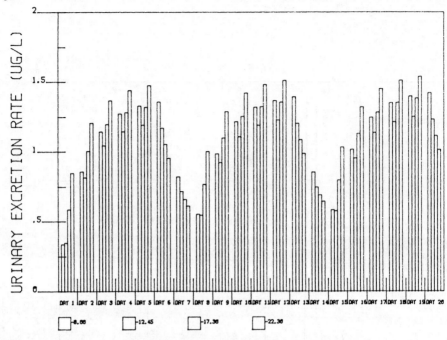

FIGURE B.7.   URINARY EXCRETION OF CADIMIUM DURING SHIFT EXPOSURE

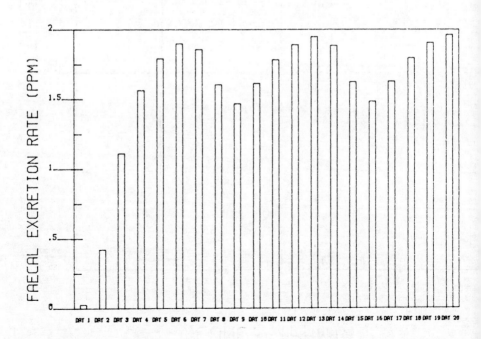

FIGURE B.8.   FAECAL EXCRETION OF CADMIUM DURING SHIFT EXPOSURE

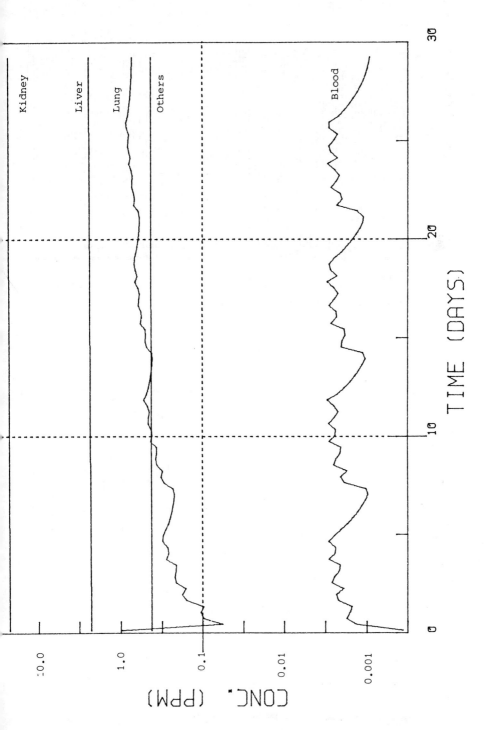

FIGURE B.9. TISSUE CADMIUM CONCENTRATIONS DURING SHIFT EXPOSURE

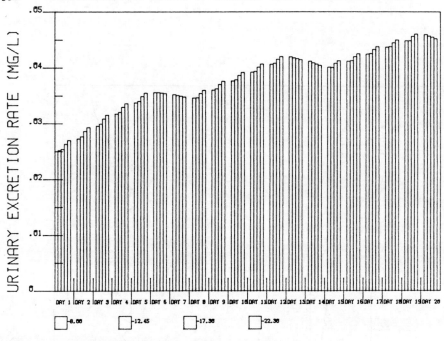

FIGURE B.10.   URINARY EXCRETION OF LEAD DURING SHIFT EXPOSURE

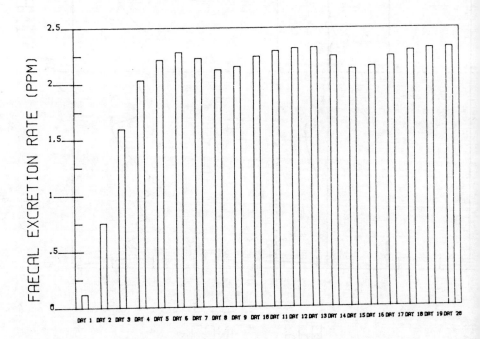

FIGURE B.11.   FAECAL EXCRETION OF LEAD DURING SHIFT EXPOSURE

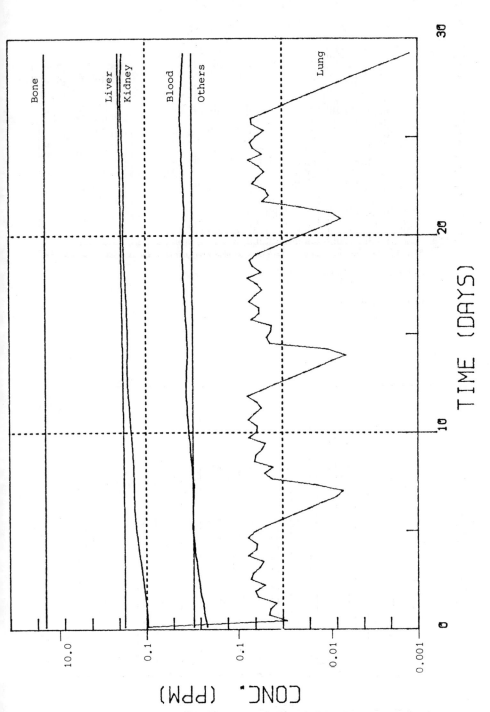

FIGURE B.12.   TISSUE CONCENTRATIONS OF LEAD DURING SHIFT EXPOSURE

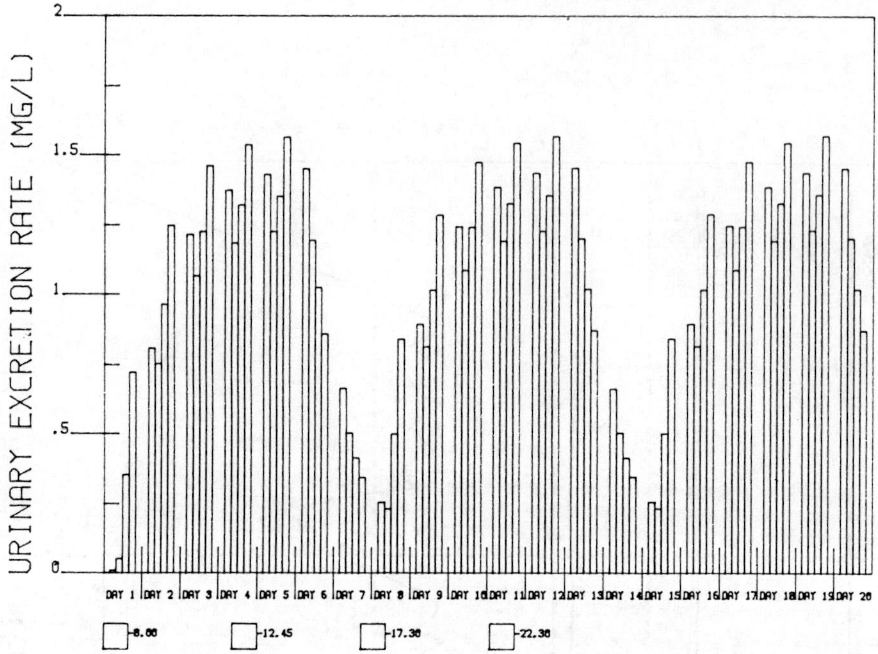

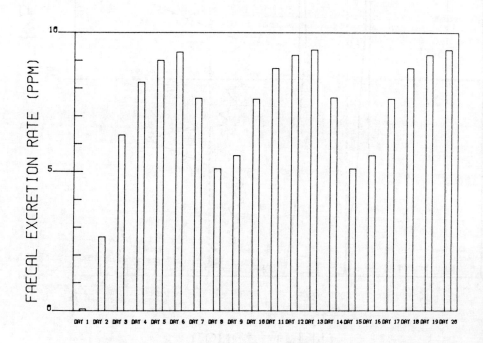

FIGURE B.13.   URINARY EXCRETION OF NICKEL DURING SHIFT EXPOSURE

FIGURE B.14.   FAECAL EXCRETION OF NICKEL DURING SHIFT EXPOSURE

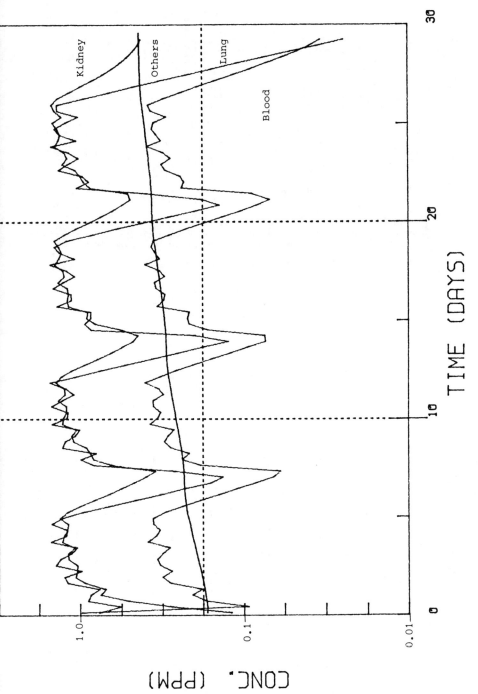

FIGURE B.15. TISSUE CONCENTRATIONS OF NICKEL DURING SHIFT EXPOSURE

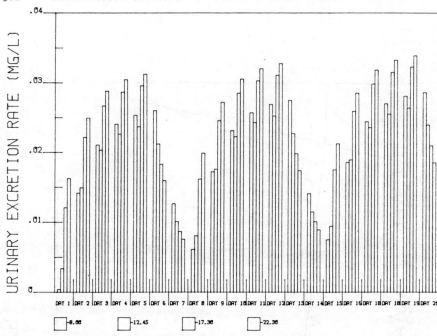

FIGURE B.16.   URINARY EXCRETION OF CHROMIUM DURING SHIFT EXPOSURE

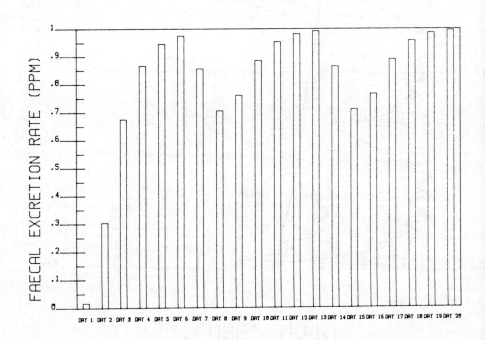

FIGURE B.17.   FAECAL EXCRETION OF CHROMIUM DURING SHIFT WORK

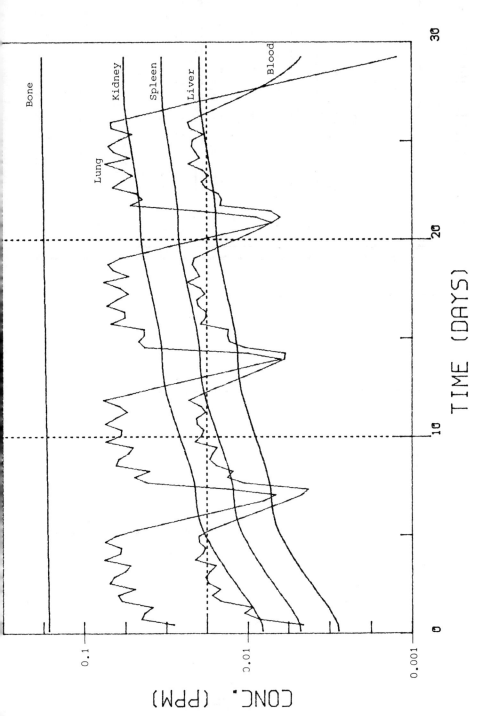

FIGURE B.18. TISSUE CHROMIUM LEVELS DURING SHIFT EXPOSURE

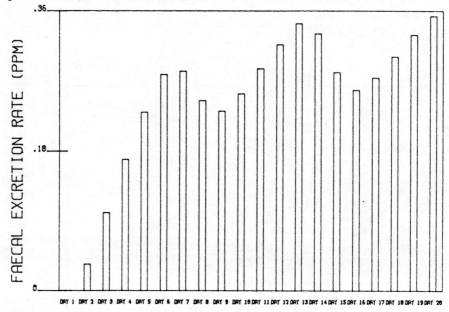

FIGURE B.19.   FAECAL EXCRETION OF ASBESTOS DURING SHIFT EXPOSURE

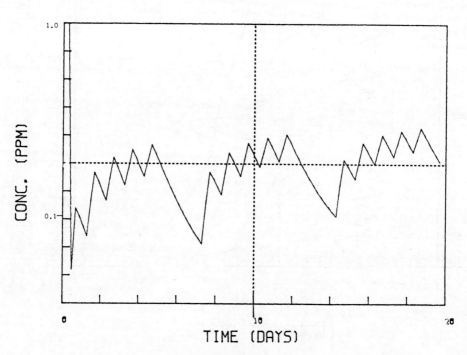

FIGURE B.20.   LUNG CONCENTRATION OF ASBESTOS DURING SHIFT EXPOSURE

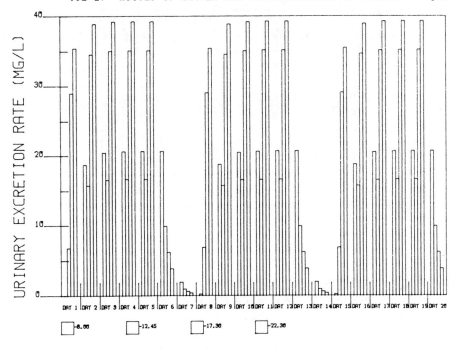

FIGURE B.21. URINARY EXCRETION OF BENZENE DURING SHIFT EXPOSURE

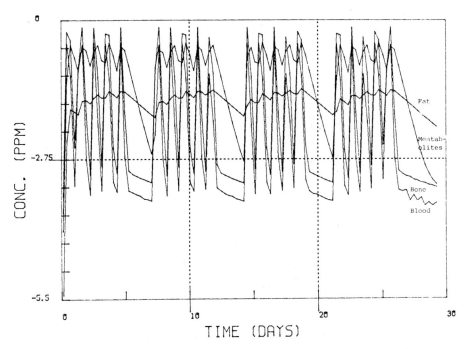

FIGURE B.22. TISSUE BENZENE CONCENTRATIONS DURING SHIFT EXPOSURE

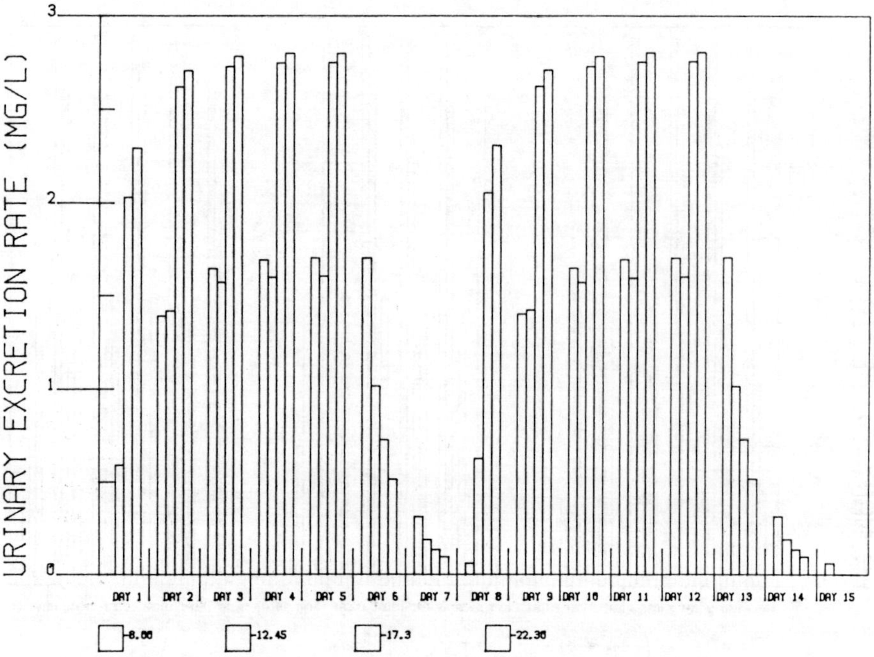

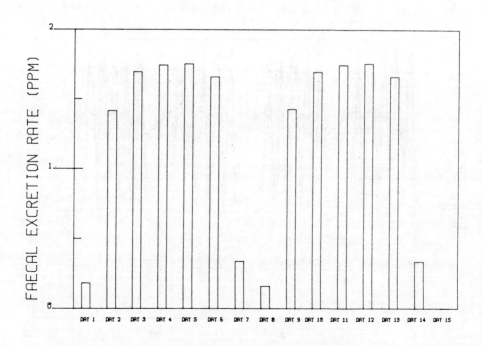

FIGURE B.23.   URINARY EXCRETION OF VINYL CHLORIDE DURING SHIFT EXPOSURE

FIGURE B.24.   FAECAL EXCRETION OF VINYL CHLORIDE DURING SHIFT EXPOSURE

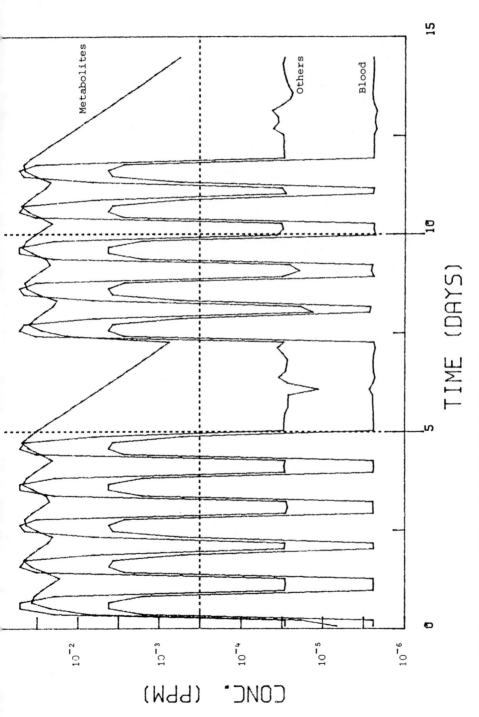

FIGURE B.25. TISSUE CONCENTRATIONS OF VINYL CHLORIDE DURING SHIFT EXPOSURE

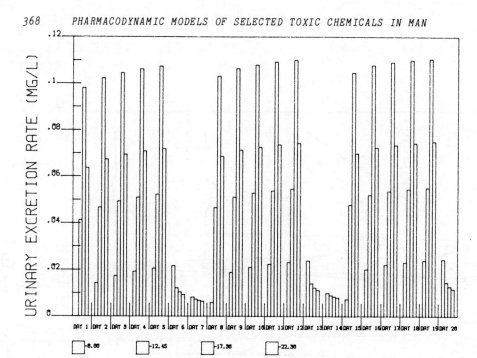

FIGURE B.26. URINARY EXCRETION OF BENZIDINE DURING SHIFT EXPOSURE

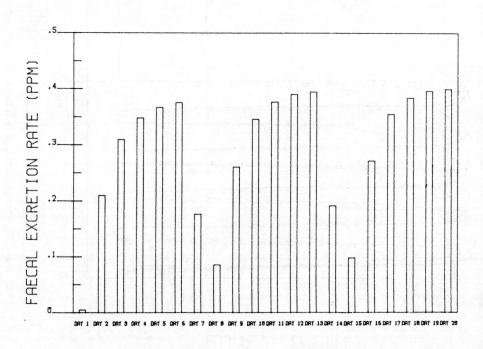

FIGURE B.27. FAECAL EXCRETION OF BENZIDINE DURING SHIFT EXPOSURE

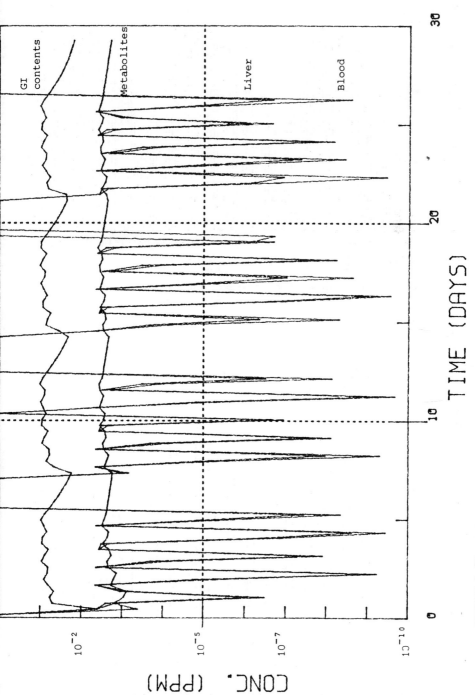

FIGURE B.28.   TISSUE CONCENTRATIONS OF BENZIDINE DURING SHIFT EXPOSURE

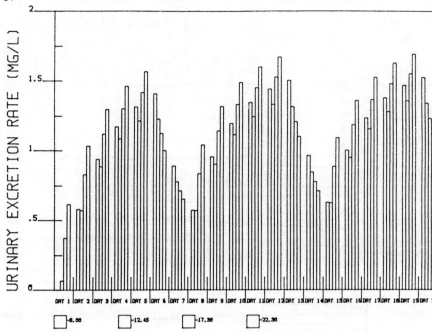

FIGURE B.29.   URINARY EXCRETION OF CARBON TETRACHLORIDE DURING SHIFT EXPOSURE

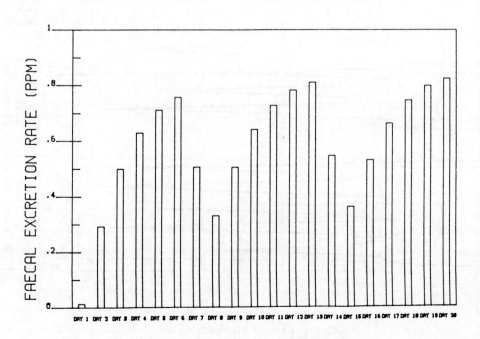

FIGURE B.30.   FAECAL EXCRETION OF CARBON TETRACHLORIDE DURING SHIFT EXPOSURE

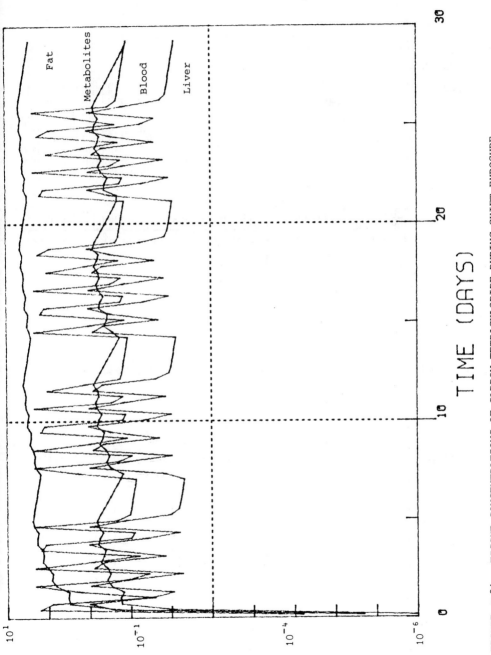

FIGURE B.31. TISSUE CONCENTRATIONS OF CARBON TETRACHLORIDE DURING SHIFT EXPOSURE

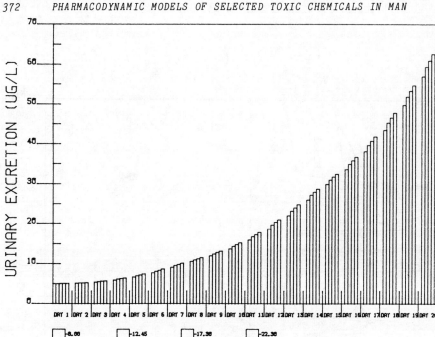

FIGURE B.32.   URINARY EXCRETION OF IODINE DURING SHIFT EXPOSURE

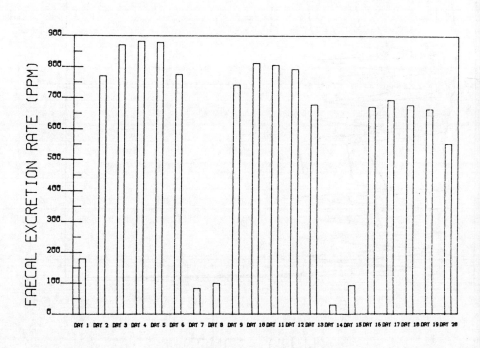

FIGURE B.33.   FAECAL EXCRETION OF IODINE DURING SHIFT EXPOSURE

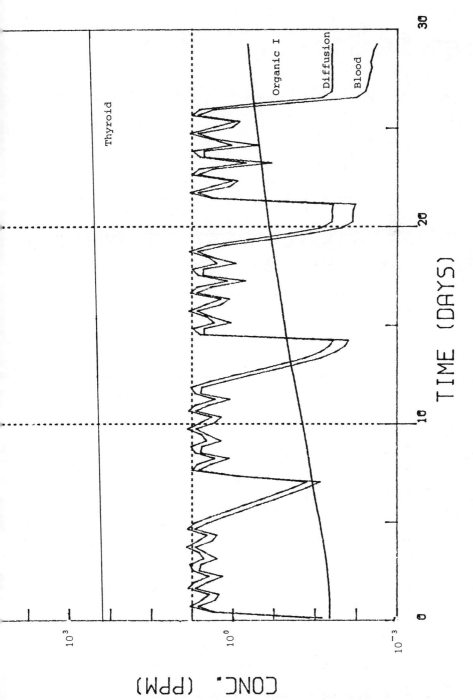

FIGURE B.34. TISSUE CONCENTRATIONS OF IODINE DURING SHIFT EXPOSURE

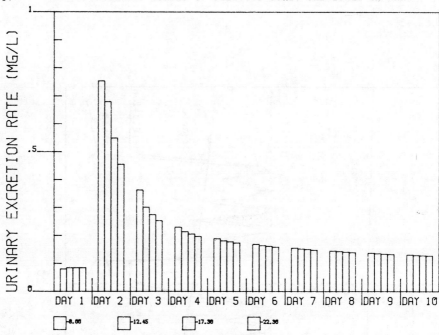

FIGURE B.35.   URINARY EXCRETION OF ARSENIC AFTER ACUTE EXPOSURE

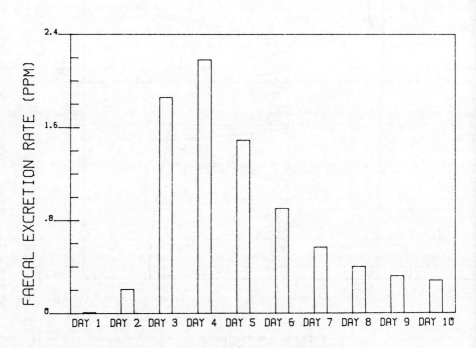

FIGURE B.36.   FAECAL EXCRETION OF ARSENIC AFTER ACUTE EXPOSURE

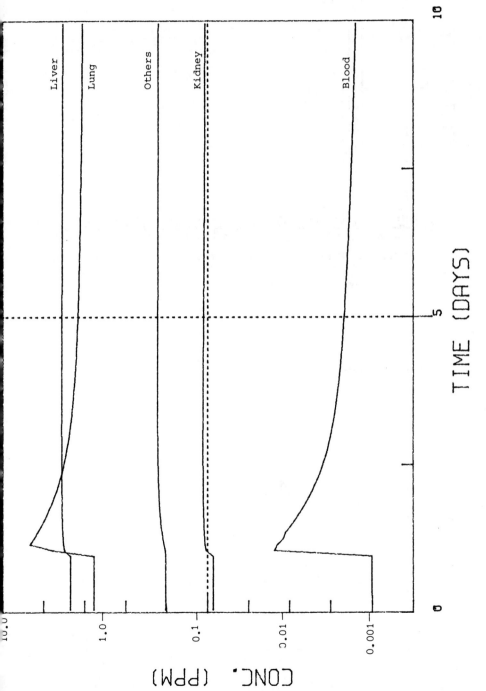

FIGURE B.37. TISSUE ARSENIC CONCENTRATIONS AFTER ACUTE EXPOSURE

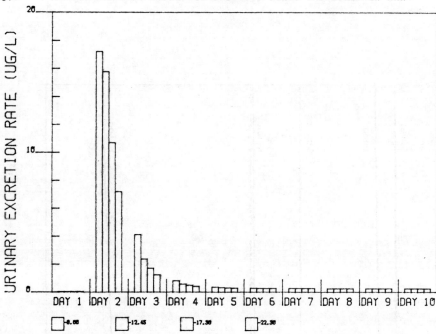

FIGURE B.38.   URINARY EXCRETION OF BERYLLIUM AFTER ACUTE EXPOSURE

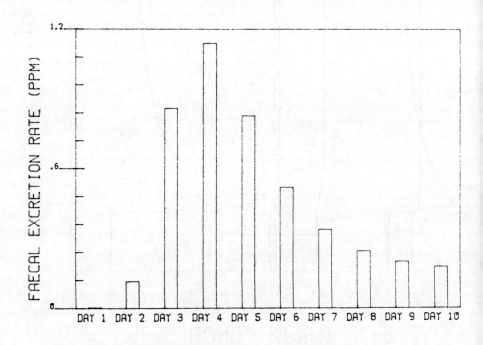

FIGURE B.39.   FAECAL EXCRETION OF BERYLLIUM AFTER ACUTE EXPOSURE

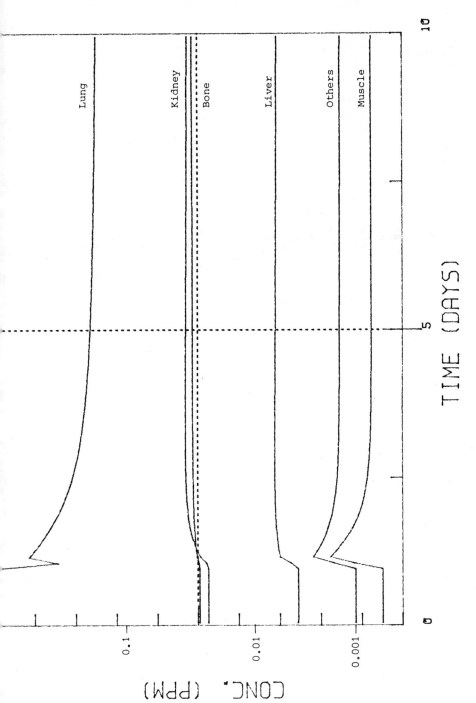

FIGURE B.40.   TISSUE CONCENTRATIONS OF BERYLLIUM AFTER ACUTE EXPOSURE

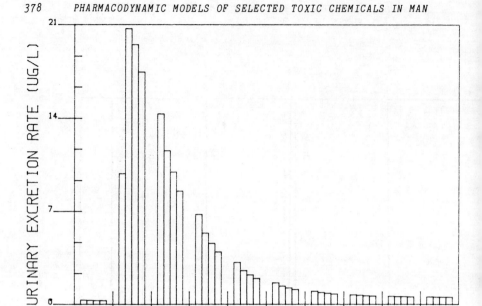

FIGURE B.41.   URINARY EXCRETION OF CADMIUM AFTER ACUTE EXPOSURE

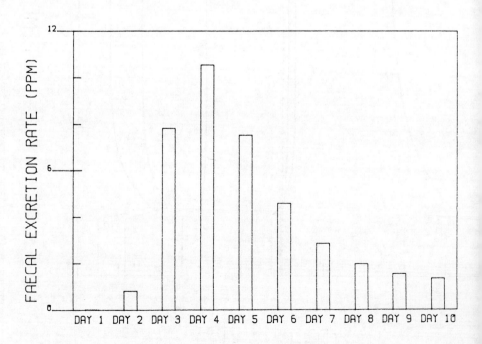

FIGURE B.42.   FAECAL EXCRETION OF CADMIUM AFTER ACUTE EXPOSURE

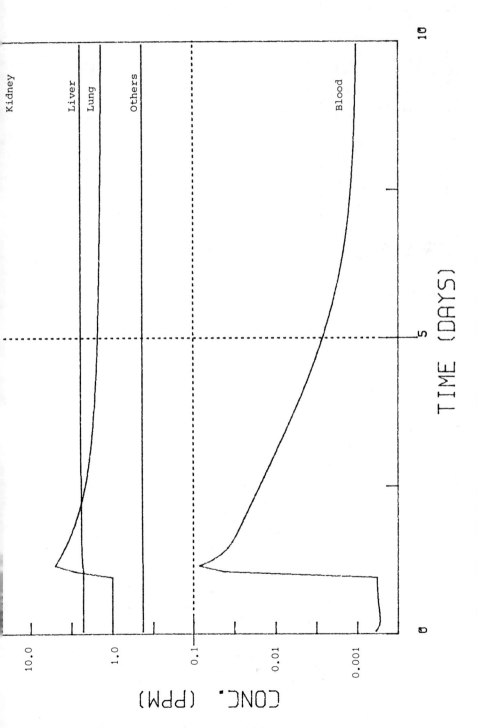

FIGURE B.43. TISSUE CONCENTRATIONS OF CADMIUM AFTER ACUTE EXPOSURE

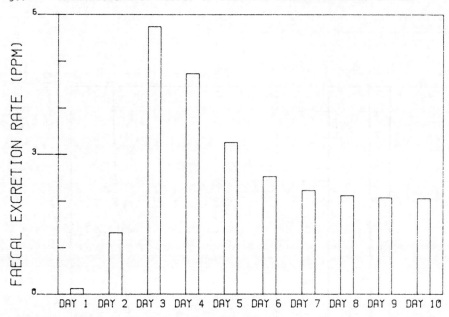

FIGURE B.45.   FAECAL EXCRETION OF LEAD AFTER ACUTE EXPOSURE

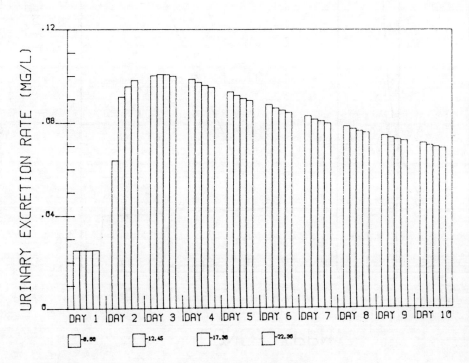

FIGURE B.44.   URINARY EXCRETION OF LEAD AFTER ACUTE EXPOSURE

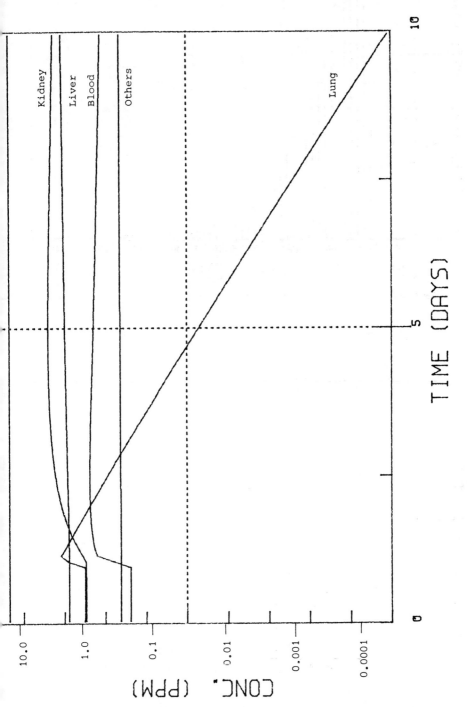

FIGURE B.46.   TISSUE CONCENTRATIONS OF LEAD AFTER ACUTE EXPOSURE

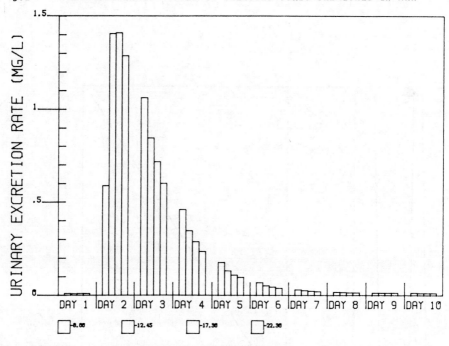

FIGURE B.47.   URINARY EXCRETION OF NICKEL AFTER ACUTE EXPOSURE

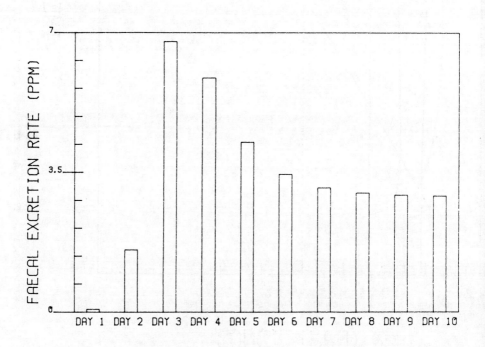

FIGURE B.48.   FAECAL EXCRETION OF NICKEL AFTER ACUTE EXPOSURE

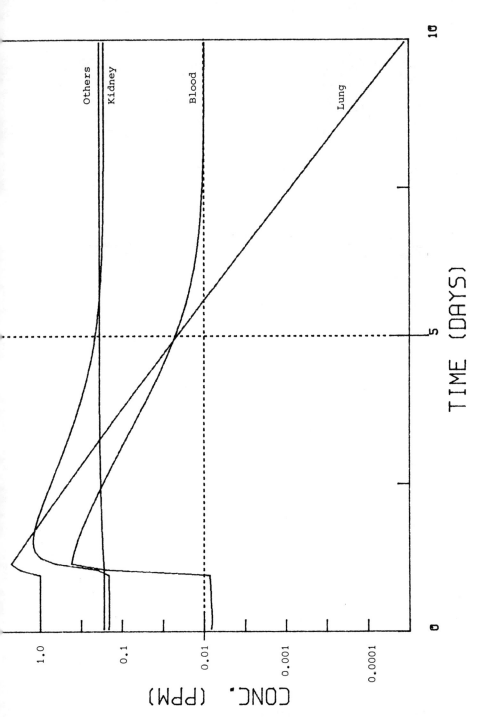

FIGURE B.49. TISSUE CONCENTRATIONS OF NICKEL AFTER ACUTE EXPOSURE

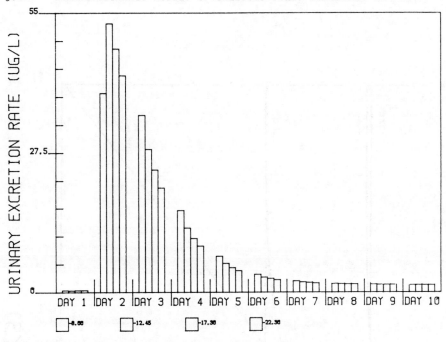

FIGURE B.50.   URINARY EXCRETION OF CHROMIUM AFTER ACUTE EXPOSURE

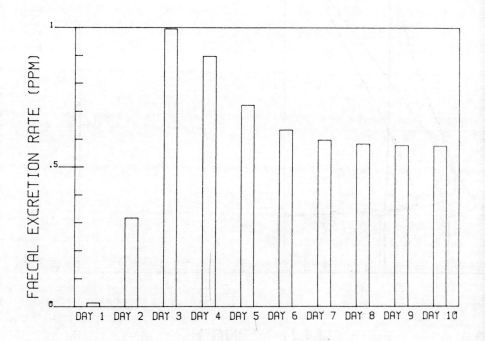

FIGURE B.51.   FAECAL EXCRETION OF CHROMIUM AFTER ACUTE EXPOSURE

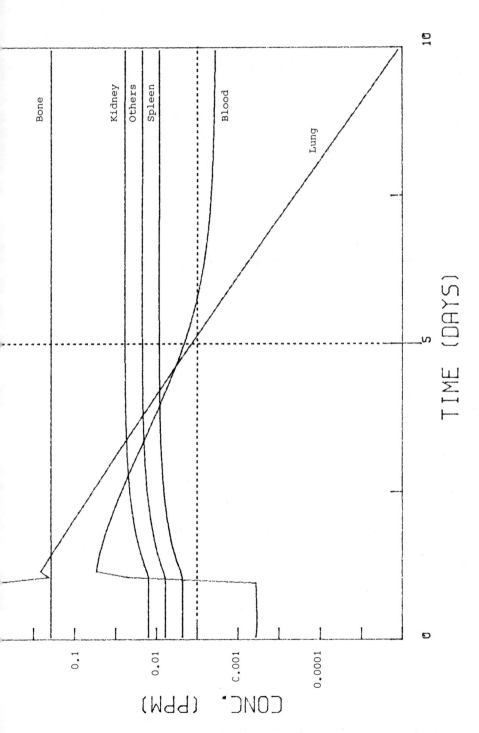

FIGURE B.52. TISSUE CONCENTRATIONS OF CHROMIUM AFTER ACUTE EXPOSURE

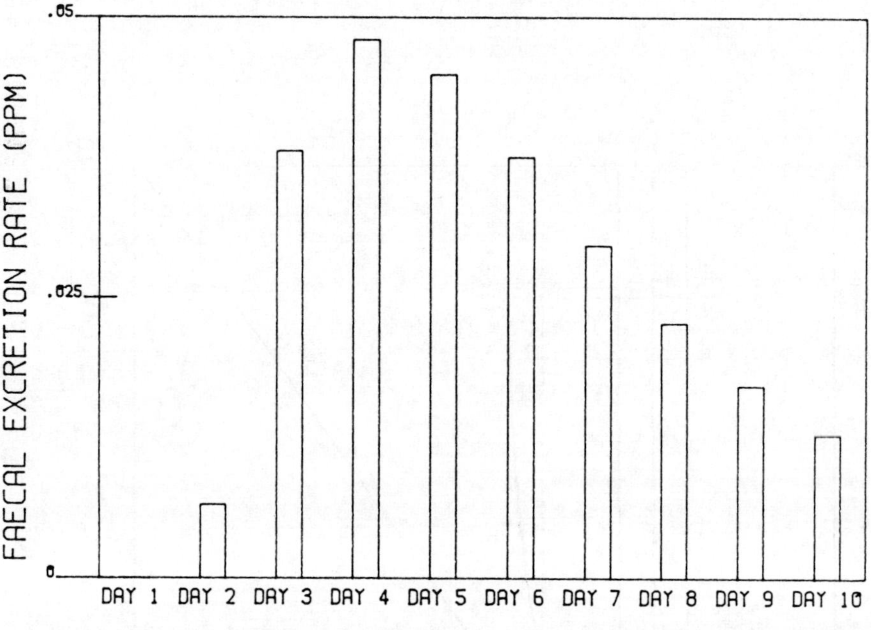

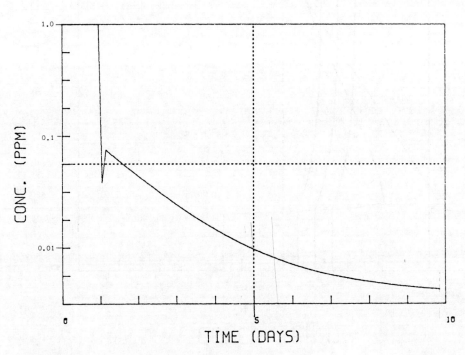

FIGURE B.53.   FAECAL EXCRETION OF ASBESTOS AFTER ACUTE EXPOSURE

FIGURE B.54.   LUNG CONCENTRATION OF ASBESTOS AFTER ACUTE EXPOSURE

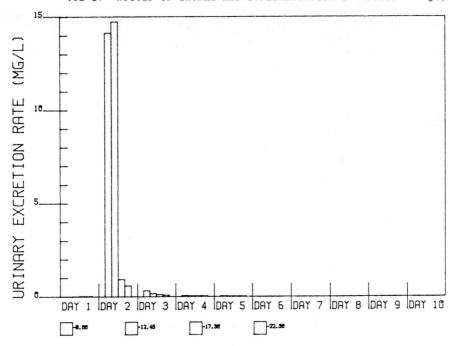

FIGURE B.55.   URINARY EXCRETION OF BENZENE AFTER ACUTE EXPOSURE

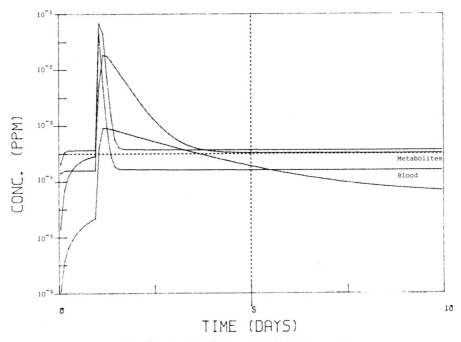

FIGURE B.56.   TISSUE CONCENTRATIONS OF BENZENE AFTER ACUTE EXPOSURE

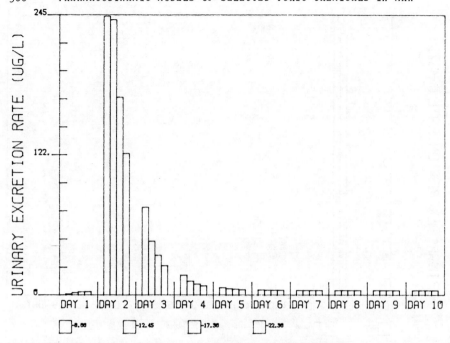

FIGURE B.57.   URINARY EXCRETION OF VINYL CHLORIDE AFTER ACUTE EXPOSURE

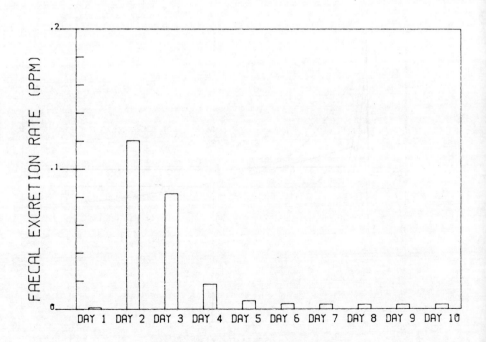

FIGURE B.58.   FAECAL EXCRETION OF VINYL CHLORIDE AFTER ACUTE EXPOSURE

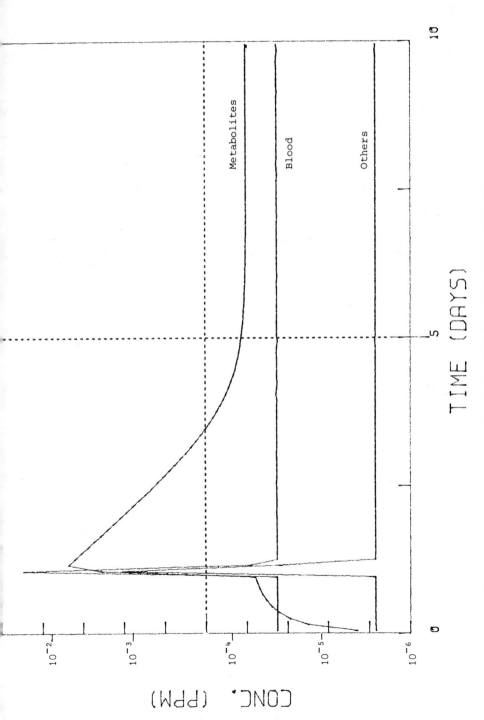

FIGURE B.59. TISSUE CONCENTRATIONS OF VINYL CHLORIDE AFTER ACUTE EXPOSURE

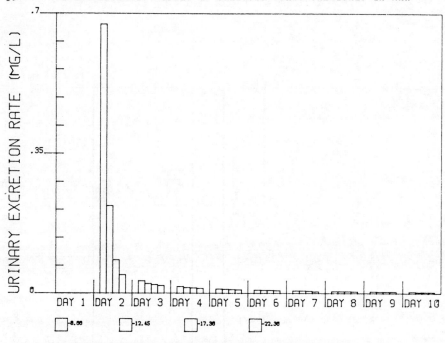

FIGURE B.60.   URINARY EXCRETION OF BENZIDINE AFTER ACUTE EXPOSURE

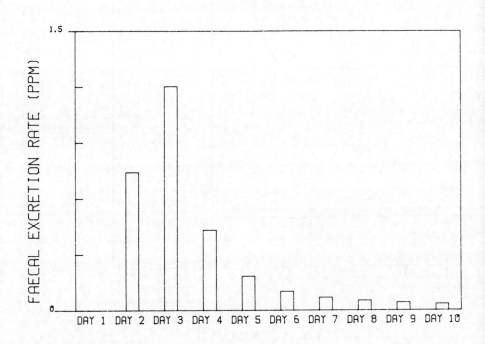

FIGURE B.61. FAECAL EXCRETION OF BENZIDINE AFTER ACUTE EXPOSURE

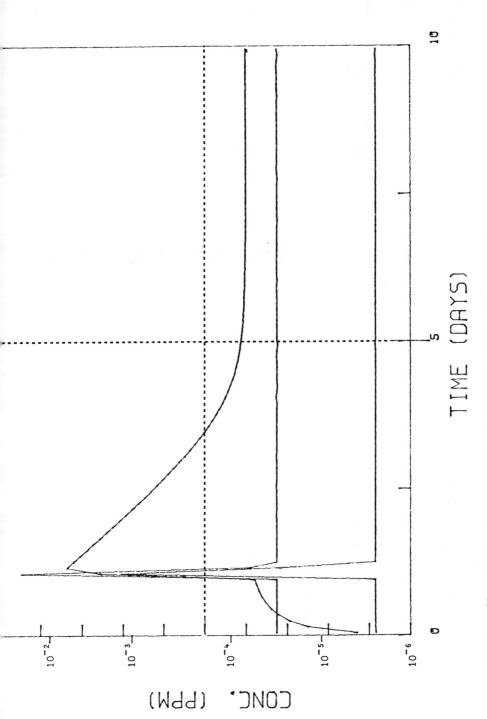

FIGURE B.62. TISSUE CONCENTRATIONS OF BENZIDINE AFTER ACUTE EXPOSURE

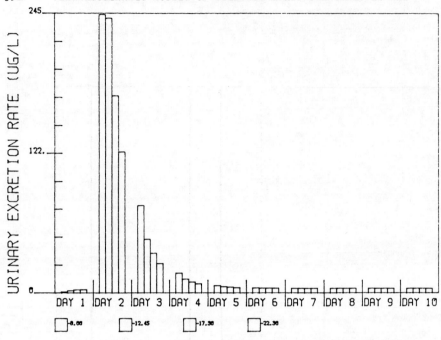

FIGURE B.63.   URINARY EXCRETION OF CARBON TETRACHLORIDE AFTER ACUTE EXPOSURE

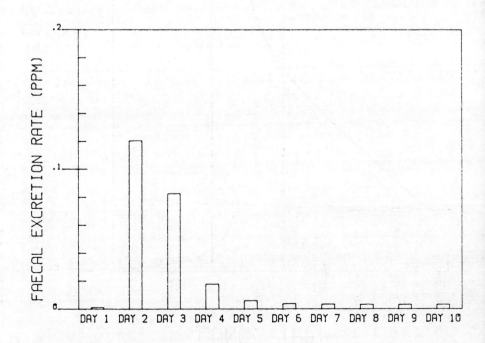

FIGURE B.64.   FAECAL EXCRETION OF CARBON TETRACHLORIDE AFTER ACUTE EXPOSURE

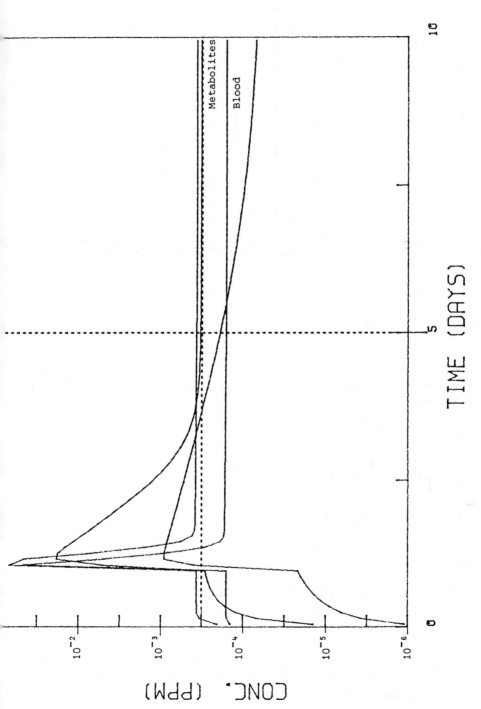

FIGURE B.65.   TISSUE CONCENTRATIONS OF CARBON TETRACHLORIDE AFTER ACUTE EXPOSURE

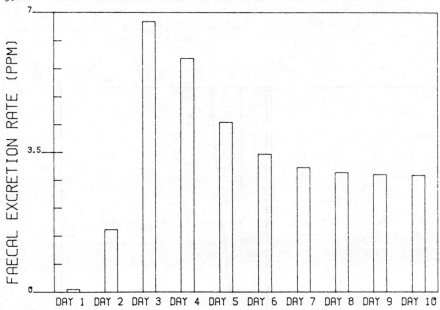

FIGURE B.67.   FAECAL EXCRETION OF IODINE AFTER ACUTE EXPOSURE

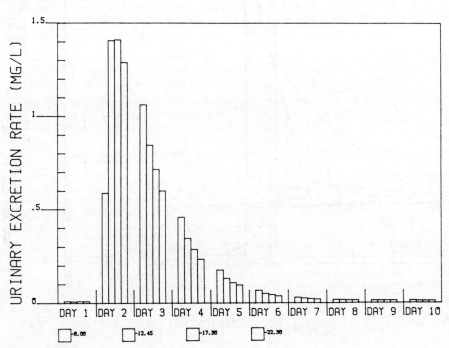

FIGURE B.66.   URINARY EXCRETION OF IODINE AFTER ACUTE EXPOSURE

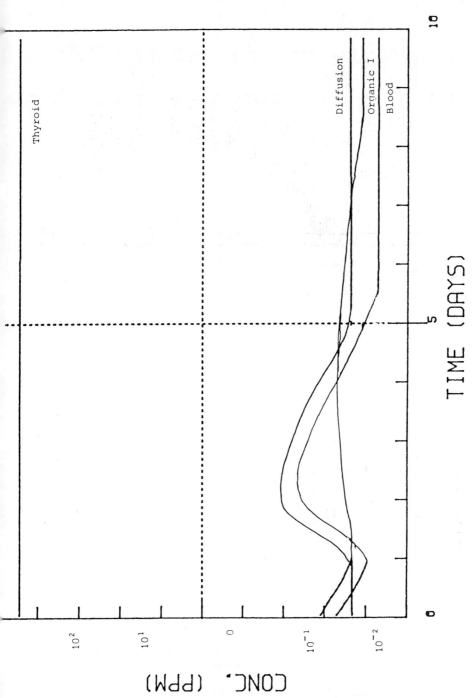

FIGURE B.68.   TISSUE CONCENTRATIONS OF METHYL IODIDE AFTER ACUTE EXPOSURE

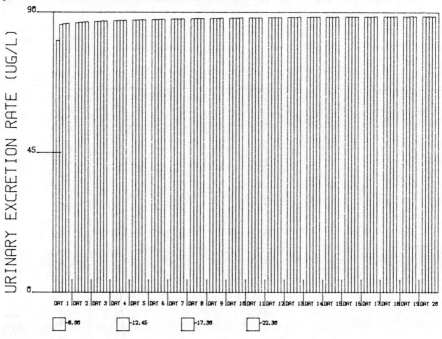

FIGURE B.69. URINARY EXCRETION OF ARSENIC DURING CHRONIC EXPOSURE

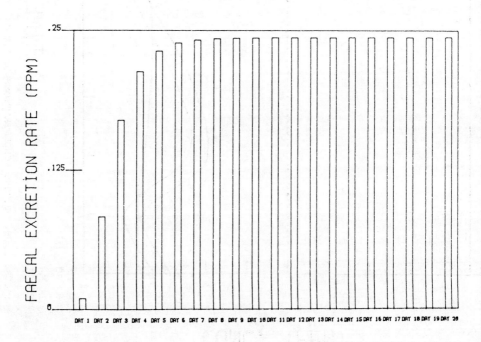

FIGURE B.70. FAECAL EXCRETION OF ARSENIC DURING CHRONIC EXPOSURE

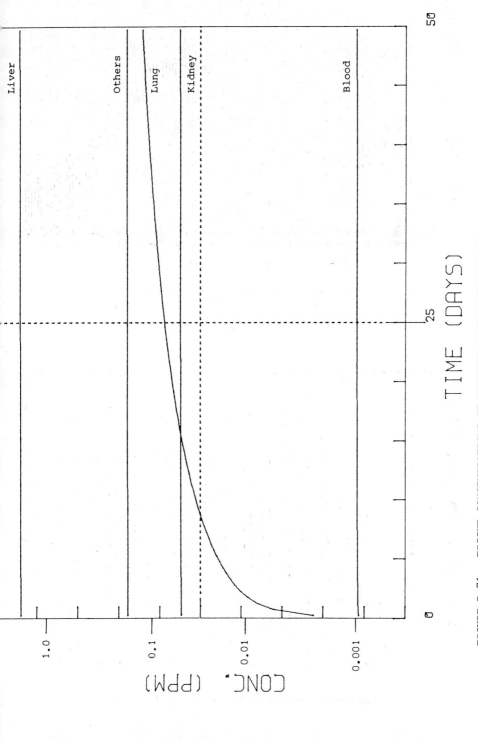

FIGURE B.71. TISSUE CONCENTRATIONS OF ARSENIC DURING CHRONIC EXPOSURE

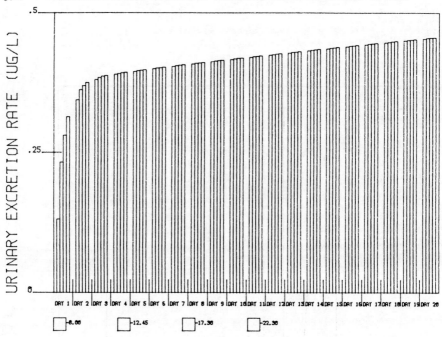

FIGURE B.72.   URINARY EXCRETION OF BERYLLIUM DURING CHRONIC EXPOSURE

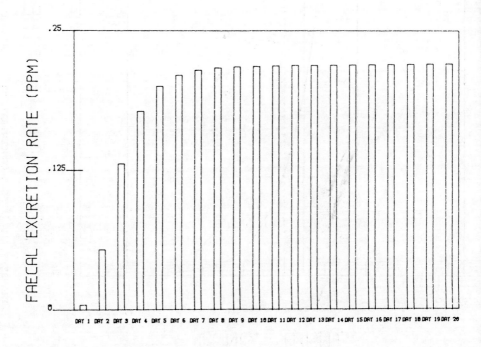

FIGURE B.73.   FAECAL EXCRETION OF BERYLLIUM DURING CHRONIC EXPOSURE

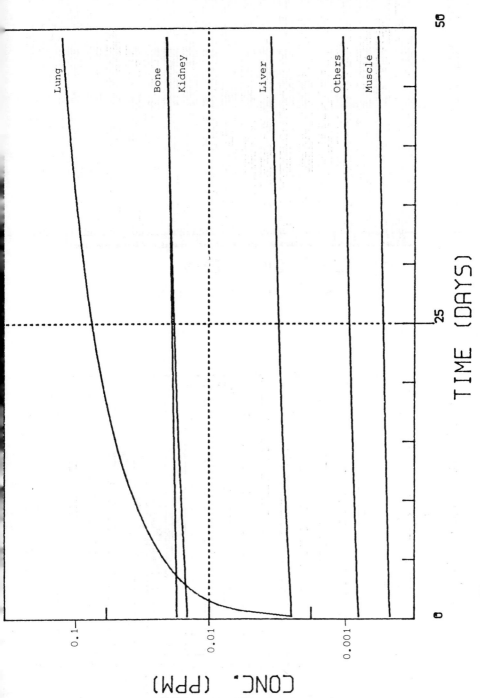

FIGURE B.74. TISSUE CONCENTRATIONS OF BERYLLIUM DURING CHRONIC EXPOSURE

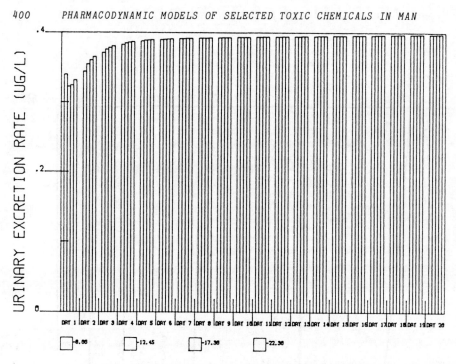

FIGURE B.75. URINARY EXCRETION OF CADMIUM DURING CHRONIC EXPOSURE

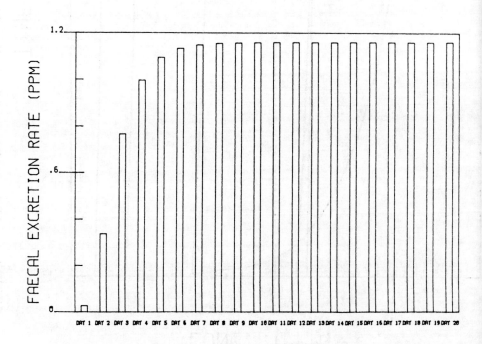

FIGURE B.76. FAECAL EXCRETION OF CADMIUM DURING CHRONIC EXPOSURE

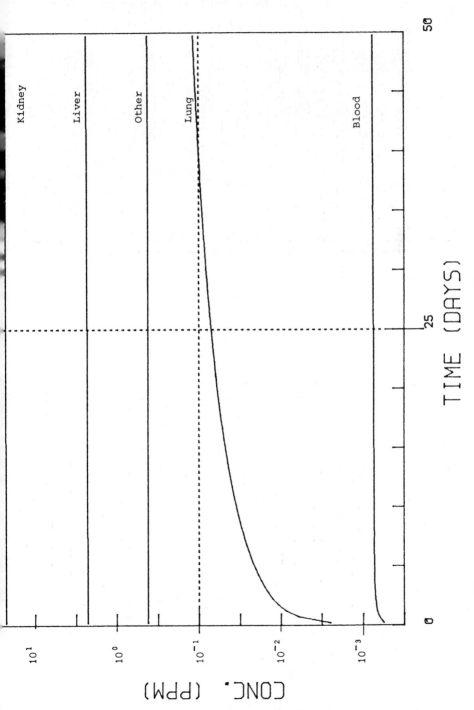

FIGURE B.77. TISSUE CONCENTRATIONS OF CADMIUM DURING CHRONIC EXPOSURE

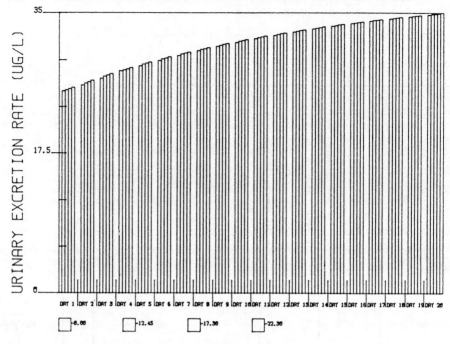

FIGURE B.78.   URINARY EXCRETION OF LEAD DURING CHRONIC EXPOSURE

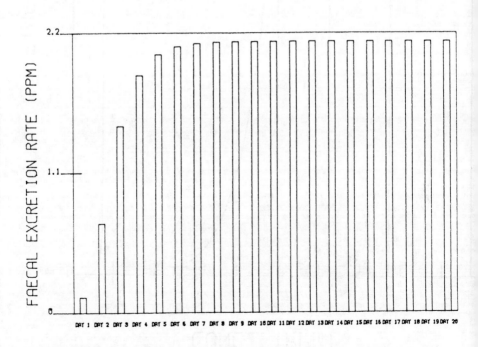

FIGURE B.79.   FAECAL EXCRETION OF LEAD DURING CHRONIC EXPOSURE

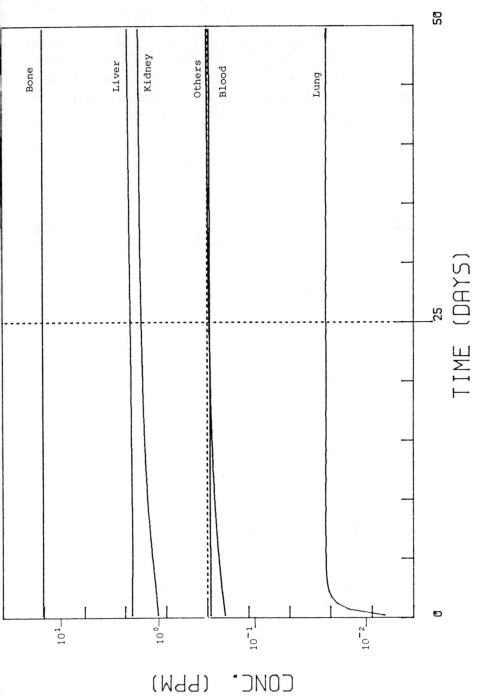

FIGURE B.80. TISSUE CONCENTRATIONS OF LEAD DURING CHRONIC EXPOSURE

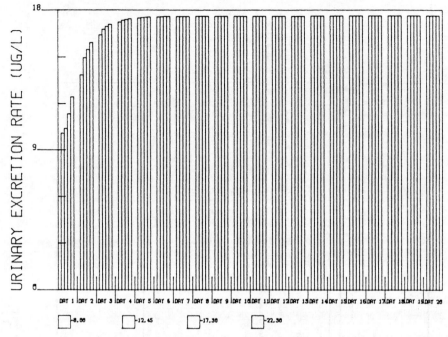

FIGURE B.81. URINARY EXCRETION OF NICKEL DURING CHRONIC EXPOSURE

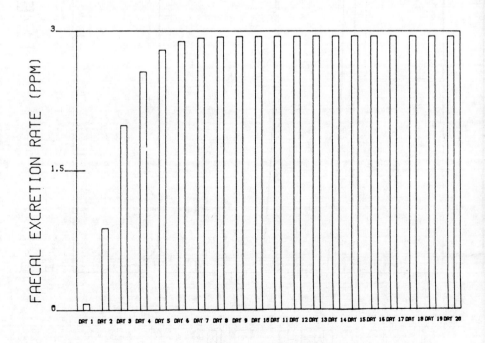

FIGURE B.82. FAECAL EXCRETION OF NICKEL DURING CHRONIC EXPOSURE

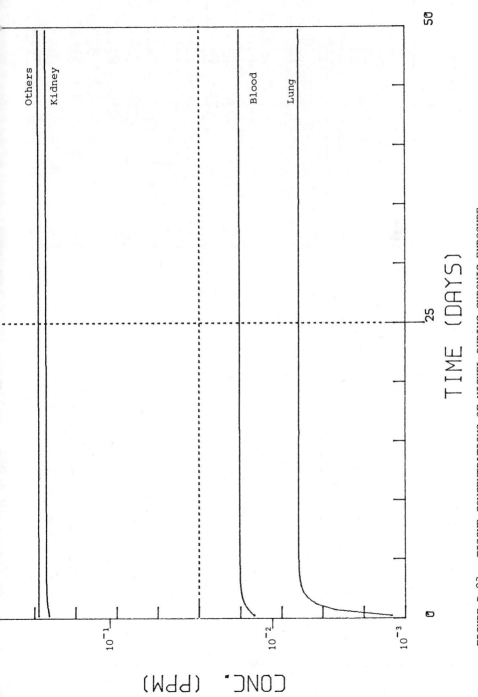

FIGURE B.83. TISSUE CONCENTRATIONS OF NICKEL DURING CHRONIC EXPOSURE

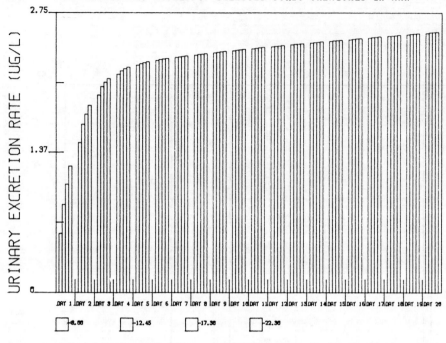

FIGURE B.84.   URINARY EXCRETION OF CHROMIUM DURING CHRONIC EXPOSURE

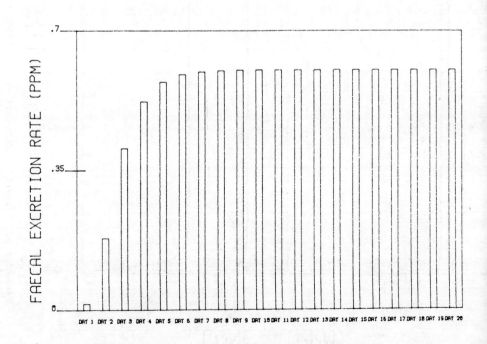

FIGURE B.85.   FAECAL EXCRETION OF CHROMIUM DURING CHRONIC EXPOSURE

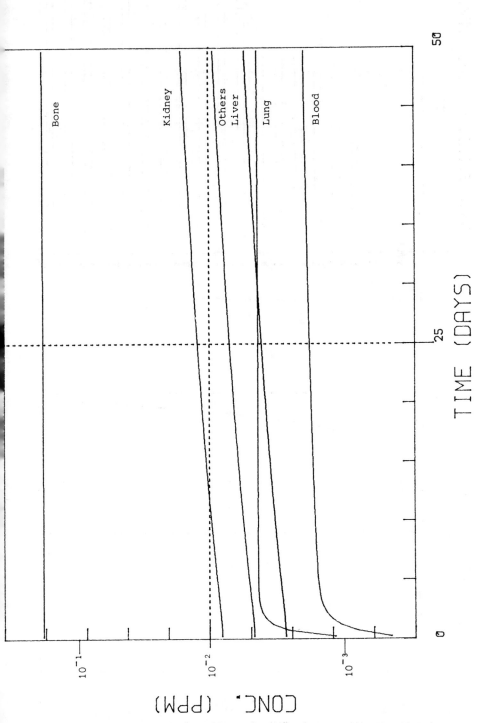

FIGURE B.86. TISSUE CONCENTRATIONS OF CHROMIUM DURING CHRONIC EXPOSURE

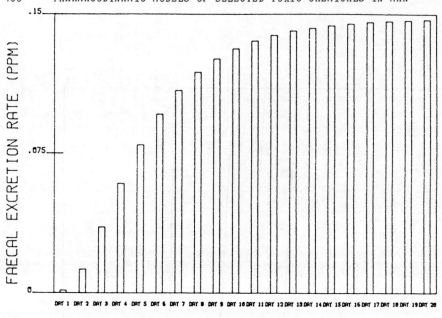

FIGURE B.87.   FAECAL EXCRETION OF ASBESTOS DURING CHRONIC EXPOSURE

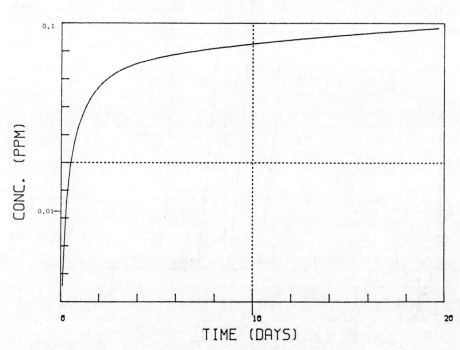

FIGURE B.88.   LUNG CONCENTRATION OF ASBESTOS DURING CHRONIC EXPOSURE

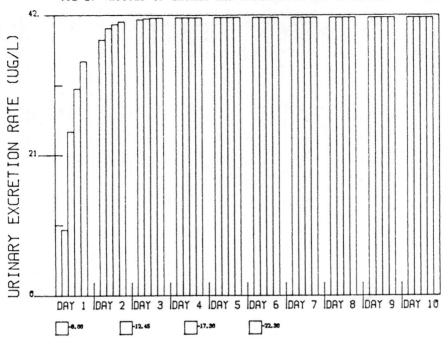

FIGURE B.89.   URINARY EXCRETION OF BENZENE DURING CHRONIC EXPOSURE

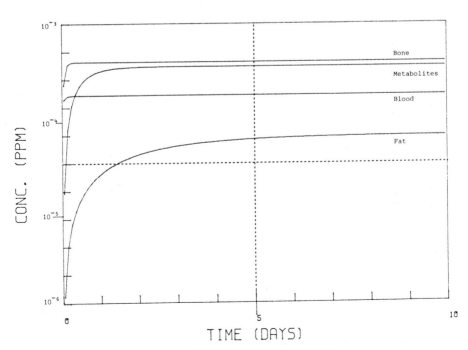

FIGURE B.90.   TISSUE CONCENTRATIONS OF BENZENE DURING CHRONIC EXPOSURE

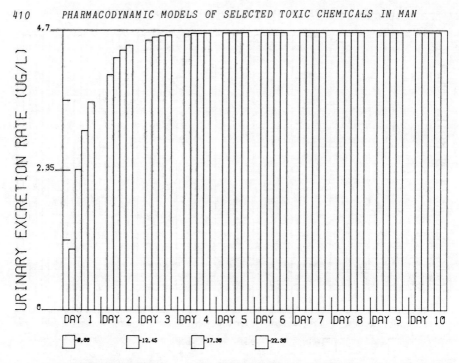

FIGURE B.91.   URINARY EXCRETION OF VINYL CHLORIDE DURING CHRONIC EXPOSURE

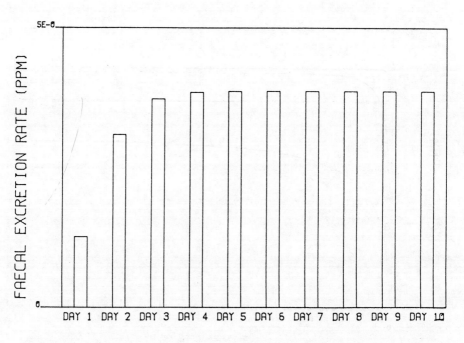

FIGURE B.92.   FAECAL EXCRETION OF VINYL CHLORIDE DUREING CHRONIC EXPOSURE

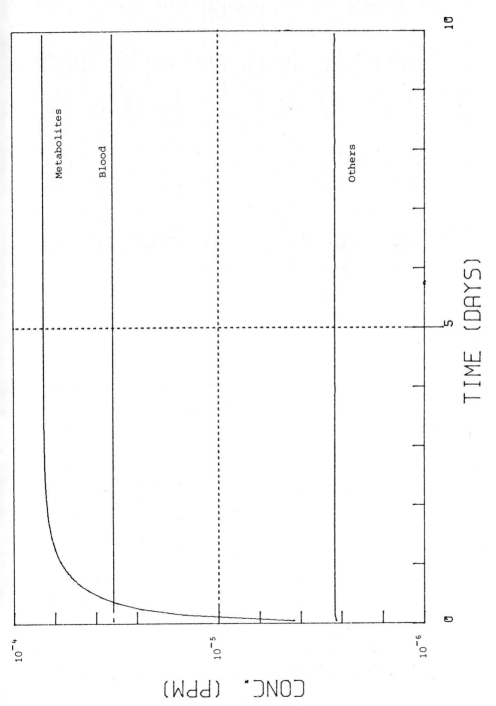

FIGURE B.93.   TISSUE CONCENTRATIONS OF VINYL CHLORIDE DURING CHRONIC EXPOSURE

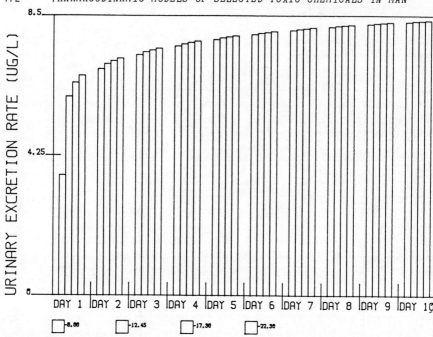

FIGURE B.94.   URINARY EXCRETION OF BENZIDINE DURING CHRONIC EXPOSURE

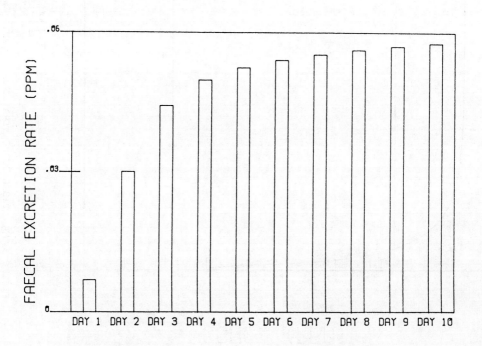

FIGURE B.95.   FAECAL EXCRETION OF BENZIDINE DURING CHRONIC EXPOSURE

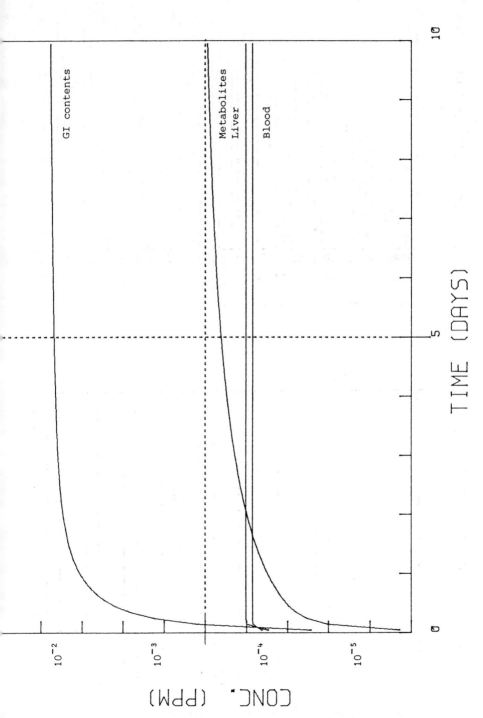

FIGURE B.96.   TISSUE CONCENTRATIONS OF BENZIDINE DURING CHRONIC EXPOSURE

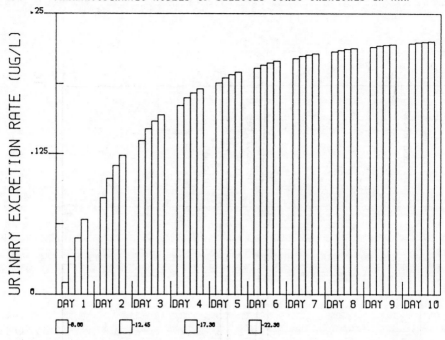

FIGURE B.97.   URINARY EXCRETION OF CARBON TETRACHLORIDE DURING CHRONIC EXPOSURE

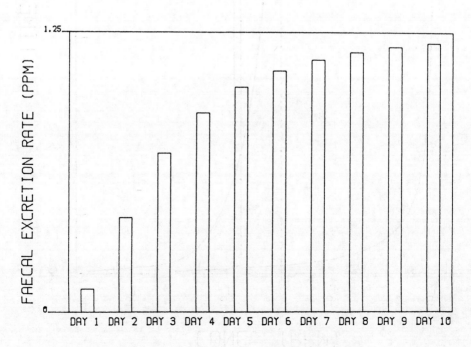

FIGURE B.98.   FAECAL EXCRETION OF CARBON TETRACHLORIDE DURING CHRONIC EXPOSURE

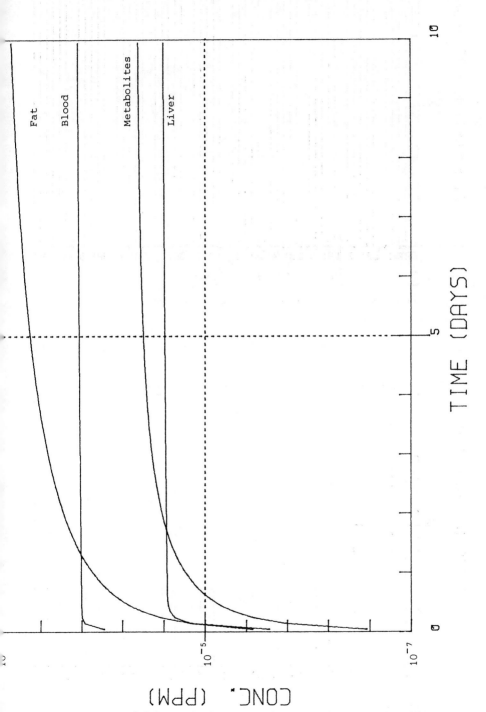

FIGURE B.99. TISSUE CONCENTRATIONS OF CARBON TETRACHLORIDE DURING CHRONIC EXPOSURE

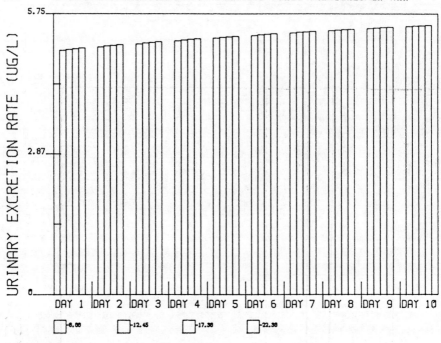

FIGURE B.100. URINARY EXCRETION OF METHYL IODIDE DURING CHRONIC EXPOSURE

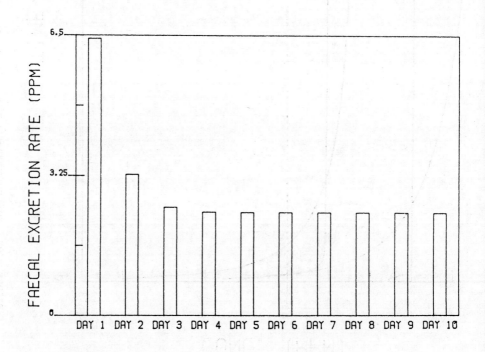

FIGURE B.101. FAECAL EXCRETION OF METHYL IODIDE DURING CHRONIC EXPOSURE

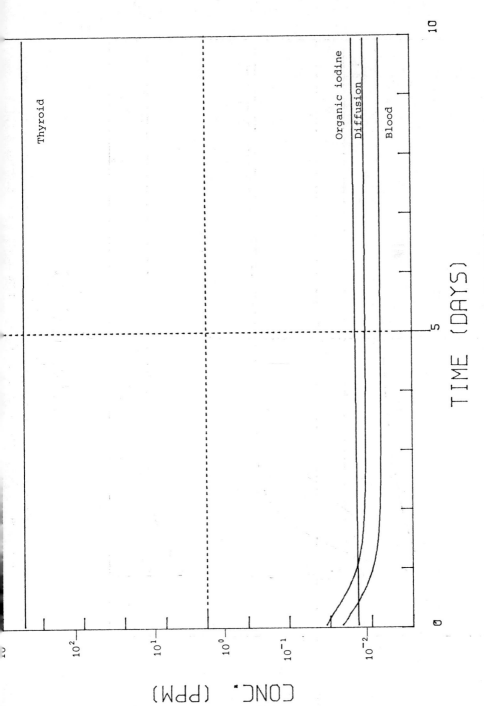

FIGURE B.102.   TISSUE CONCENTRATIONS OF METHYL IODIDE DURING CHRONIC EXPOSURE

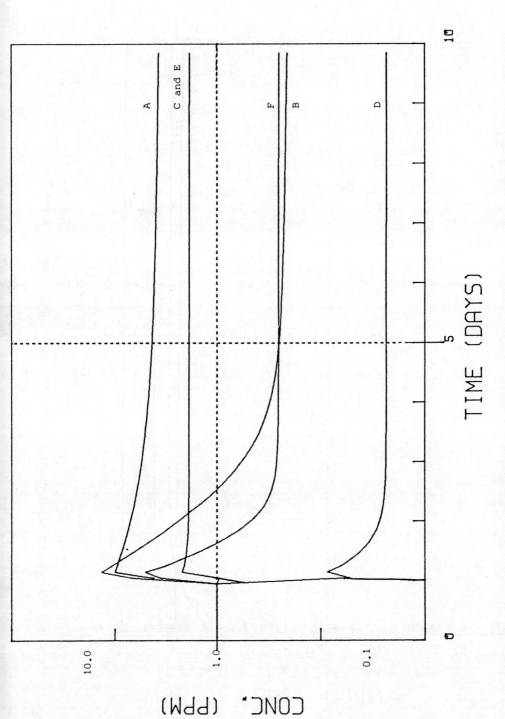

FIGURE B.103.   LUNG CONCENTRATIONS OF CADMIUM AFTER ACUTE EXPOSURE IN ORDER TO COMPARE THE ICRP LUNG MODEL WITH THE MODEL PROPOSED IN SECTION 6.   FOR SYMBOLS SEE SECTION 8.2.4